Computational Neuroendocrinology

Computational Neuroendocrinology

EDITED BY

Duncan J. MacGregor and Gareth Leng

Centre for Integrative Physiology, The University of Edinburgh, UK

WILEY Blackwell

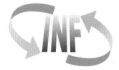

Contents

List of Contributors, vii

Series Preface, ix

Preface, xi

About the Companion Website, xv

1 Bridging Between Experiments and Equations: A Tutorial on Modeling Excitability, 1
   David P. McCobb and Mary Lou Zeeman

2 Ion Channels and Electrical Activity in Pituitary Cells: A Modeling Perspective, 80
   Richard Bertram, Joël Tabak, and Stanko S. Stojilkovic

3 Endoplasmic Reticulum- and Plasma-Membrane-Driven Calcium Oscillations, 111
   Arthur Sherman

4 A Mathematical Model of Gonadotropin-Releasing Hormone Neurons, 142
   James Sneyd, Wen Duan, and Allan Herbison

5 Modeling Spiking and Secretion in the Magnocellular Vasopressin Neuron, 166
   Duncan J. MacGregor and Gareth Leng

6 Modeling Endocrine Cell Network Topology, 206
   David J. Hodson, Francois Molino, and Patrice Mollard

7 Modeling the Milk-Ejection Reflex, 227
   Gareth Leng and Jianfeng Feng

8 Dynamics of the HPA Axis: A Systems Modeling Approach, 252
   John R. Terry, Jamie J. Walker, Francesca Spiga, and Stafford L. Lightman

9 Modeling the Dynamics of Gonadotropin-Releasing Hormone
   (GnRH) Secretion in the Course of an Ovarian Cycle, 284
   Frédérique Clément and Alexandre Vidal

   Glossary, 305

   Index, 315

List of Contributors

Richard Bertram
Department of Mathematics and Program in
Neuroscience
Florida State University
Tallahassee, FL, USA

Frédérique Clément
INRIA Paris-Rocquencourt Research Centre
Domaine de Voluceau
Le Chesnay, France

Wen Duan
Department of Mathematics
University of Auckland
Auckland, New Zealand

Jianfeng Feng
Department of Computer Science
University of Warwick
UK

Allan Herbison
Department of Physiology
University of Otago
Otago, New Zealand

David J. Hodson
CNRS, Institut de Génomique Fonctionnelle
Montpellier, France
INSERM, Montpellier, France
Universités de Montpellier 1 & 2
Montpellier, France
Department of Medicine
Imperial College London
London, UK

Gareth Leng
Centre for Integrative Physiology
University of Edinburgh
Edinburgh, UK

Stafford L. Lightman
Henry Wellcome Laboratories for Integrative
Neuroscience and Endocrinology
University of Bristol
Bristol, UK

Duncan J. MacGregor
Centre for Integrative Physiology
University of Edinburgh
Edinburgh, UK

David P. McCobb
Department of Neurobiology and Behavior
Cornell University
Ithaca, NY, USA

Patrice Mollard
CNRS, Institut de Génomique Fonctionnelle
Montpellier, France
INSERM, Montpellier, France
Universités de Montpellier 1 & 2, Montpellier,
France

Francois Molino
CNRS, Institut de Génomique Fonctionnelle
Montpellier, France
INSERM, Montpellier, France
Universités de Montpellier 1 & 2
Montpellier, France
Centre National de la Recherche Scientifique,
Unité Mixte de Recherche
University Montpellier 2
Montpellier, France

Arthur Sherman
Laboratory of Biological Modeling
NIDDK, National Institutes of Health
USA

James Sneyd
Department of Mathematics
University of Auckland
Auckland, New Zealand

Francesca Spiga
Henry Wellcome Laboratories for Integrative
Neuroscience and Endocrinology
University of Bristol
Bristol, UK

Stanko S. Stojilkovic
National Institute of Child Health and Human
Development
National Institutes of Health
Bethesda, MD, USA

Joël Tabak
Department of Mathematics and Program in
Neuroscience
Florida State University
Tallahassee, FL, USA

John R. Terry
College of Engineering
Mathematics and Physical Sciences
University of Exeter
Exeter, UK
Henry Wellcome Laboratories for Integrative
Neuroscience and Endocrinology
University of Bristol
Bristol, UK

Alexandre Vidal
Laboratoire de Mathématiques et Modélisation
d'Évry (LaMME)
Universite´ d'Évry-Val-d'Essonne
Évry, France

Jamie J. Walker
Henry Wellcome Laboratories for Integrative
Neuroscience and Endocrinology
University of Bristol
Bristol, UK

Mary Lou Zeeman
Department of Mathematics
Bowdoin College
Brunswick, ME, USA

Series Preface

This series is a joint venture between the International Neuroendocrine Federation and Wiley-Blackwell. The broad aim of the series is to provide established researchers, trainees, and students with authoritative up-to-date accounts of the present state of knowledge and prospects for the future across a range of topics in the burgeoning field of neuroendocrinology. The series is aimed at a wide audience as neuroendocrinology integrates neuroscience and endocrinology. We define neuroendocrinology as the study of the control of endocrine function by the brain and the actions of hormones on the brain. It encompasses the study of the normal and abnormal functions, and the developmental origins of disease. It includes the study of the neural networks in the brain that regulate and form neuroendocrine systems. It includes the study of behaviors and mental status that are influenced or regulated by hormones. It necessarily includes the understanding and study of peripheral physiological systems that are regulated by neuroendocrine mechanisms.

Clearly, neuroendocrinology embraces many current issues of concern to human health and well-being, but research on these issues necessitates reductionist animal models.

Contemporary research in neuroendocrinology involves the use of a wide range of techniques and technologies, from subcellular to systems and the whole organism level. A particular aim of the series is to provide expert advice and discussion about experimental or study protocols in research in neuroendocrinology and to further advance the field by giving information and advice about novel techniques, technologies and interdisciplinary approaches.

To achieve our aims, each book is based on a particular theme in neuroendocrinology, and for each book, we have recruited an editor, or pair of editors, experts in the field, and they have engaged an international team of experts to contribute chapters in their individual areas of expertise. Their mission was to give an update of knowledge and recent discoveries, to discuss new approaches, "gold-standard" protocols, translational possibilities, and future prospects. Authors were asked to write for a wide audience to minimize references, and to consider the use of video clips and explanatory text boxes; each chapter is peer-reviewed and has a *Glossary*, and each book has a detailed index. We have been guided by an Advisory

Editorial Board. The Masterclass Series is open-ended: books in preparation include *Neuroendocrinology of Neuroendocrine Neurons, Neuroendocrinology of Stress, Computational Neuroendocrinology, Molecular Neuroendocrinology,* and *Neuroendocrinology of Appetite.*

Feedback and suggestions are welcome.

John A Russell, University of Edinburgh, and William E Armstrong, University of Tennessee

Advisory Editorial Board:

Ferenc A Antoni, Egis Pharmaceuticals PLC, Budapest

Tracy Bale, University of Pennsylvania

Rainer Landgraf, Max Planck Institute of Psychiatry, Munich

Gareth Leng, University of Edinburgh

Stafford Lightman, University of Bristol

International Neuroendocrine Federation – www.isneuro.org

Preface

I started wondering about the brain when I was walking up and down the road to school. I was amazed by vision, how we are able to sense light with our eyes and turn it into electrical signals that are somehow reconstructed into conscious experience and the ability to interact with the world. Despite being a teenager, I didn't think much about hormones. I pursued these wonderings by becoming interested in philosophy, and then because I was already into computers, artificial intelligence. In the pre-internet age I gleaned as much as I could mostly from magazine articles, reading of the wonders of neural networks and robotics. The desire to pursue these things was great enough to go and study artificial intelligence and philosophy at university.

How do you pursue the brain? Artificial intelligence teaches you most of all just how difficult all the things that our brains can do are. So marvelous, and potentially powerful that they seem almost impossible, and yet we do them all the time, and the answers to how are in here somewhere. By the end of my first degree, it became clear that if I really wanted answers then I should be a neuroscientist, and an opportunity came along to do modeling in 'neuroendocrinology'. It was a neatly packaged masters (to turn me into a neuroscientist) and a PhD, on exactly the path I wanted to follow, and I didn't worry too much that I didn't know what 'neuroendocrinology' was. When I eventually looked it up I was somewhat disappointed to find out it was hormones. This seemed rather unglamorous besides topics such as vision, motor control, and learning and memory. I had no idea how fortunate I was.

Among neuroscientists, we are remarkably privileged in neuroendocrinology, because we have measurable outputs that we can directly relate to measurable neural activity. And beyond this, we know the purpose of these outputs, how these hormonal signals interact with the body and the greater world. We have access to a complete system to study.

How do we pursue this? First comes the anatomy, discovering the location and physical nature of the elements involved in the system. Then the physiology, measuring these elements, detecting their activity, and relating this to function. The hard-won knowledge comes in many small pieces and at many levels, higher level measurements such as hormone concentration in blood plasma, and lower levels such as changes in mRNA content in some component of a cell. Occasionally, these results are easily built into a more complete understanding of how the systems work, but more often there are large gaps and apparent contradictions. We are also not good at combining knowledge from different levels. A common mistake in neuroscience is the attempt to interpret any result directly in the context of high level system behavior. Every experiment and result must be justified by purpose, and given context, but we often struggle to build the structures to do this, and fall back on lazy reductionism.

What we need are the tools to structure our knowledge and to ask better questions. Many of us have a model of some sort in our heads, written as a hypothesis, or drawn as diagram, but with the skills to formalize these models, and turn them into testable living things, they can be much more powerful. Building models also brings discipline, forcing us to consider what we know and don't know, and most importantly what we *need* to know. In an ideal modelers' world every piece of work would be centered on building a model. The model would be used to plan experiments, interpret results, and ultimately, demonstrate and document the working understanding of a system, as the final product of the research.

The basic skill required for modeling is to be able to translate physiological mechanisms into a mathematical form. There are many well-established techniques for doing this. Mostly they use very simple high-school-level mathematics. More complex analysis is often applied, but this is not necessary to do useful modeling. One basic form is the Hill equation. This models the activation of some element due to binding of a ligand to a receptor. It has two parameters, one for threshold, and one for gradient, and generates a *sigmoid* curve, of the familiar form often seen in dose-response data. Another classic and very successful technique, which features in several chapters of this book, is the Hodgkin–Huxley model. It represents the currents that sum together to generate a neuron's membrane potential. It is able to very accurately reproduce electrophysiological data, bridging our knowledge at the level of individual ion channels and their mechanisms to action potentials and all their variations in shape and patterning. It is successful because both its low-level elements and parameters, and its high-level output can be directly compared to experimental data.

The detail we include in a model will be determined partly by the knowledge we have from which to build it, but also at what level we hope to understand a system, and what data we will test the model against. A guiding principle is that the model should be as simple as possible in order to explain the observed behavior. The Hodgkin–Huxley model is powerful, but it is more difficult to apply to neurons studied *in vivo* where we have less direct access to detailed electrophysiological properties. The alternative is integrate-and-fire type models of action potential generation, where more simple equations with fewer parameters reduce the complex changes in membrane potential to just the essential changes in neuronal excitability. The more complex models help us to know what elements should be in the simpler model, but we can simplify these elements so that they are easier to work with, and easier to interpret in the context of the behavior of the model.

When we want to study an entire system, such as the HPA axis or the activity of GnRH neurons in the context of an ovarian cycle, we will use a much more abstract representation. A single variable in the model might represent the activity and secretory output of an entire population of neurons. We can use such models to understand how the major elements of the system must interact in order for the system to function and explain the behavior we observe, such as pulsatile hormone output. We will only add more complexity to the model when we determine that more elements are necessary to its functioning. Sometimes these new elements will be based on mechanisms we already know, and sometimes they will be entirely new predictions, to test experimentally.

The objective of this book is to make these techniques accessible to interested experimental neuroendocrinologists and other neuroscientists, and perhaps also to draw those already with the skills for modeling into neuroendocrinology, because hormones are glamorous! All the essential and wonderful elements of life depend on hormones. And as a general way to pursue intelligence and the brain, neuroendocrinology gives us one of the best paths to be able to understand neurons (and glia) and how they process information to drive function.

Our authors are some of the very best in the field of computational neuroendocrinology. They come from diverse backgrounds: mathematics, computing, biology, and medicine, and many of them do both theoretical and experimental work. All of the chapters present examples where modeling has been successfully applied; however, they also tell the story of how they got there, and will hopefully show experimentalists how they can think like modelers, with a view to making use of models and even developing their own.

About the Companion Website

This book is accompanied by a companion website:

www.wiley.com/go/leng/computational

The website includes:
- PowerPoint figures and PDF tables from the book
- A glossary of keywords
- Videos and data sets

CHAPTER 1

Bridging Between Experiments and Equations: A Tutorial on Modeling Excitability

David P. McCobb[1] and Mary Lou Zeeman[2]
[1] Department of Neurobiology and Behavior, Cornell University, Ithaca, NY, USA
[2] Department of Mathematics, Bowdoin College, Brunswick, ME, USA

The goal of this chapter is to empower collaboration across the disciplines. It is aimed at mathematical scientists who want to better understand neural excitability and experimentalists who want to better understand mathematical modeling and analysis. None of us need to be expert in both disciplines, but each side needs to learn the other's language before our conversations can spark the exciting new collaborations that enrich both disciplines. Learning is an active process:

> *Tell me and I will forget; show me and I may remember; involve me and I will understand.*

> – Proverb

We have, therefore, written this chapter to be highly interactive. It is based on the classic model of excitability developed by Morris and Lecar (1981), and built around exercises that introduce the freely available dynamical systems software, XPP (Ermentrout, 2012), to explore and illustrate the modeling concepts. An online graphing calculator, such as Desmos (www.desmos.com), is also used occasionally. The modeling and dynamical systems techniques we develop are extremely versatile, with broad applicability throughout the sciences and social sciences. In the chapters of this volume, they are applied to systems at scales ranging from individual cells to entire neuroendocrine axes. We recommend that you work on the exercises as you read, with plenty of time, and tea and chocolate in hand. It is a great way to learn.

Outline. In Section 1.1, we introduce excitability, encompassing the diversity of action potential waveforms and patterns, recurrent firing, and bursting. We also describe the voltage clamp, the essential tool for dissection of excitability used by Hodgkin and Huxley (1952)

Computational Neuroendocrinology, First Edition. Edited by Duncan J. MacGregor and Gareth Leng.
© 2016 John Wiley & Sons, Ltd. Published 2016 by John Wiley & Sons, Ltd.
Companion Website: www.wiley.com/go/Leng/Computational

in their foundational work. In Section 1.2, we introduce the classic, two-dimensional Morris–Lecar model, developed originally from barnacle muscle data to expose the minimal mathematical essence of excitability (Morris and Lecar, 1981). In Sections 1.3 and 1.4, we introduce the software package XPP (see Section 1.3 and Ermentrout (2012)) for download instructions), and use it to explore the model behavior, thereby introducing the language and graphics of dynamical systems and phase-plane analysis. This provides a platform for extending the model and including data from naturally occurring ion channels to dissect the excitability of diverse and more complex cells.

In Sections 1.5–1.10, we follow the seminal paper by Rinzel and Ermentrout (1989) to explore the surprising richness of behavior the Morris–Lecar model can exhibit in response to sustained current injection at various levels. We use three different parameter sets, differing only in the voltage dependence and kinetics of potassium channel gating. For each parameter set, we simulate a current clamp experiment in which sustained current is applied to a cell at rest. In all the three cases, sufficiently high levels of applied current induce tonic spiking, but the onset of spiking occurs through different mechanisms with different properties. With the first parameter set ("Hopf" in Table 1.1), tonic spiking is restricted to a narrow frequency range, as in Hodgkin's Class II, typically resonator, neurons (Hodgkin, 1948). The second parameter set ("SNIC" in Table 1.1) exhibits tonic spiking with arbitrarily low frequency, depending on the applied current, as in Hodgkin's Class I, typically integrator, neurons. The final parameter set ("Homoclinic" in Table 1.1) generates tonic spiking with a high baseline between the spikes. In Section 1.10, we exploit the high baseline to illustrate how adding a slow variable to the model can generate bursting behavior. Our tour of the Morris–Lecar model owes much to Rinzel and Ermentrout (1989) and many others, including Ellner and Guckenheimer (2006), Izhikevich (2007), Morris and Lecar (1981), and Sherman (2011).

Mathematically, a qualitative change in system behavior, such as the onset of spiking arises through a bifurcation. Different mechanisms for the onset of spiking correspond to different bifurcations. We work through each of these bifurcations carefully, as they typify the mechanisms for generating oscillations in two-dimensional systems, they can underlie mechanisms in higher dimensional systems, and they recur throughout the text.

Our interdisciplinary conversations have led to a route through the mathematical material that may seem unusual. We have not begun with local linear stability theory, because our experience suggests that, while many experimentalists have excellent intuition about rates of change at their fingertips, the abstraction of eigenvalues presents a road block. (This is a natural consequence of the typical mathematics requirements for a biology degree.) We have chosen, instead, to harness the intuition about rates, and the visual intuition afforded by XPP, to develop an insight into the global nonlinear dynamics and bifurcations of the system. Only then we conclude with a discussion of the role eigenvalues play in determining local stability, and thereby signalling bifurcations. References are provided for the interested reader to learn more.

1.1 Introducing excitability

Action potentials: Decisive action and "information transportation". Cellular excitability is defined as the ability to generate an action potential (or spike): an explosive excursion in a cell's membrane potential (Figure 1.1). Its all-or-nothing aspect makes it decisive. Its propensity to propagate in space enables signal transmission in biological "wires" that are too small and electrically leaky to transmit a passive electrical signal over more than a millimeter or 2. Most cells have strong ionic gradients that are nearly, but imperfectly counterbalanced: a higher concentration of potassium ions (K^+) inside than out, versus higher sodium (Na^+), calcium (Ca^{++}) and chloride (Cl^-) concentrations outside than in. Higher "resting" permeabilities of the cell membrane to K and Cl result in a significant inside-negative *resting potential* (for largely historical reasons this is referred to as a *hyperpolarized* state). Action potentials are explosive excursions in the positive (*depolarizing*) direction from the resting potential, often reversing the polarity substantially (but still referred to as depolarizing).

The explosive mechanism uses positive feedback to produce a spatially regenerative event that propagates along a nerve axon, muscle fiber, or secretory cell's membrane. Positive feedback arises from the fact that the opening of either sodium (Na) or calcium (Ca) ion channels (small selective and gated pores in the cell membrane) is (1) promoted by depolarization and (2) leads to further depolarization, as Na or Ca ions enter through the opened channels. The explosive depolarization can propagate at rates anywhere from 1 to 200 m/s (Xu and Terakawa, 1999) depending on cell specifics. This is very slow compared to the passive spread of a voltage signal in a metal wire (on the order of the speed of light!). It is limited by the time required for channels to respond to voltage, together with the effects of membrane capacitance and leak. Nevertheless, it is much faster than any other form of chemical or biochemical signal propagation, and fast enough to support animal life, including the transmission of information over some 2 million miles of axons in the human body.

The explosive, roughly all-or-nothing nature of the action potential also serves as a decisively thresholded regulator of Ca entry. It thereby regulates many precisely timed and scaled cellular events, including neurotransmitter and hormone secretion, muscle contraction, biochemical reactions, and even gene regulatory processes. Membrane voltage thus underlies rapid signal integration in the "biological computer," including the regulation of neuroendocrine function.

For a cell to recover from the excursion from negative resting potential and prepare to fire another action potential, repolarization has to occur. This is achieved by combatting the positive feedback with slightly delayed negative feedback, or feedbacks. An essentially identical mechanism of depolarization-triggered opening of ion channels as described for Na or Ca, but now involving a channel type that selectively conducts K, quickly restores the hyperpolarized state. In response, the Na- or Ca-channel gates can now relax back to the closed state (as do the K-channel gates), a process referred to as *deactivation*. In most cases, the K-channel restorative mechanism is backed up by the closing of a separate *inactivation* gate within the body of the Na or Ca channel, which would prevent prolonged depolarization (and flooding of Na or Ca into the cell) even without the K channel. Together these events speed repolarization, deactivation and *deinactivation* (the reversal of inactivation). The separability of these gating events provides raw material for very sophisticated and sometimes subtle differences in firing and consequent signal integration.

Action potential shape and timing in information processing. Synaptic transmission is well known to play important roles in information processing. The details of intrinsic excitability of neuroendocrine cells are at least as important as in neurons, and even more so in cells like those in the anterior pituitary that are not directly driven by synaptic inputs. Thus, the variety, subtlety and susceptibility to modulatory changes of ion channels underlying excitability are critical to the nuances of neuroendocrine signalling. See Hille (2001), Chapter 7 in Izhikevich (2007) and Figure 1.1. Details of the rising phase control threshold and rise time, and influence frequency. The details of repolarization, recovery, and preparation for subsequent signalling events are even more nuanced and diverse, as indicated by the enormous diversity of K channels (at least an order of magnitude greater than that of Na and Ca channels). Action potential threshold, differing between cells, and depending on recent events and modulatory factors within a cell, determines whether a response is transmitted or squelched. It also contributes, as do ensuing features of the action potential, to the encoding of the stimulus strength as firing frequency. Spike amplitude shapes calcium channel activation and calcium entry, as well as K-channel activation. These in turn sculpt ensuing features, and, especially through calcium influx, sculpt the transduction from electrical response to output, including, for example, transmitter, modulator, hormone release, or muscle contraction. The latency of the rising phase is critical to encoding or integration, and can serve as a temporal filter. So, too, can the timing of repolarization

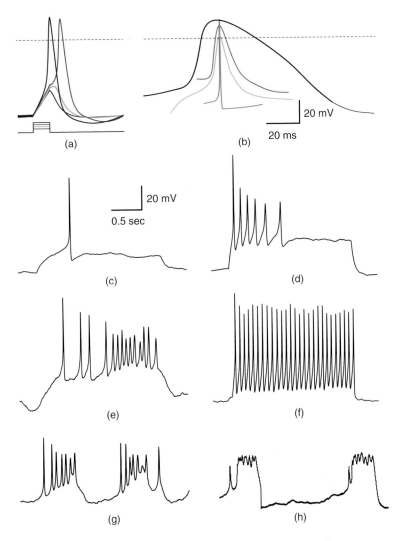

Figure 1.1   Variety of natural excitability. (a) Voltage responses of a mouse
adrenal chromaffin cell to 10 ms current steps, recorded with whole-cell current clamp
(McCobb Lab data). Action potential (AP) amplitudes were nearly invariant, and rise
times varied modestly with stimulus amplitude. Voltage scale as in (b). (b) AP
waveforms vary widely between cell types, ranging in duration from 180 μs for a
purkinje cell (orange; Bean (2007)) to > 80 ms for a cardiac muscle AP (black). Shown
for comparison are spikes from a barnacle muscle cell (blue; Fatt and Katz (1953)) and a
chromaffin cell (purple; McCobb Lab). (c–f) Patterns of spikes elicited with sustained
current steps vary even between mouse chromaffin cells (McCobb Lab). Cell (c) would
not fire more than one spike, (d) fired a train with declining frequency, amplitude, and
repolarization rate, (e), an irregular volley, and (f), a very regular train at high
frequency. (g, h) Pituitary corticotropes fire spontaneous bursts with features that vary
between bursts and between cells, including spike amplitudes and patterns, as well as
burst durations (McCobb Lab). Scale bars in (c) apply to (c–h).

and recovery. These can confer a resonance on the system that makes it selectively responsive to timing of input, and potentially, as responsive to hyperpolarizing as depolarizing input. Timing and the interplay between the channel mechanisms together pattern the timing of spikes. They can also confer intrinsic firing, exemplified by the beautifully complex rhythms of burst firing. In addition to influencing reactivity to inputs, intrinsic firing makes a neuron a potential source of action (or maintenance or inaction). Together the dimensions of complexity and variability that have evolved in electrical signalling contribute enormously to the intelligence of biological systems, including (but not exclusive to) the brain function.

Dissecting action potential mechanisms with voltage clamp. Hodgkin and Huxley (1952) used the *voltage clamp* to dissect the action potential in the squid giant axon. (The axon is a milimeter or more in diameter, roughly 100 times the diameter of the largest human fibers). This clever device measures the opening and closing of ion channels, as follows: the voltage difference between the inside and outside of an axon is measured, and compared to a desired or "command" voltage. Any discrepancy between measured and command potentials is then immediately eliminated by injecting current into the axon through a second internal electrode. The amount of current required to clamp the voltage depends on the membrane conductance (inverse of resistance), and thus changes as ion channels open or close (see Figure 1.2). While useful for studying any channels, the voltage clamp is especially important for voltage-gated channels. By varying the voltage itself in stepwise fashion, Hodgkin and Huxley were able to prove that the membrane had conductances that were directly gated by voltage. Then by removing Na and K ions independently, they resolved distinct inward and outward components, and noted their dramatically different kinetics. The inward (Na) current responded more rapidly, but terminated quickly, while the outward (K) current was slower but persisted. Recognizing that this voltage sensitivity might provide the feedback underlying the action potential, they carefully measured voltage- and time-dependent features, including activation and deactivation of inward and outward components, and inactivation and deinactivation of the inward component. They then constructed a mathematical model and solved it numerically for the response to a stimulus, with the similarity between the theoretical voltage response and a recorded action potential supporting the view that they had explained the basic mechanism.

So why do we need to continue modeling action potentials and excitability? Hodgkin and Huxley (1952) predated the identification of ion channel proteins,

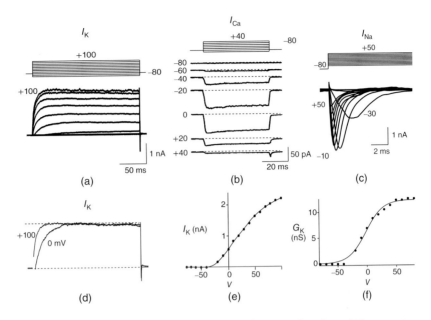

Figure 1.2   Voltage clamp data. (a, b, and c) Voltage-gated K, Ca, and Na currents, respectively, elicited with voltage steps in whole-cell voltage clamp mode applied to mouse chromaffin cells (McCobb Lab data). Outward currents are positive (upward), and inward currents are negative (downward). The K and Ca currents shown here exhibit little inactivation, though both types can inactivate in some chromaffin cells. The Na currents inactivate rapidly, and the current amplitude reverses sign when the test potential crosses the Na reversal potential. (d) K-current activation is faster at more depolarized potentials, as shown by normalizing the K currents at 0 and +100 mV from (a). (e) Current–voltage (I–V) plot for K currents from the cell in (a); peak current values are plotted against the corresponding test potential. (f) Conductance–voltage (G–V) plot; current values from (e) are divided by the driving force ($V_{test} - V_{reversal}$) and plotted against test potential. The G–V curve gives a summary of the voltage dependence of gating without the confounding effect of driving force.

but their results implied sophisticated voltage-sensing and gating nuances, and gave birth to structure-function analysis with unprecedented temporal resolution. Action potentials in barnacle muscle, another early preparation, were shown to depend on Ca rather than on Na influx (Keynes *et al.*, 1973). This laid the foundation for the Morris–Lecar model, in which one (excitatory) Ca current and one (repolarizing) K current interact to generate excitability (Morris and Lecar, 1981). Moreover, with glass electrodes enabling recordings in many more cell types, it became ever clearer that there was enormous variation on the general theme, begging further dissection. Every quantifiable feature of action potentials, from threshold to rise-time, duration, ensuing dip (*afterhyperpolarization*) and size, number, frequency, and pattern of additional action potentials elicited by various stimuli could be shown to vary from cell to cell. It is now clear that this variety sculpts signal input–output relationships for neurons and networks in almost limitless fashion. Meanwhile, a vast array of ion channel genes, accessory proteins, and modulatory mechanisms contributing to excitability has been identified (Coetzee *et al.*, 1999; Dolphin, 2009; Hille, 2001; Jan and Jan, 2012; Jegla *et al.*, 2009; Lipscombe *et al.*, 2013; Zakon, 2012). A wealth of questions arise. How do structural elements and combinations encode functional nuances appropriate to physiological, behavioral, and ecological contexts in diverse animals? How did they arise through evolution? How they are coordinated in development? And how does event-sensitive plasticity contribute to adaptive modification of excitability-dependent computations? Relevant hypotheses clearly depend on theoretical dissection via mathematical modeling.

Why work with a model originating in barnacle muscle? Throughout the chapter, we will work with the Morris–Lecar model, which was originally developed for barnacle muscle and includes only two voltage-gated channel types (Ca and K), neither of which inactivates. Moreover, based on observations that showed the activation rate for the excitatory Ca current to be about 10-fold faster than that for the repolarizing K current and 20-fold faster than that for charging the capacitor (Keynes *et al.*, 1973), Morris and Lecar (1981) simplified the model even further, reducing dimension by treating the Ca-channel activation as instantaneous.

You may ask why a neurobiologist or endocrinologist should spend time on such a simple system, so obviously peripheral to sophisticated neural computation. Or how simplification and omission justify the trouble of learning mathematical "hieroglyphics". These questions raise the issue of what a mathematical model is good for. A powerful use of models is to help test hypotheses and design experiments about putative biological mechanisms underlying observed behaviors. To that end, minimal models, built from the ground up, allow for thorough dissection and attribution of mechanisms. For example, see Izhikevich (2007, Chapter 5) for a summary of six minimal models of excitability. After studying the Morris–Lecar model in this chapter, we hope that you will agree that what may at first look like an extremely limited system turns out to be capable of a surprisingly rich repertoire of waveforms and firing dynamics. Without studying such a minimal model, one might assume that more channel types or more complex gating mechanisms were needed to generate such a variety. After developing modeling confidence, it is easy to adjust parameters, or add inactivation, other channel types or gating mechanisms, as detailed in Chapter 2. The comparison between Morris–Lecar, Hodgkin–Huxley, and other model behaviors then helps to clarify the interactive mechanisms at play, and the roles of specific terms and parameters.

The reduced dimension of the Morris–Lecar model also provides an excellent starting point for model analysis. It allows us to explore and dissect the model behavior in a two-dimensional *phase plane* (detailed in Section 1.4), where, with the help of graphical software, we can harness our visual intuition to understand the concepts and language of dynamical systems. The dynamical systems approach is extremely versatile, generalizing to more complex models and higher dimensions, and highlighting similarities among mechanisms in a wide range of applications. Throughout this volume, we will see how dynamical analysis of minimal models, designed with the scale and complexity of the specific neuroendocrine question in mind, yields new biological insights.

1.2   Introducing the Morris–Lecar model

The Morris–Lecar model is discussed in many texts in mathematical biology and theoretical neuroscience. See, for example, Ellner and Guckenheimer (2006), Ermentrout and Terman (2010), Fall *et al.* (2005), Izhikevich (2007), and Koch (1999).

What is in the Morris–Lecar model? The model structure is represented by the circuit diagram in Figure 1.3a (Morris and Lecar, 1981). A system of Ca and K gradients with selective conductances provides "batteries" defining equilibrium or reversal potentials. There is also a "leak" of undefined (probably composite) conductance, with a measurable reversal potential. For our purposes, the chemical gradients do not change appreciably: ion pumps and exchangers work in the background to ensure this. Currents applied through the current electrode travel in parallel across the capacitor and any open ion channels or other leaks. Internal and external solutions offer no resistance to flow, so that the voltage across the capacitor and resistors/conductors in the membrane is equivalent. Moreover, the system is assumed to be spatially uniform; voltage over the entire membrane changes in unison. This fits well with data from compact neuroendocrine cells (Bertram *et al.*, 2014; Liang *et al.*, 2011; Lovell *et al.*, 2004; Stojilkovic *et al.*, 2010; Tian and Shipston, 2000). The approach is also useful for membrane patches in most neuronal contexts. Spatial nonuniformity and spatio-temporal propagation of signals are not addressed here.

What makes this an "excitable" membrane and an interesting dynamical system, is (1) feedback: the proportion of channels open (for both Ca and K channels) depends on voltage and (2) reactions of the channel gates to changes in voltage take time. Reaction rates also vary with voltage; but while this influences the voltage waveform, it is not essential for excitability.

Ion channel openings and closings are stochastic events, but their numbers are large enough that the currents associated with each type can be modeled as smooth functions. Thus, four variables interact dynamically:

- The voltage (transmembrane potential), V, typically in millivolts, mV.
- The proportion of open channels, M, for the voltage-gated Ca channel that drives the rising phase of the action potential. Since M is a proportion, it ranges between 0 and 1, and has no units.
- The proportion of open channels, W, for the voltage-gated K channel that terminates the action potential. Like M, W is a proportion, so ranges between 0 and 1.
- Time, t, the independent variable, typically in milliseconds, ms.

Again, the dependent variables are functions of one another; they interact, and do so with time dependence. The rules by which they interact are translated into differential equations, as discussed below.

What is a differential equation? The only mathematical background we assume is that you have taken a calculus course sometime in the past (perhaps long ago) and remember (perhaps dimly) that the *derivative* represents instantaneous rate of change, or the slope of a graph. For example, Figure 1.1 shows several graphs of voltage, $V(t)$ versus time. Consider the detailed action potentials shown in Figure 1.1b. During the rising phase of each action potential, the slope of the graph is positive. So the derivative, $\frac{dV}{dt}$, is positive. This is just another way of saying that V is increasing or depolarizing. During the hyperpolarizing (decreasing) phase of each action potential, the graph is heading "downwards," with a negative slope, so $\frac{dV}{dt} < 0$. At the peak of each action potential, a line tangent to the graph would be horizontal, with zero slope. So $\frac{dV}{dt} = 0$ as the graph turns from increasing to decreasing. Similarly, $\frac{dV}{dt} = 0$ as the graph turns from decreasing to increasing.

(1.2.1) This is where the interactive part of the tutorial begins. This first exercise is designed to help cement the concepts of slope and derivative, and does not require any software. Choose one of the graphs in Figure 1.1 and track $\frac{dV}{dt}$ as you move along the graph. When is $\frac{dV}{dt}$ positive? When is it negative? How many times is it zero? When is $\frac{dV}{dt}$ greatest? When is it most negative? Try sketching the graph of $\frac{dV}{dt}$ below your graph of $V(t)$ (it helps to have the time axes lined up).

A *differential equation* is just an equation with a derivative in it somewhere. Equation (1.1) is a differential equation relating the rate of change of voltage to the currents flowing through the cell membrane. The differential equation does not tell us about V directly, in the sense that it is not of the form

$$V(t) = \text{"something"}$$

But if we can measure the value of V at one *initial* moment in time, Equation (1.1) tells us how V will change, so that we can use it to predict all future values of $V(t)$. Adding up all the incremental changes in V over time is called *numerical simulation*. It can be hard to do by hand, but is a job well suited to a computer. This is one of the reasons that mathematical modeling in biology has flourished with the computer revolution of recent decades, and why this tutorial is designed to be interactive, using the numerical simulation software XPP (Ermentrout, 2012).

A word of warning: the derivative is a fundamental concept in mathematics, so has earned many names; $\frac{dV}{dt}$ ("dV by dt"), V' ("V prime"), and $\dot{V}$ ("V dot") are all equivalent in this context, and not to be confused with plain V.

The differential equation for voltage change over time. According to Kirchoff's current law, if a current I is applied across the membrane (through an electrode, say), it is balanced by the sum of the capitative and ionic currents:

$$I = C\frac{dV}{dt} + I_{Ca} + I_K + I_L$$

If there is no applied current, then $I = 0$. Here, I_{Ca} and I_K denote the Ca and K currents respectively; I_L denotes a leak current (a voltage independent current that may or may not be selective); C denotes the capacitance, and $C\frac{dV}{dt}$ represents the capacitive current. The fact that capacitive current is proportional to how quickly voltage changes $\left(\frac{dV}{dt}\right)$ is what makes this a differential equation. Rearranging to bring the derivative to the left-hand side,

$$C\frac{dV}{dt} = I - I_{Ca} - I_K - I_L$$

Thus,

$$C\frac{dV}{dt} = I - g_{Ca}M(V - V_{Ca}) - g_K W(V - V_K) - g_L(V - V_L) \qquad (1.1)$$

where the ionic currents are modeled by

$$I_{Ca} = g_{Ca}M(V - V_{Ca}) \qquad (1.2)$$

$$I_K = g_K W(V - V_K) \qquad (1.3)$$

$$I_L = g_L(V - V_L) \qquad (1.4)$$

Let us walk through these equations term by term, to understand the notation, and how the ionic currents are represented. To fix ideas, consider the K current. In Equation (1.3), I_K is modeled as the product of:

- The maximal K conductance, g_K, that can be measured at any voltage (see Figure 1.2).
- The K-channel activation variable, W, which changes over time (so is written $W(t)$, or W for short). There is no K-channel inactivation in the model, so, relative to maximal conductance, $W(t)$ represents the proportion of K channels that are open at time t, and the instantaneous probability that an individual K channel is in its open state. In other words, $W(t)$ represents the normalized K conductance at time t (taking values between 0 and 1), and $g_K W(t)$ represents the absolute K conductance. Expressions for the voltage dependence and kinetics of W are formulated in Equations (1.6), (1.9), and (1.10).
- The driving force, $(V - V_K)$, on K current through the K channels. This is the difference between V of the moment and V_K, the K reversal potential. The larger the difference, the larger the driving force; and as V changes over time, the driving force changes accordingly.

Thus, Equation (1.3) is simply a mathematical translation of the fact that K current is given by K conductance multiplied by K driving force. Clear translation between the biology and the mathematics is at the heart of mathematical modeling.

The Ca and leak currents are treated similarly, with the Ca-channel activation variable denoted by M in Equation (1.2). Equation (1.4) for the leak current looks slightly different, because leak conductance is assumed to be independent of voltage, so it does not need an activation variable. Thus, the leak has constant conductance, g_L. In this tutorial, we set the conductances at $g_{Ca} = 4$, $g_K = 8$ and $g_L = 2$ (see Table 1.1).

(1.2.2) In this exercise, let us think about the impact of the K current on V, to help understand the signs in Equation (1.1). If $V > V_K$, is I_K positive or negative? It helps to remember that g_K and W are both positive. You should find that I_K is positive. So, when you check the signs in Equation (1.1), you see that the K current contributes *negatively* to $\frac{dV}{dt}$. That is, the K current promotes change in the negative direction. In the absence of other currents, what impact would this have on V? Would it increase V or decrease V? So, is the K current driving V towards V_K, or away from V_K? (Remember that we started by assuming $V > V_K$.)

(1.2.3) What happens if $V < V_K$? Explain how the K current drives V towards V_K in this case, too.

The reversal potential for a purely selective channel is equal to the Nernst equilibrium potential for the ion carrying the current. For a current representing multiple permeabilities (such as leak), the reversal potential is calculated using the Goldman–Hodgkin–Katz equation if the relative permeabilities and ionic gradients are known, or measured in voltage clamp if the current species can be isolated (Hille 2001). In this tutorial, we set the reversal potentials at $V_{Ca} = 120$ mV, $V_K = -84$ mV, and $V_L = -60$ mV (see Table 1.1.)

Looking back at Equation (1.1), we can think of the three ionic currents competing with each other and with the applied current, each trying to drive V to its own reversal potential as in Exercises 1.2.2 and 1.2.3. Over the course of an action potential, the different voltage dependence of Ca- and K-channel gating changes the relative sizes of M and W, allowing different terms in Equation (1.1) to dominate. When the Ca term dominates, V is driven toward the high Ca reversal potential and the cell depolarizes. And when the K term dominates, V is driven back down toward the low K reversal potential and the cell hyperpolarizes (see Figure 1.4a).

The voltage dependence of steady-state conductance. K-channel activation, W, is assumed to have kinetics and voltage dependence. Both aspects are measured using the voltage clamp, as illustrated in Figure 1.2. In these experiments, the voltage is stepped instantaneously to each of a series of test voltages and held there, while the current reaches a new steady state (Figure 1.2a). Arrival at the steady state is not instantaneous, but defines the kinetics of channel activation, which is itself voltage dependent (Figure 1.2d). We return to the kinetics presently.

The amount of current at the steady state for a test voltage reflects the conformational stability of open states of the K channel; the greater the stability, the more channels open and the greater the conductance. To characterize the voltage dependence of steady-state conductance, the steady-state values of current are first plotted against test voltage to give the current–voltage (*I–V*) plot (Figure 1.2e). Since the measured current is assumed to be the product of driving force and conductance, the current is divided by the driving force to give the conductance–voltage (*G–V*) plot (Figure 1.2f). To estimate the maximal conductance, g_K, the *G–V* curve is fit with a Boltzmann function (Figure 1.2f), then g_K is given by the maximal value, or upper asymptote, of the Boltzmann curve. The Boltzmann function is then normalized (divided) by g_K to yield the proportion, $W_\infty(V)$, of (activatable) channels that are open at the steady state, as a function of V.

Equations (1.5) and (1.6) define the steady-state open probabilities, $M_{\infty(V)}$ and $W_{\infty(V)}$, for the Ca and K channels, respectively, in our Morris–Lecar model (see Figure 1.3b):

$$M_\infty(V) = \frac{1}{1 + e^{-2(V-V_1)/V_2}} = 0.5\left(1 + \tanh\left(\frac{V - V_1}{V_2}\right)\right) \qquad (1.5)$$

$$W_\infty(V) = \frac{1}{1 + e^{-2(V-V_3)/V_4}} = 0.5\left(1 + \tanh\left(\frac{V - V_3}{V_4}\right)\right) \qquad (1.6)$$

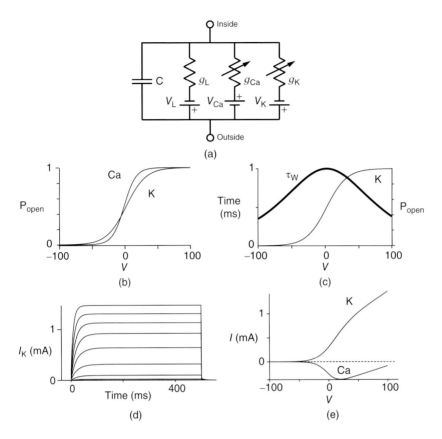

Figure 1.3   Morris–Lecar model. (a) Equivalent electrical circuit representation of the Morris–Lecar model cell. Membrane capacitance is in parallel with selective conductances and batteries (representing driving forces arising from ionic gradients). Arrows indicate variation (with voltage) for Ca and K conductance. (b) Normalized G–V curves, W_∞ and M_∞, assumed for model K and Ca conductances, respectively. (c) The kinetics of voltage-dependent activation of K channels is also voltage dependent, with the normalized time constant, τ_W, assumed to peak (i.e., channel gating slowest) at the midpoint of the G–V curve, where channel conformational preference is weakest. (d) Simulated voltage clamped K currents at 20 mV increments up to $V=100$ mV. Voltage clamp simulated in XPP by removing the equation for dV/dt and, instead, setting V as a fixed parameter. (e) Model I–V plots for K and Ca currents. Different reversal potentials for the two conductances ($V_K = -84$, $V_{Ca} = 120$ mV) make the current traces look very different, despite similar activation functions in (b). (b)–(e) Use Hopf parameter set.

In the next exercises, we will graph $W_\infty(V)$ to cement intuition for the role of V_3 and V_4. $M_\infty(V)$ is similar. In Exercise 1.2.7, we will confirm that the two different forms of the equations are, indeed, equal. The exercises are written with the online graphing calculator *Desmos* in mind, but any graphing calculator will do. We choose Desmos because it is fun to work with, and for the ease of setting up sliders to explore the way parameters shape the graph. See Table 1.1 for the values of $V_1, V_2, V_3,$ and V_4 used in later sections of this tutorial.

(1.2.4) Open Desmos in a browser (www.desmos.com). You enter functions in the panel on the left, and watch them appear on the axes on the right. For example, click on the left panel, and type in $y = e^x$. You should see the familiar exponential function appear. Now click on the next box on the left, and enter $y = e^{(x-c)}$. Click on the "button" to accept the offer to add a slider for c. Slide the value of c (by hand, or by clicking the "play" arrow) and watch your graph shift to the left or right accordingly. Now, try $y = d + e^{(x-c)}$. You can add a new slider for d. What is the effect of sliding d? Notice how the old c slider now works for both the functions. You can temporarily hide a graph by clicking on the colored circle next to its equation, or permanently erase it by clicking on its gray X. There is also an edit button to explore.

(1.2.5) As we have seen, Desmos uses x and y for variables, and single letters for other parameters. So, to graph $W_\infty(V)$, you will need to re-write Equation (1.6) with x playing the role of V, y playing the role of W_∞, a playing the role of V_3 and b playing the role of V_4. In other words, working with the Boltzmann form of Equation (1.6) first, enter

$$y = \frac{1}{1 + e^{(-2(x-a)/b)}} \tag{1.7}$$

(being careful with your parentheses!), and accept the sliders for a and b. You should see a typical (normalized) G–V curve ranging between 0 and 1, as shown in Figures 1.2f, 1.3b, and 1.3c. Slide a and b to see what role they play in shaping the curve. You can change the limits of the sliders if you like. For example, click on the lower limit of b and set it to zero, to keep b positive.

(1.2.6) Translating back to the language of Equation (1.6), confirm that V_3 is the half-activation voltage of W_∞, and V_4 determines the "spread" of W_∞. As V_4 increases, the spread increases. In other words, as V_4 increases, the slope at half-activation decreases. In fact, differentiating Equation (1.6) at $V = V_3$ shows that the slope at half-activation is given by $\frac{1}{2V_4}$. Confirm this with Desmos, by graphing the line $y = \frac{1}{2} + \frac{1}{2b}$ (which has slope $\frac{1}{2b}$) together with Equation (1.7), setting $a = 0$, and sliding b.

(1.2.7) Use Desmos to plot

$$y = 0.5 \left(1 + \tanh\left(\frac{x-a}{b}\right)\right) \tag{1.8}$$

and confirm that this second form of Equation (1.6) is equivalent to the first. In other words, it has exactly the same graph. This second form is also commonly used, and you will see it in the XPP code provided. If you are unfamiliar with the hyperbolic tangent function, $\tanh x$, develop your intuition by building up the graph of Equation (1.8) in parts. First graph $y = \tanh x$, then $y = \tanh(x - a)$, etc. (Recall that the more familiar $\sin x, \cos x$, and $\tan x$ are defined using a point on the unit circle $x^2 + y^2 = 1$. The hyperbolic functions $\sinh x, \cosh x$, and $\tanh x$ have analogous definitions using a point on the hyperbola $x^2 - y^2 = 1$.)

Voltage-dependent kinetics of voltage gating. Now we return to the kinetics of K-channel gating, governing the rate of approach to the steady state. The channels are trying to reach the steady state for conductance at a particular voltage, but during the process the voltage is typically changing. As a result, the channels are always playing catch-up. Moreover, the rate at which the channels respond to voltage is itself a function of voltage. These kinetics are modeled by the differential equation

$$\frac{dW}{dt} = \frac{\phi}{\tau_W(V)}(W_\infty(V) - W) \tag{1.9}$$

Here, ϕ and $\tau_W(V)$ are both positive, and together define the time scale (or time constant) of K kinetics. The voltage dependence of the time scale is captured by the equation for $\tau_W(V)$

$$\tau_W(V) = \frac{1}{\cosh((V - V_3)/2V_4)} \tag{1.10}$$

See Figure 1.3c. We will develop intuition for Equations (1.9) and (1.10) in the following exercises. See Table 1.1 for the values of ϕ, V_3, and V_4 used in later sections of this tutorial.

(1.2.8) First let us focus on the $(W_\infty(V) - W)$ term in Equation (1.9). It is reminiscent of the $(V - V_K)$ term in Equation (1.3), and can be analyzed in a similar way. Recall that V and W change over time. So, at a given time t, V and W will have values $V(t)$ and $W(t)$. What happens if, at time t, $W(t) > W_\infty(V(t))$? Will W increase or decrease in the next increment of time? Remember that ϕ and $\tau_W(V)$ are both positive. So, if you keep track of the signs, you should find that if $W(t) > W_\infty(V(t))$, then $dW/dt < 0$, so W is driven down, toward $W_\infty(V(t))$.

(1.2.9) What happens if $W(t) < W_\infty(V(t))$? Explain how the conductance is driven towards steady state in this case, too. As time marches on, V changes. So the voltage-dependent steady-state conductance, $W_\infty(V)$, also changes. Thus, the $(W_\infty(V) - W)$ term in Equation (1.9) ensures that W adjusts course accordingly, in its tireless game of catch-up.

(1.2.10) Now, let us focus on $\tau_W(V)$ to prepare us for understanding its role in Equation (1.9). Use Desmos to graph $\tau_W(V)$, as shown in Figure 1.3c. Recall that you will need to rewrite the equation for $\tau_W(V)$ with x playing the role of V, y playing the role of τ_W, and single letters playing the role of V_3 and V_4. For example, you could graph

$$y = \frac{1}{\cosh((x - a)/2b)} \tag{1.11}$$

with sliders for a and b. Here, $\cosh x$ stands for hyperbolic cosine, the analog of cosine for the hyperbola. If you are unfamiliar with hyperbolic cosine, then build up Equation (1.11) in parts: first graph $y = \cosh x$, then $y = \cosh(x - a)$, etc. What role does a play in the graph of Equation (1.11)? What role does b play? What is the maximum value of τ_W? What is the minimum value? Translating this back to the language of Equation (1.10), you should find that $\tau_W(V)$ reaches a peak value of 1 at $V = V_3$, and decays down to zero on either side of V_3. The rate of decay is governed by V_4: the greater the value of V_4, the greater the "spread" of τ_W.

(1.2.11) Recall that V_3 and V_4 are also the shape parameters for $W_\infty(V)$. Use Desmos to plot the graph of $W_\infty(V)$ on the same axes as your graph of $\tau_W(V)$ (see Figure 1.3c). Use a to represent V_3 in both equations, and b to represent V_4. Then, when you slide a and b, you can see their effect on both equations simultaneously. What do you notice? τ_W and W_∞ have similar spreads, and τ_W has its maximum at the half-activation voltage of K conductance.

(1.2.12) Now, look back at Equation (1.9). Does W change faster when $\tau_W = 1$ or when $\tau_W = 0.1$? In other words, does W change faster at half-activation, or far from half-activation? Does that make sense?

Recapping, Equations (1.9) and (1.10) model the voltage-dependent kinetics of K$^+$ conductance. The time constant $\frac{\tau_W(V)}{\phi}$ governs the rate at which W catches up with the ever-changing $W_\infty(V)$. The kinetics are slowest around the half activation voltage where the probabilities of K$^+$ channel opening or closing balance.

Fast calcium kinetics reduce the dimension of the model. Equations similar to (1.9) and (1.10) could be used to model the kinetics of Ca conductance. However, as described in Section 1.1, Morris and Lecar (1981) used the time-scale separation observed between the Ca and K kinetics to reduce the dimension of their model. Instead of including an additional differential equation to follow the very fast approach of Ca conductance to its steady state, they made the assumption that Ca-channel activation occurs immediately, relative to the time scale of K kinetics. In other words, they assume that Ca activation, M, is always "caught-up" to $M_\infty(V)$. So, $M_\infty(V)$ can be substituted for M in Equation (1.1), yielding Equation (1.12).

Summarizing. The Morris–Lecar model is given by the system of two coupled nonlinear differential equations

$$C\frac{dV}{dt} = I - g_{Ca}M_\infty(V - V_{Ca}) - g_K W(V - V_K) - g_L(V - V_L) \tag{1.12}$$

$$\frac{dW}{dt} = \frac{\phi}{\tau_W(V)}(W_\infty(V) - W) \tag{1.13}$$

where

$$M_\infty(V) = 0.5\left(1 + \tanh\left(\frac{V - V_1}{V_2}\right)\right) \tag{1.14}$$

$$W_\infty(V) = 0.5\left(1 + \tanh\left(\frac{V - V_3}{V_4}\right)\right) \tag{1.15}$$

$$\tau_W(V) = \frac{1}{\cosh((V - V_3)/2V_4)} \tag{1.16}$$

The variables, parameters, and parameter values we use are summarized in Table 1.1.

Table 1.1 Variables and parameter values used.

Variable or parameter	Definition	Units	Hopf values	SNIC values	Homo values
t	Time	ms			
$V(t)$	Membrane voltage at time t	mV			
$W(t)$	Proportion of K channels open at time t				
$M_\infty(V)$	Proportion of Ca channels open at steady state at voltage V				
$W_\infty(V)$	Proportion of K channels open at steady state at voltage V				
I	Applied current*	μA cm^{-2}			
C	Capacitance*	μF cm^{-2}	20	20	20
V_{Ca}	Ca reversal potential	mV	120	120	120
V_K	K reversal potential	mV	−84	−84	−84
V_L	Leak reversal potential	mV	−60	−60	−60
g_{Ca}	Maximal Ca conductance*	mS cm^{-2}	4	4	4
g_K	Maximal K conductance*	mS cm^{-2}	8	8	8
g_L	Leak conductance*	mS cm^{-2}	2	2	2
V_1	Voltage at half-activation of Ca channels	mV	−1.2	−1.2	−1.2
V_2	Spread (steepness $^{-1}$) of $M_\infty(V)$	mV	18	18	18
V_3	Voltage at half-activation of K channels	mV	2	12	12
V_4	Spread (steepness $^{-1}$) of $W_\infty(V)$	mV	30	17	17
ϕ/τ_W	Rate constant for K-channel kinetics	ms^{-1}			
$\tau_W(V)$	Voltage dependence of K-channel kinetics	ms			
ϕ	Rate constant for K-channel kinetics at half-activation voltage		0.04	0.04	0.22

*Throughout the tutorial, we suppress the cm^{-2} on current, capacitance, and conductance.

What does the model tell us? Now, we have equations for how V and W change! In the rest of the tutorial, we use numerical simulation and graphical analysis to gradually uncover the richness of behavior the minimal mechanisms included in this model cell can exhibit.

The model is autonomous. Notice that the independent variable, time, does not appear explicitly in the right-hand sides of Equations (1.12)–(1.16). So the system is *autonomous*, or self-governing, meaning that the rates of change, $\frac{dV}{dt}$ and $\frac{dW}{dt}$ depend only on the state of V and W, and not on when they achieve that state. In Section 1.4, we will see how this autonomous structure is key to the phase-plane approach used throughout the text.

1.3 Opening XPP and triggering an action potential

From here on, you will need a dynamical systems software package to work the interactive exercises. The main tools used in this tutorial are: (1) numerical integration of systems of two and three differential equations, and plotting solutions against time, and (2) phase-plane plots and calculations for systems of two differential equations, including trajectories, direction fields, nullclines, equilibria, limit cycles, and eigenvalues. We will define these terms as we come to them.

There are many good software packages available for simulating differential equations, each with its own strengths and weaknesses. We have written this tutorial to work directly with XPP (also called XPP-Aut), by Bard Ermentrout (2012). We have chosen XPP for several reasons. It is freely available, widely used in the computational neuroendocrine community, and works on many platforms, including Mac, Windows, and Linux machines, all with the same menu system and graphical user interface. We find that it has a good balance of computational power, user friendliness, and modeling freedom. The combination of two-dimensional phase-plane graphics and the capability of simulating higher dimensional models is particularly useful, especially if your goal is to develop more complex models of your own, involving several coupled differential equations. XPP can also simulate many types of differential equation, and a wide range of examples from biology, chemistry, and physics are included with the download.

There are also XPP apps for the iPad and iPhone. The interface is different for these apps, since it makes use of the touch-sensitive screen. Thus, to work this tutorial on an iPad or iPhone, you will need to learn the interface and modify our menu instructions. Similarly, if you prefer a different software package, it should be straightforward to translate the exercises accordingly. For example, PPLANE (MATLAB or Java based, http://math.rice.edu/ dfield) and Berkeley Madonna (www.berkeleymadonna.com) both have user friendly two-dimensional phase-plane graphics. Or you may prefer the independence of Matlab (www.mathworks.com), R (http://www.r-project.org), or Mathematica (http://www.wolfram.com/mathematica). See the online supplementary materials to Ellner and Guckenheimer (2006) for Matlab and R-tutorials, and R-based PPLANE.

Download XPP. At the time of writing, the following steps work to download the Mac, Windows, or Linux versions of XPP.
- Visit Bard Ermentrout's XPP-Aut page at: http://www.math.pitt.edu/ bard/xpp/xpp.html There is online documentation, an interactive tutorial, and much more. Read the information for your platform below the *DOWNLOAD* link, then click on *DOWNLOAD*.
- Go to *Assorted Binaries*, then *Latest* to find the latest binary file for your platform. Mac versions are "dmg" files with "mac" or "osx" in the title somewhere, windows versions are "zip" files with "win" in the title somewhere.
- Download a version for your platform, then open the file *install.pdf*. Carefully follow the instructions that tell you where to put the files, how to download an "X server," if necessary, and how to fire up XPP. (If you run into trouble trying to quit XPP, look ahead a couple of pages to the paragraph headed *Essential XPP tips.*)

ODE files. XPP is a tool for simulating differential equations. It reads the equations from an *ODE file* written by the user. There is a lot of helpful information about the structure of ODE files, and a wealth of examples, on the XPP website. Example ODE files are also included in the files downloaded with XPP, together with a manual (*XPP_doc*) and a succinct summary of commands (*XPP_sum*) in PDF and postscript (ps) formats. XPP was written for applications to neuroscience, and the manual and online tutorial use neural models throughout. It is well worth learning to read and write ODE files, as it gives you control over the nuances of the model, and the freedom to experiment with new models of your own. The components of the ODE file given below will be explained as we work with it in XPP.

Download the ODE file for this tutorial. For the interactive exercises, you will need the file BridgingTutorial-MLecar.ode reproduced below. Electronic copies are available on the website for this volume and from the authors. We recommend downloading an electronic copy, to save yourself the trouble of re-typing it and, more importantly, the possibility of mis-typing.

As stated in the XPP manual: "ODE files are ASCII readable files that the XPP parser reads to create machine usable code." This means that it is important to use a plain text editor for ODE files, because complex editors (such as word) add invisible extra characters to your document that render it unreadable to XPP. Use an editor like Textedit (on a Mac) or NotePad or WordPad (in Windows). Be sure to save the file as plain text such as ASCII, or UTF-8.

```
# BridgingTutorial–MLecar.ode
# From 'Bridging Between Experiments and Equations' by McCobb and Zeeman
# Adapted from online examples by Bard Ermentrout and by Arthur Sherman

# differential equations
dV/dt = (I – gca*Minf(V)*(V–Vca) – gk*W*(V–Vk) – gl*(V–Vl))/C
dW/dt = phi*(Winf(V)–W)/tauW(V)

# functions
Minf(V)=.5*(1+tanh((V–V1)/V2))
Winf(V)=.5*(1+tanh((V–V3)/V4))
tauW(V)=1/cosh((V–V3)/(2*V4))

# default initial conditions
V(0) = −60
W(0)=0

# default parameters
param I=0,C=20
param Vca=120,Vk=−84,Vl=−60
param gca=4,gk=8,gl=2
param V1=−1.2,V2=18

# uncomment the parameter set of choice
param V3=2,V4=30,phi=.04
# param V3=12,V4=17,phi=.04
# param V3=12,V4=17,phi=.22

# choose a parameter set using '(F)ile' then '(G)et par set' in XPP menu
set hopf  {Vca=120,Vk=−84,Vl=−60,gca=4,gk=8,gl=2,C=20,V1=−1.2,V2=18,V3=2, V4=30,phi=.04}
set snic  {Vca=120,Vk=−84,Vl=−60,gca=4,gk=8,gl=2,C=20,V1=−1.2,V2=18,V3=12,V4=17,phi=.04}
set homo {Vca=120,Vk=−84,Vl=−60,gca=4,gk=8,gl=2,C=20,V1=−1.2,V2=18,V3=12,V4=17,phi=.22}

# track some currents and conductances
aux Ica = gca*Minf(V)*(V–Vca)
aux Ik = gk*W*(V–Vk)
aux Il = gl*(V–Vl)
aux CaCond = gCa*Minf(V)
aux KCond = gk*W
aux POpenCa = Minf(V)
aux POpenK = W

# Open XPP with (t,V) voltage–trace window or (V,W) phase–plane window.
@ xp=t,yp=V,xlo=0,xhi=200,ylo=−80,yhi=50
# @ xp=V,yp=W,xlo=−75,xhi=70,ylo=−0.2,yhi=1

# some numerical settings
@ dt=.25,total=200,bounds=10000,maxstore=15000

done
```

Reading the ODE file. Lines beginning with a # symbol are not read by XPP. They can be used for comments, or to make choices between options by inactivating the unwanted options.

(1.3.1) Find the differential equations and associated functions in *BridgingTutorial-MLecar.ode*, and check that they agree with Equations (1.12)–(1.16). The notation is slightly different in XPP, because there are fewer symbols available and no subscripts, but the translation from Equations (1.12)–(1.16) is fairly straightforward. For example, *Minf(V), Winf(V), tauW(V),* and *phi* correspond to $M_\infty(V), W_\infty(V), \tau_W(V),$ and ϕ, respectively.

(1.3.2) Confirm that the parameter values listed in the ODE file agree with those in Table 1.1.

Initial conditions. Recall from Section 1.2 that the differential equations for V and W tell us the rate of change of V and W. So, if we know the values of V and W at one *initial* moment in time, we (or preferably XPP) can numerically predict the future values of $V(t)$ and $W(t)$ by adding on the incremental changes over time. Thus, in order to simulate the time course of V and W, XPP needs *initial conditions* $V(0)$ and $W(0)$.

(1.3.3) Find the default initial conditions in the ODE file. What does the initial condition $W(0) = 0$ tell you about the K channels?

(1.3.4) The initial membrane voltage is $V(0) = -60$. What does this tell you about the Ca channels? Hint: Use the equation for the voltage dependence of Ca-channel gating (Equation (1.14)), with the parameter values from the ODE file (see also Figure 1.3b).

Notice, again, the difference in the way Ca and K channels are treated in the model. The assumption of "instantaneous" kinetics of Ca-channel gating means that the state of the Ca channels at any given time can be deduced directly from the membrane voltage at that time. In particular, the initial state of the Ca channels follows from that of the membrane voltage, as in Exercise 1.3.4. By contrast, the slow response of K channels to changing voltage is tracked by $W(t)$, which, in turn, depends on their initial state, $W(0)$.

(1.3.5) Confirm that the applied current, I, is set to a default value of zero in the ODE file. In the absence of applied current, and with the default initial conditions, how do you expect this cell to behave?

The rest of the ODE file will be explained as we work with XPP. For more information, see the XPP manual *XPP_doc* (included with the download and available online (Ermentrout, 2012)).

Opening XPP. Methods for firing up XPP depend on the platform you are using and are described in the file *install.pdf* included with the download. In all cases, XPP has a console window, and is fired up from the console using an ODE file. On a Mac and Windows computer, the install instructions describe how to set up a shortcut to the XPP console. XPP can be started by dragging an ODE file onto the icon, or into the open console window. On a Linux computer, the install instructions describe how to set up the path and fire up ODE files from the command line (the terminal window then functions as the console). The console reports errors and other useful information.

(1.3.6) Fire up XPP using the ODE file *BridgingTutorial-MLecar.ode*. The console will report XPP's progress on reading the ODE file and, if all is well, an XPP command window will open up. The command window includes a graphics window, a menu down the left-side buttons and a command line along the top, and sliders along the bottom. If the menu and sliders are overlapping, enlarge the window by dragging the bottom right corner. Let us graph the voltage time course of our model cell. Click on the ICs button at the top of the command window. A small window should open, showing the initial condition $V = -60$ and $W = 0$. Click *Go*. An unremarkable voltage trace appears on the graph, showing a cell at rest, close to $V = -60$. Is this what you expected?

Essential XPP tips. We will use XPP to trigger action potentials, explore and dissect the model behavior, and learn some of the concepts and language of dynamical systems. But first a few essential tips to help give you immediate XPP independence.

- Quitting XPP. There are several ways to quit XPP, none of them quite obvious. In the command window menu, click *File* then *Quit* in the submenu, then *Yes* on the tiny pop-up window. Alternatively, depending on your operating system, you may be able to click *Cancel* on the console (bottom right), then click *Quit* in the same place.
- To close a pop-up window, use the *close* button within the window. The usual way of closing windows (e.g., red button on a mac) may not work.
- The capital letter in the name is the shortcut to each menu item. Within each submenu, there are similar shortcuts, shown in parentheses. For example, typing *FQY* is a shortcut for quitting XPP. Henceforth, we will show the short cuts in parentheses.
- When you hover over a menu item with the mouse, a brief description is given in the skinny text line along the bottom of the command window.
- Sometimes you need to press the *escape* key to escape the mode you have put XPP into. For example, the *(N)umerics* menu is unlike the others: if you enter it, you need to press *escape* to exit.

- Sometimes XPP needs your input before it can run your command. For example, if you click on *(X)i* versus *t* in the menu, it may appear that nothing has happened. In fact, the skinny command line along the top of the command window is asking you which variable you want to plot against time, *t*. Enter your choice (e.g., *W*), then press return.
- So, if XPP seems unresponsive, check to see if it is asking a question in the command line or in a tiny pop-up window (possibly hidden behind other windows). If not, try pressing escape a few times.
- Some menu items only apply to some types of graph. For example, the *(D)ir. field/flow* menu only works when you are plotting two dependent variables against each other (e.g., *V* versus *W*, see Section 1.4). Otherwise, nothing happens when you try it.
- Succinct information about all the main menu and submenu commands is listed in the manual *XPP_doc* that is downloaded with XPP, and in the *Online Documentation* on the XPP homepage (Ermentrout, 2012).

Triggering an action potential. Returning to our model cell, imagine applying a short pulse of positive current, as in a current clamp experiment designed to characterize the cell's excitability. During the pulse, the membrane voltage will rapidly depolarize (increase), with the amount of depolarization depending on the magnitude and duration of the applied current. The K channels will, in turn, respond to the voltage change, but on a slower time scale. A useful way to think about this, from the modeling point of view, is that the brief stimulus has the effect of resetting the initial values of *V* and *W*, where the word "initial" now refers to the moment of termination of the stimulus (initiation of the post-stimulus response). In other words, we can think of the initial values of *V* and *W* as reflecting the recent history of the cell. In the case of our stimulus pulse, if it is very brief relative to the time scale of the K channels, then *W* does not have time to change much during the pulse, so, roughly speaking, only *V* is reset. The subsequent effect on *W* is seen in the post-stimulus response.

Figure 1.4a shows model voltage responses during and after a range of 2 ms stimulus pulses (amplitudes in Figure 1.4b). Before each pulse, the cell is at rest at $V = -60$. During the pulse, $I = I_{stim} > 0$ in Equation (1.12), and the voltage rises rapidly. Thus, at the end of the pulse, when *I* returns to zero, *V* has been "reset." After the pulse, the cell responds with classic threshold behavior: firing an action potential only if the reset *V* is sufficiently high.

In the next exercises, we will use XPP to explore the cell's post-stimulus response. Instead of modeling the stimulus pulse itself, we will reset the initial value of *V* directly – as a proxy for the cell's stimulus history – and plot *only* the post-stimulus response. In Section 1.4, we will see how

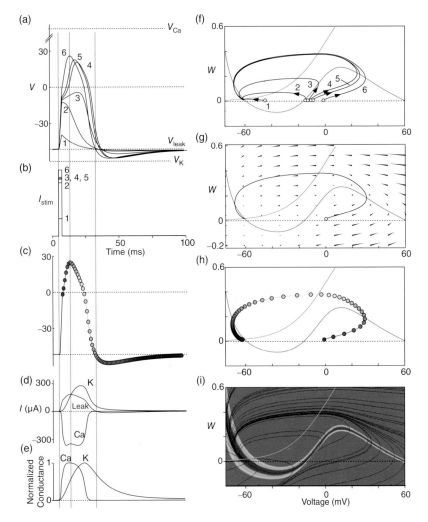

Figure 1.4 Model action potentials. Simulated response to a stimulus pulse, using Hopf parameter set. (a) Sub- and super-threshold voltage responses to the brief current steps in (b). Current amplitudes 1–6 were 150, 460, 480, 490, 500, and 570 µA, respectively. Responses 1 and 2 are below, 3 is near, and 4–6 are above firing threshold. (c) Voltages at 1 ms intervals for time course 6 in (a) (colored circles). (d) Model currents, and (e) normalized voltage-dependent conductances underlying response 6. Note the slower kinetics of K-current activation, despite similar G–V curves (Figure 1.3b), due to the different kinetic assumptions in the model. (f–i) Trajectories and nullclines (red and green, marking where V and W turn, respectively) in the phase plane. The intersection of the nullclines is a stable equilibrium; the ultimate destination of all trajectories after the brief stimulus pulse. (f) Trajectories corresponding to the voltage time courses in (a). An action potential corresponds to a counterclockwise excursion around the phase plane. (g) Trajectory 6 plotted with the direction field; vectors indicate the direction and rate of movement at any point in the phase plane. (h) Trajectory 6 plotted at 1 ms intervals, as in (c), indicating the speed of motion around the trajectory. The motion slows where V turns on the red nullcline, and where V approaches equilibrium. (i) The flow, represented by trajectories from many initial values in the phase plane. Color indicates speed of motion around the phase plane, from blue (slow) to orange (fast).

this approach lends itself to simultaneously plotting the cell's response to *all* possible histories on one graph, called the *phase plane*. (Note: if you wish to also explore the response during stimulus, an ODE file *BridgingTutorial-StimPulse.ode* is available on the website for this volume, or from the authors.)

(1.3.7) Continuing from Exercise 1.3.6, activate the XPP command window by clicking on it. Then click *(E)rase* to clear the graph. Click the *ICs* button, if necessary, to re-open the small window showing the initial conditions for V and W. Reset V to the depolarized value -30 (you may need to click once or twice in the box before you can erase or type in it). Leave W unchanged at 0, and click the *Go* button. How does the cell respond?

(1.3.8) The depolarization in the last exercise was evidently not strong enough to trigger an action potential, since the cell returned directly to rest. Try resetting the initial V to the more depolarized value -10, to represent a stronger stimulus. Now what happens?

(1.3.9) We saw in the last exercise that the cell fires an action potential if the stimulus is strong enough to reset V to -10 mV. Experiment with the initial V to see the decisive, all-or-nothing nature of the response, and reproduce the post stimulus responses of Figure 1.4a. Where is the firing threshold? In other words, approximately what is the smallest value of V that can trigger an action potential?

Dissecting the action potential. In the next exercises we will plot the post-stimulus time courses of the currents, conductances, and K-channel activation, W, that contribute to the action potential. Then, in Section 1.4, we will analyze the action potential from the phase-plane point of view, as in Figure 1.4f–i.

(1.3.10) To see the slow K-channel response, let us plot the post-stimulus time course of W. Click on the command window to activate it, then click on *(M)akewindow* in the menu, followed by *(C)reate* in the submenu. A new, small graphics window should open, showing a copy of the most recent V time course plotted. Notice that the new window does not have its own menu system. Instead, the command window menu applies to whichever graphics window is activated. A tiny black square in the upperleft corner of a graphics window indicates it is active. Activate the new window by clicking in it, and resize it to your taste. Click on *(V)iewaxes* in the menu, then *(2)D* in the submenu. Replace V with W for the *Y-axis*, and, since W is a proportion, set the Y range from a minimum of 0 to a maximum of 1. Note that you can also set the axis labels: t for the X label and W for the Y label. Then click the *OK* button. A W time course should appear in the new graphics window.

(1.3.11) The *W* time course you have plotted corresponds to the initial values of *V* and *W* currently displayed in the small *ICs* window (headed *Initial Data*). In case you have a confusion of too many plots at this point, you can clear each graphics window by activating it, and then clicking *(E)rase* in the menu. When both windows are clear, choose an initial condition just above firing threshold (e.g., $V = -13$), then click the *Go* button after activating each graphics window in turn.

(1.3.12) Resize and line up the *W* time course graphics window below the original *V* time course. Do you see how the K channels are slow, lagging behind the changes in *V*?

(1.3.13) You can also activate all the open graphics windows simultaneously. Click on *(M)ake window*, followed by *(S)imPlot On*. Click *(E)rase*, and notice that both the graphics windows are erased. (Recall that in Exercise 1.3.11 you had to erase one window at a time.) Now click the *Go* button, to see the *V* and *W* time courses plotted simultaneously in the two graphics windows. This can be very convenient, but it does slow XPP down, so remember to turn *(S)imPlot* off when you do not need it.

(1.3.14) In our ODE file *BridgingTutorial-MLecar.ode*, we define several *auxiliary quantities* (labeled *aux* in the ODE file), representing different components of the model response. Click on the *Equations* button at the top of the command window. A small window will pop up listing all the equations from the ODE file. You cannot edit the equations in this small window, but it is useful for reminding you of the names of the auxiliary quantities, and the roles of the parameters. Confirm that the auxiliary equations for the individual currents, conductances, and channel open probabilities agree with those developed in Section 1.2.

(1.3.15) Now click on the *Data* button at the top of the command window. A large window will pop up, in which the simulated data for each variable and auxiliary quantity are shown. This data can be exported to a space-delimited *dat* file using the *Write* button. Navigate around the data set using the *PgDn, PgUp, Right,* and *Left* buttons at the top of the window. Confirm that there are columns for all the auxiliary quantities. Also, confirm that the time increments are 0.25 ms and the total run time is 200 ms. Look back at the ODE file to see how these internal numerical parameters (*dt* and *total*) were pre-set, using the @ symbol.

(1.3.16) Each column in the data viewer can be plotted against time, or the columns can be plotted against each other. One way to plot a time course is by using *(V)iewaxes*, as in Exercise 1.3.10. A quick alternative is to click *(X)i versus t* in the menu, then enter the name of the variable or auxiliary quantitity to be plotted in the command line (using the name as it appears in the *Eqns* and *Data* windows). When you use *(X)i versus t*, the axes are automatically scaled to fit the data. The scale can then be adjusted using *(V)iewaxes*, if desired. Make three new graphics windows (using *(M)akewindow*, then *(C)reate*). Line the new windows up underneath each other, and use *(X)i* versus *t* to plot the K conductance, the K driving force, and the K current (with initial V above firing threshold, at $V = -13$).

(1.3.17) Confirm that the graph of K conductance, given by $g_{Ca}W$, is the same shape as the graph of W, scaled by g_{Ca}.

(1.3.18) Why does the K driving force, given by $(V - V_K)$, start at 71 mV? Confirm that the graph of K driving force is an upward shift of the graph of V.

(1.3.19) The K current is given by $I_K = g_{Ca}W(V - V_K)$. Describe how the properties of the graph of the K-current result from the properties of the graphs of conductance and driving force. For example, why does the graph of I_K start at 0 µA? why does it peak at approximately 250 µA? and why does it drop more suddenly than the graph of K conductance?

(1.3.20) Let us plot the Ca conductance in the same window as the K conductance. Activate the window, then click on *(G)raphic stuff* in the menu, followed by *(A)dd curve* in the submenu, and enter CaCond for the *Y-axis* (the *Z-axis, Color*, and *Line type* can be ignored). Click Ok. Next, use *(V)iewaxes* to set the *Y*-axis range from 0 to 4 mS, so both graphs are visible. Confirm that, once again, the Ca channels lead the K channels. (In Figure 1.4e, we plot the normalized conductances, to help compare the kinetics.) Use the equation for Ca conductance in the *Equations window*, and the initial value of V, to explain the initial Ca conductance shown on your graph and in the data set.

(1.3.21) Next, plot the Ca driving force in the same window as the K driving force, using *(G)raphic stuff* and *(A)dd curve* again, after activating the appropriate window. At first, nothing new appears on the driving force graph. Explain why not. It might help to look at the data, or the value of V_{Ca}. Use *(V)iewaxes* to set the *Y*-minimum to −200 mV. Once again, the driving force is a vertical shift of the graph of V, but this time V is shifted down, representing an inward current.

(1.3.22) Now plot the Ca current on the same graph as the K current, and confirm that it is an inward current, adjusting the axis range as needed (see Figure 1.4d). As before, describe how the properties of the graph of the Ca current result from properties of the graphs of conductance and driving force.

In *silico experiments with XPP*. We hope that you are inspired to experiment independently. You could plot the currents and conductances for an initial V just *below* firing threshold; you could adapt the building blocks developed in the Morris–Lecar model to include more channels or more complex gating properties (see Chapter 2 for inspiration); or you could include calcium dynamics (see Chapters 3 and 4 for inspiration). You could then compare model behaviors to clarify the roles of different channels, gating nuances, and your model assumptions.

Hodgkin–Huxley and Fitzhugh–Nagumo models. The XPP download comes with ODE files for several models of excitability. The Hodgkin–Huxley model (Hodgkin and Huxley, 1952), includes both activation and inactivation, and the kinetics are more realistic, reflecting the number of gating domains required to be in the corresponding state. In the Fitzhugh–Nagumo model (Fitzhugh, 1961; Nagumo *et al.*, 1962), the terms have been abstracted to capture, as simply as possible, the essential geometric features of the nullclines (defined in the next section) that underlie excitability. These and other models recur throughout the text, illustrating the art of letting the biological question determine the level of model complexity to use. They are discussed in most texts on theoretical neuroscience, such as Edelstein-Keshet (2005), Ermentrout and Terman (2010), Fall *et al.* (2005), Izhikevich (2007), Keener and Sneyd (2008), or Koch (1999).

1.4 Action potentials in the phase plane

In this section, we take a different view of the action potential. We exploit the fact that the Morris–Lecar model has only two dependent variables (V and W) to plot them against each other instead of plotting each against time. Then we see how graphical analysis of the resulting *phase plane* yields surprisingly many insights into the behavior of the model, through an appeal to our geometric intuition.

(1.4.1) Let us start afresh. If XPP is not already open, then fire it up with *BridgingTutorial-MLecar.ode*. If you still have XPP open with lots of graphics windows from the last section, then clean up by clicking *(M)akewindow*, then *(K)ill all* (a tiny pop-up window will ask if you are sure). If you have been experimenting with different values for the parameters, then click on *(F)ile*, followed by *(G)et par set* and select *hopf* to restore the default parameters of the Hopf column of Table 1.1. (Look back at the ODE file to see how the parameter set choices available in *(F)ile, (G)et par set* are coded using the *set* command.) Set the initial V and W to −13 and 0, respectively. Plot an action potential in the graphics window, and open the data viewer (*Data* button in the command window).

Trajectories in the phase plane. The first three columns of simulated data are time, voltage (V), and K-channel activation (W). The familiar voltage trace (or time course) is graphed by plotting the time and voltage columns against each other, but there are many other ways of visualizing the same data.

A *trajectory* in the *phase plane* is graphed by plotting the V and W columns against each other.

(1.4.2) Let us plot the trajectory corresponding to the action potential in Exercise 1.4.1. Make a new window *((M)akewindow, (C)reate)*, and use *(V)iewaxes, (2)D* to choose V for the *x*-axis and W for the *y*-axis, setting the *Xlabel* and *Ylabel* accordingly. Set V to range from -80 to 60, and W to range from -0.2 to 0.6. (Note that channel activation cannot, in reality, be negative. Our reason for including the negative range is to make it easier to see what's going on when $W = 0$).

(1.4.3) At first glance the trajectory does not look much like an action potential. We will examine it more closely, to recognize the familiar components of excitability embedded within it. The first row in the data viewer corresponds to time 0 ms, so $V = -13$ mV and $W = 0$ (the initial conditions we chose in Exercise 1.4.1). Locate the corresponding point $(V, W) = (-13, 0)$ in the phase plane. This is where the trajectory starts.

(1.4.4) Each subsequent row in the data viewer represents a small step forward in time, and each corresponding (V, W) point is plotted in the phase plane. The resulting curve is the *trajectory with initial condition* $(V, W) = (-13, 0)$. Use the *Down* button at the top of the data window to confirm that when $t = 10$ ms, V is approximately 8.3 mV and W is approximately 0.13. Locate the corresponding point on the trajectory.

(1.4.5) As time progresses, the cell continues around the trajectory. What is the peak voltage reached? When does it peak? What proportion of K channels are open when it peaks? Which of these questions can be answered using: (i) the phase plane? (ii) the voltage trace? (iii) the data viewer? Confirm that they give the same answers, where applicable.

Translating between a time course and the phase plane. It takes some practice to relate the "vertical" voltage axis of the time course to the "horizontal" voltage axis of the phase plane. Figure 1.4c and h illustrates how motion around the phase-plane trajectory corresponds to the action potential time course. The dots mark equal time intervals of 1 ms. There is no time axis in the phase plane. Instead, the progression of time is captured by progression around the trajectory. (The solid red and green curves in the phase plane are the *nullclines*, defined later in this section.) During the rapid depolarization and hyperpolarization segments of the spike in the voltage trace, voltage (V) is changing much faster than K-channel activation (W), thus yielding the rapid, roughly "horizontal" segments of the trajectory in the phase plane. Around the peak of the voltage trace, and during hyperpolarization, the voltage changes more slowly, so the K channels have time to open (close, respectively), and the motion around the phase plane has more "vertical" component. As voltage gradually returns to rest, W also stabilizes, and the trajectory approaches an *equilibrium point* in the phase plane. In summary, the explosive action potential characteristic of excitability corresponds to a large counterclockwise excursion around the phase plane before returning to equilibrium.

(1.4.6) Figure 1.4f shows six trajectories in the same phase plane, corresponding to the post-stimulus components of the six voltage traces in Figure 1.4a. Each trajectory has a different initial condition, as set by the pulsatile stimuli shown in Figure 1.4b. Which of the trajectories has initial condition $(V, W) \approx (-13, 0)$? And which has the initial condition $(V, W) \approx (-14, 0)$? Explain how you know.

(1.4.7) More generally, any point (V, W) in the phase plane can be used as initial data for the model. XPP allows you to select initial points with the mouse as follows. Activate the phase plane, then click *(I)nitialconds* in the side menu of the command window (not the *ICs* window we have used so far.) Select *m(I)ce* in the submenu. A tiny pop-up window appears with instructions. Experiment with initial points all over the phase plane. Press the *escape* key to exit this mode of choosing initial points when you are ready. Recall that we can view the initial condition of our model cell as reflecting its recent history. What history could lead to each initial point you chose? Some of them are more physiologically meaningful than others. Do the corresponding trajectories make sense? Remember you can turn *(S)implot* on (in the *(M)akewindow* menu), if you would like to see the corresponding voltage traces simultaneously, and you can click *(E)rase*, for a fresh start.

(1.4.8) The family of all trajectories is called the *flow* of the system. Erase everything, and turn *Simplot* off (it is off if the menu toggle offers to turn it on). To plot a representative sample of the flow, called a *phase portrait*, activate the phase plane and click on *(D)ir. field/flow*, followed by *(F)low*. Press *return* to accept the suggestion, in the command line, of a 10×10 grid of initial points, and watch the beautifully flowing dynamics emerge. Try experimenting with different sized grids.

The phase portrait shows the full range of behavior. A powerful feature of the phase plane is that it shows the cell's response to all possible histories, all at once. It gives immediate intuition for the full range of responses this cell can exhibit. The cell can fire at most one action potential and all trajectories eventually settle at the same rest point. The "all-or-nothing" quality of the response is captured by the very thin threshold region dividing trajectories that take the large, counterclockwise excursion from those that return directly to rest, and we see that there is, in fact, some variability in the amplitude of the excursion (or spike). In later sections, we will explore how a sustained stimulus expands this range of behaviors.

Trajectories never cross. Another powerful feature of the phase plane is that trajectories may flow toward each other, but they never cross. This has profound consequences for two-dimensional systems, because it means each trajectory imposes a spatial barrier to all the others, trapping them in different regions of the phase plane. This fundamental geometric fact that one-dimensional curves form barriers in a two-dimensional plane explains why geometric phase-plane analysis is so powerful, and can lead to qualitative predictions with relative ease. To understand why trajectories cannot cross each other, it is helpful to relate our model equations (1.12)–(1.16) directly to the phase plane:

(1.4.9) Equations (1.12) and (1.13) govern the time course of V and W for our model cell. Using $(V, W) = (-13, 0)$, and the parameter values in the Hopf column of Table 1.1, do the calculations to confirm that $M_\infty(V) \approx 0.21$, $W_\infty(V) \approx 0.27$ and $\tau_W(V) \approx 0.97$. Thus, the rate of change of V is $\frac{dV}{dt} \approx 0.95$ mV/ms, and the rate of change of W is $\frac{dW}{dt} \approx 0.01$ ms^{-1}.

(1.4.10) At the rates given in Exercise 1.4.9, in 1 ms, V would increase by 0.95 mV to -12.05 mV and W would increase from 0 to 0.01. Carefully sketch, on paper, the arrow, or *vector*, pointing from the initial point $(V, W) = (-13, 0)$ to the new point $(V, W) = (-12.05, 0.01)$. Your vector has components $\left(\frac{dV}{dt}, \frac{dW}{dt}\right) = (0.95, 0.01)$, and shows the instantaneous direction of motion that a trajectory passing through the point $(V, W) = (-13, 0)$ *must* follow. Use XPP to plot the trajectory with initial condition $(-13, 0)$, and confirm your direction vector agrees with the direction of the trajectory at $(-13, 0)$. (You may need to adjust the scale on the axes to make the comparison.)

(1.4.11) The *direction field* of the system consists of the vectors $\left(\frac{dV}{dt}, \frac{dW}{dt}\right)$ representing the direction of motion all over the phase plane. To plot a representative sample of direction vectors, as shown in Figure 1.4g, activate the phase plane and click on *(D)ir. field/flow*, followed by *(D)irect Field*, and press *return* to accept a 10×10 grid of initial points.

(1.4.12) Revisit Exercises 1.4.9 and 1.4.10 to confirm that the different lengths of the direction vectors indicate the relative speed of motion around the phase plane. (In contrast, *(D)ir. field/flow*, followed by *(S)caled Dir. Fld*, shows all the direction vectors scaled to the same length.)

(1.4.13) Choose initial conditions (using *(I)nitialconds, m(I)ce*) to superimpose individual trajectories on the direction field (as shown in Figure 1.4g). Alternatively, you can superimpose the flow (as demonstrated in Exercise 1.4.8). Notice that trajectories always travel in the direction of motion dictated by the direction field. This is not a coincidence. This is what it means for trajectories to be *solutions* of the system of differential equations (1.12) and (1.13). Now, it is clear why trajectories cannot cross each other. They have to follow the direction field. And the direction field cannot point in two different directions at once.

Autonomous systems. This is a good moment to emphasize that the argument we just used, and the entire phase-plane viewpoint, depends on the fact that our model equations (1.12)–(1.16) are *autonomous*. Recall from Section 1.2 that this means that the independent variable, time, does not appear explicitly on the right-hand side of the equations. So the direction vector through a given point (V, W) does not change over time, and can only point in one direction.

Nullclines. Recapping, we have seen that the range of behaviors our model cell can exhibit is predicted by the flow in the phase plane. The flow, in turn, follows the direction field, which is given by the differential equations. We now introduce the *nullclines* of the system, which give a quick guide to how the direction field is organized.

(1.4.14) Erase everything and plot the flow with a 10×10 grid (*e, d, f,* then *return,* via shortcut keys). Now plot the nullclines by clicking on *(N)ullcline,* and then *(N)ew.* (Recall that you can hover over each menu item for a description along the bottom of the command window, if you wish). There are two nullclines, one red and one green, as in Figure 1.4f–i. How can you tell the nullclines are *not* trajectories? (Hint: trajectories do not cross.)

(1.4.15) So what are the nullclines? Let us uncover their meaning from the XPP plot, starting with the red nullcline. What do you notice about the direction of the trajectories as they cross the red nullcline? And what would that correspond to on the associated voltage traces? It may help to make your graphics window huge, and redraw everything.

Nullclines mark turning points. The trajectories always "turn back" on themselves at the red nullcline. Below the red nullcline, trajectories flow to the right (as well as flowing "up" or "down" the phase plane). At the nullcline they turn, so that above the red nullcline trajectories flow to the left. Those that reach the red nullcline again, at the far left of the graph, turn again, flowing gently rightwards towards the equilibrium point. This observation yields the definition. Rightward and leftward flow in phase space correspond to increase and decrease in voltage, respectively. Thus, the red nullcline marks the points in the phase plane where the voltage turns. In more biological words it marks the peaks and troughs of the corresponding voltage trace. In more mathematical words, it marks the points where the graph of V against t has a maximum or minimum (or inflection point). So the red nullcline marks the points where $\frac{dV}{dt} = 0$, and is, therefore, called the *V-nullcline.*

(1.4.16) Recall from Exercises 1.4.9 to 1.4.11 that the direction field consists of the vectors $\left(\frac{dV}{dt}, \frac{dW}{dt} \right)$ evaluated at each point. Use this to explain as to why the flow is parallel to the W axis as it crosses the V-nullcline. (Hint: $\frac{dV}{dt} = 0$ on the *V-nullcline*.)

(1.4.17) The (green) W-nullcline is defined analogously. Use your XPP plot to confirm that $\frac{dW}{dt} = 0$ on the green nullcline. In other words, flow across the W-nullcline is parallel to the V axis, and the nullcline marks the points where trajectories turn from increasing W (K channels opening) to decreasing W (K channels closing), or vice versa.

Nullclines organize the direction field. Presently, we will examine how the shape of the nullclines is derived from the model equations. First, we will explore how the nullclines mark equilibria and organize the direction field, giving a rough, but immediate, guide to the dynamics of the system.

(1.4.18) Erase everything, and plot the direction field with a 10×10 grid (*e, d, d* then *return*). If the nullclines do not redraw automatically, plot them again (*n, n*). The nullclines divide the phase plane into regions. Confirm that, in each region, the direction vectors all point in roughly the same direction or *quadrant* (e.g. upward and rightward, or upward and leftward, etc.) Explain why. (Hint: nullclines mark turning points).

(1.4.19) What happens at the point where the two nullclines meet? Let us call it point P. Try choosing initial conditions exactly at P (using *i,i*). Nothing appears to happen. Why? (Remember to *escape* from *i,i* mode when you are done.)

Equilibria lie at the intersection of nullclines. The point P lies on both null-clines, so both $\frac{dV}{dt} = 0$ and $\frac{dW}{dt} = 0$ at P. Thus, from initial point P, there is no change in V or W, the direction vector reduces to $(0,0)$, and the trajectory is fixed at P for all time. We call P an *equilibrium* or *fixed point* of the system. By the same argument, every intersection of the two nullclines yields an equilibrium, and every equilibrium lies at an intersection of the nullclines.

(1.4.20) Try choosing initial conditions close to P (using *i,i* again). Confirm that trajectories from all nearby initial conditions converge to P. In other words, P represents rest, where our model cell stabilizes. Thus, we call P a *stable* equilibrium or *attractor*.

Stable versus unstable equilibria. We classify the stability of an equilibrium according to the behavior of the system *near* the equilibrium. If nearby initial conditions are all attracted to an equilibrium, it is *stable*. If they are generally repelled from the equilibrium, it is *unstable*. The very fact that systems settle down at stable equilibria makes them easy to observe in nature and experimentally, while unstable equilibria are much more difficult to observe. In the next sections, we will see how stable and unstable phenomena interact to shape both the transient and long-term dynamics of the system.

What determines the shape of the nullclines? We will use a combination of algebra and XPP experiments to develop intuition for the nullcline shape. Algebraically, each nullcline can be viewed as the graph of some equation of the form $W = f(V)$ in the $V-W$ phase plane. We will find these equations, to see which model parameters influence each nullcline.

W-nullcline. We will start with the W nullcline, because the algebra is simpler. Recall that the W component of direction vectors in the phase plane is given by Equation (1.13)

$$\frac{dW}{dt} = \frac{\phi}{\tau_W(V)}(W_\infty(V) - W)$$

Also, recall that the W-nullcline marks the points where $\frac{dW}{dt} = 0$. Thus, points on the W-nullcline satisfy the equation

$$0 = \frac{\phi}{\tau_W(V)}(W_\infty(V) - W) \tag{1.17}$$

From our model assumptions, we know the time scale $\frac{\phi}{\tau_W(V)}$ is positive and non-zero. So Equation (1.17) can be simplified and rearranged to yield the desired equation for the W-nullcline

$$W = W_\infty(V) \tag{1.18}$$

In other words, the green, W-nullcline is the familiar graph of steady-state K-channel activation $W_\infty(V)$ given by Equation (1.15), shown in Figures 1.3b and c, and explored in Exercises 1.2.4–1.2.7. Thus, points on the W-nullcline satisfy the equation

$$W = 0.5\left(1 + \tanh\left(\frac{V - V_3}{V_4}\right)\right) \tag{1.19}$$

In retrospect, this makes sense: we developed the K-channel kinetic model so that K-channel activation, W, is always playing catch-up to the voltage-dependent, "steady" state, $W_\infty(V)$. If, at a point (V, W) in the phase plane, W is lower than the corresponding $W_\infty(V)$, then W will increase to catch up. In other words, below the graph of $W_\infty(V)$, W increases. Above the graph of $W_\infty(V)$, W decreases. Thus, the graph of $W_\infty(V)$ is the W-nullcline, marking the points in the phase plane where W turns in its quest to follow the elusive $W_\infty(V)$.

(1.4.21) Using *(V)iewaxes, (2)D*, expand the V axis to range from -100 mV to 100 mV, and the W axis to range from -0.2 to 1.2. Erase everything *(e)*, and redraw the nullclines *(n,n)* to confirm that the green, W-nullcline is, indeed, the graph of $W_\infty(V)$.

(1.4.22) Click on *Par/Var* in one of the slider bars at the bottom of the command window to set up a slider, ranging from -50 to 50 mV for the half-activation (V_3) of steady-state K-channel activation. (Note that *SimPlot* slows down the slider bars considerably, so it is helpful to turn if off (in the *Makewindow* menu) if not needed.) What happens to the W-nullcline as you slide V_3? Explain why.

(1.4.23) Shift the W-nullcline to the right, so that it crosses the V-nullcline again and there are three equilibria. Plot trajectories starting close to each of the equilibria *(i,i)* to determine whether each equilibrium is stable or unstable. Confirm that the stability of the rightmost equilibrium depends on how much V_3 has been shifted. Also, plot the flow *(d, f* then *return)* to see how the local behavior, close to the equilibria, is globally connected. Describe the overall behavior of the model cell. It may help to plot the voltage traces for some trajectories. Does the change in behavior as V_3 increases make physiological sense?

(1.4.24) Set up another slider for the spread (V_4) of steady-state K-channel activation, ranging from 10 to 50 mV. Confirm that, for intermediate values of V_3, changing V_4 can also change the number of equilibria and overall behavior of the system.

V-nullcline. It takes more work to develop intuition for the "folded" (or roughly "cubic") shape of V-nullcline, because more of the parameters play a role in the associated differential equation. Nevertheless, we can follow the same approach we used for the W-nullcline. Recall that the V component of direction vectors is given by Equation (1.12)

$$C\frac{dV}{dt} = I - g_{Ca}M_\infty(V - V_{Ca}) - g_K W(V - V_K) - g_L(V - V_L)$$

The V-nullcline marks the points where $\frac{dV}{dt} = 0$. Thus, points on the V-nullcline satisfy

$$0 = I - g_{Ca}M_\infty(V - V_{Ca}) - g_K W(V - V_K) - g_L(V - V_L) \tag{1.20}$$

Bringing the K-current term to the left-hand side, we have

$$g_K W(V - V_K) = I - g_{Ca}M_\infty(V - V_{Ca}) - g_L(V - V_L) \tag{1.21}$$

Then, rearranging to isolate W on the left-hand side yields the equation for the V-nullcline in the $V–W$ plane

$$W = \frac{I - g_{Ca}M_\infty(V - V_{Ca}) - g_L(V - V_L)}{g_K(V - V_K)} \tag{1.22}$$

(1.4.25) Reset your initial condition close to threshold, and experiment with different values of the model parameters appearing in Equation (1.22), including those hidden in Equation (1.14) for M_∞, to see their role and effect on the V-nullcline, equilibria, direction field, flow and voltage traces. Parameter values can be changed using the parameter window (click on the *param* button at the top of the command window, then enlarge the window to see all the parameters), or by using the slider bars. You can reset the parameters to their default values using *(F)ile, (G)et par set* then *hopf*. As you experiment, pay particular attention to:

- The way the shape and position of the nullclines dictate the number of equilibria (intersections). The number of equilibria is typically 1 or 3. Why is it so rare to have exactly two equilibria?
- The way the nullclines and direction field change together, so that trajectories always turn at the nullclines, and in each region defined by the nullclines, direction vectors point into the same quadrant.
- Changes to the firing threshold and overall behavior. Do they make physiological sense for your parameter changes?

Summarizing. With the help of XPP, we have seen how the Morris–Lecar model, with its minimal mechanism of one excitatory and one depolarizing current, qualitatively reproduces some basic characteristics of excitable cells; firing an action potential when the stimulus is sufficient to cross firing threshold. We can plot the voltage trace and the currents contributing to the action potential, and translate between these traditional time courses and the phase plane; an action potential in the voltage trace corresponds to an excursion around the phase plane, and resting potential corresponds to an equilibrium. We can also use these plots in concert to gain a fuller understanding of the model cell's behavior. The time courses show the detailed response to a single stimulus history or initial condition, while the phase plane shows the qualitative response to all initial conditions at once. Within the phase plane, the direction field indicates how the flow is generated from the differential equations, and the nullclines are useful for locating the equilibria and showing how the flow is organized.

Many of these ideas generalize to the concept of *phase space* for autonomous systems in higher dimensions, which is useful as we add more variables to our models. As the number of variables increases, the geometry gets harder to visualize, so we have to introduce more mathematical formalism to describe the model dynamics. The geometric nature of the phase plane makes it an excellent point of contact, where experimentalists and theoreticians can learn enough about each others' language to spark collaborations about more complex biological systems modeled in higher dimensions.

For more about the phase plane and its generalizations, see any introductory text on dynamical systems, such as Blanchard *et al.* (2011), Hirsch *et al.* (2012), or Strogatz (1994).

1.5 Model response to sustained current injection

In the next few sections, we take a tour through parameter space, following the route mapped out by Rinzel and Ermentrout (1989), to explore the surprising richness of behavior the Morris–Lecar model cell exhibits in response to a simulated current clamp experiment in which sustained current is applied to a cell at rest.

Recall that in Sections 1.3 and 1.4, we discussed a current clamp experiment in which a brief stimulus current was applied to set the cell's initial condition. The applied current, I, was then returned to zero, and the cell's post-stimulus response was analyzed in the phaseplane corresponding to $I = 0$. Henceforth, the simulated current clamp experiments are different, in that the applied current is sustained indefinitely. Each different current amplitude corresponds to a different phaseplane, and the model behavior changes accordingly.

Most of the time the behavior changes gradually as I changes. But occasionally a small change in applied current leads to a qualitatively dramatic change in behavior. Mathematically, these qualitative changes arise through *bifurcations*, which are most easily understood in the phaseplane. Different bifurcation mechanisms correspond to different characteristics of excitability, and our tour through parameter space will introduce us to the bifurcations that occur most commonly in two-dimensional systems. We continue, in this section, with the parameter set "Hopf" from Table 1.1.

(1.5.1) From now on, it will be convenient to have the phaseplane as the default graph in the command window, and to open a secondary voltage trace window. So quit XPP *((F)ile,(Q)uit,(Y)es)*, and look back at the ODE file (*BridgingTutorial-MLecar.ode*) to see how the default axes and their ranges were set, using the @ symbol. Edit the ODE file to comment out the line that sets the *x*- and *y*-axes as *t* and *V*, respectively, and uncomment the line that sets the *x*-axis as *V* and the *y*-axis as *W*. Also, in the line headed *some numerical settings*, reset the *total* (run time) from 200 to 500.

(1.5.2) Re-open XPP. Now the command window should show the phase plane, with V ranging from −75 to 70 mV on the *x*-axis, and W ranging from −0.2 to 1 on the *y*-axis. Open a second window for the voltage trace using *(M)akewindow, (C)reate* then set *t* from 0 to 500 ms on the *x*-axis, and *V* from −80 to 60 mV on the *y*-axis using *(V)iewaxes, (2)d*.

Open the parameter window (using the *param* button at the top of the XPP window) and check that the parameters agree with the Hopf column of Table 1.1. If not, select the Hopf parameter set using *(F)ile, (G)et par set.*

(1.5.3) Let us explore the impact of sustained current on the voltage trace first, then we will take the phase-plane view. Set up a slider for *I* ranging from 0 to 275 using one of the slider bars at the bottom of the command window. Activate the voltage trace window by clicking on it (recall that a tiny black dot in the top left corner of a graphics window tells you which window is active), then use the slider to gradually increase *I*. Notice the sudden changes in the voltage trace, and compare your simulations with Figure 1.5. The cell starts at rest. Small values of the applied current increase the resting potential. Around $I = 73$, a single action potential is triggered. As you continue to increase *I*, the applied current pushes the "resting potential" across firing threshold so that there is a sudden onset of repetitive spiking just before $I = 96$. The spiking behavior continues as *I* is increased, until it suddenly disappears around $I = 239$, and the voltage settles to a plateau level.

(1.5.4) Now let us take the phase-plane viewpoint. Return the slider to $I = 0$, activate the phase-plane window and plot the nullclines *((N)ullcline, (N)ew)*. Gradually increase *I*, and notice how changes in the trajectory in the phase plane correspond to changes in the voltage trace, as in Figure 1.5. What phase-plane behavior corresponds to tonic spiking? (Note, if you turn simplot on *((M)ake window, (S)implot on)*, then the slider applies to both graphs at once, but operates more slowly. Alternatively, you can keep simplot off, and switch between graphs by activating the window you want, erasing the old graph (*e*), restoring a plot of the most recent simulation (*r*), and replotting the nullclines if in the phaseplane (*n,n*)).

Tonic spiking corresponds to a limit cycle. The sudden appearance of tonic spiking in the voltage trace corresponds to the appearance of a *limit cycle* (or closed loop, or *periodic orbit*) in the phaseplane. The trajectory no longer settles at an equilibrium (or rest point), but instead travels endlessly round and round the limit cycle, tracing out repeated action potentials. In the next exercises, we will consider the role of the nullclines and equilibrium in shaping the voltage waveform.

(1.5.5) What happens to the each of the nullclines as you increase *I*? Look back at the role of *I* in the nullcline equations (1.19) and (1.22) to explain why the (red) *V*-nullcline moves upwards, while the (green) *W*-nullcline stays fixed. Recall that the equilibrium is at the intersection of the two nullclines. Slide *I* up and down again, and watch how the equilibrium gradually travels up and down the *W*-nullcline at the same time as it

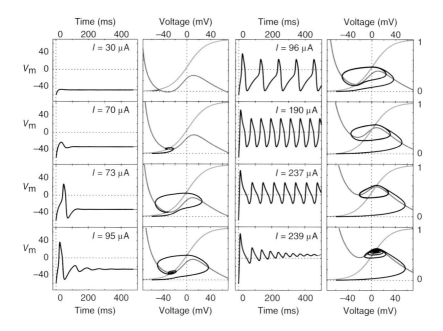

Figure 1.5 Sustained current injection with the Hopf parameter set. Model responses to a progressive series of sustained current stimuli (amplitudes indicated), showing voltage traces in time and the corresponding phase-plane trajectories and nullclines. As stimulus amplitude begins to increase, single action potentials are elicited. At a sharply defined value close to $I = 96$ μA, repetitive trains of action potentials are elicited, corresponding to the sudden appearance of a stable limit cycle in the phase plane. At this point, the firing frequency is immediately at a characteristic non-zero value (determined by the speed around the cycle), from which it increases only modestly over a wide range of stimulus currents, as in Hodgkin's Class II neurons. At another sharply defined stimulus amplitude, just below $I = 239$ μA, the stable cycle and corresponding spike train are suddenly lost, and voltage damps to a stable equilibrium at relatively positive potential.

travels back and forth along the V-nullcline. Pay close attention to the cycling behavior of the trajectory as the equilibrium travels past the local maximum and minimum (turning points) of the V-nullcline. Do you see a pattern? Roughly speaking, when the equilibrium is on the middle branch of the V-nullcline, between the turning points, there is tonic spiking. When the equilibrium is outside the middle branch the voltage settles down to the equilibrium value.

(1.5.6) For another insight into the role of the nullclines, plot the scaled direction field (*(D)ir. field/flow, (S)caled Dir.Fld*). Click the *return* key to accept the default 10×10 direction field grid suggested in the XPP command line. Recall, the arrows show the direction of motion of a trajectory as it travels around the phase plane. On the W-nullcline, there is no motion in the W direction, so arrows with "feet" on the W-nullcline are perfectly horizontal (the dots represent the arrowheads). Similarly, arrows with feet on the V-nullcline are perfectly vertical. Use these facts to explain why the left and right extremes of a limit cycle lie on the V-nullcline. What do these extremes correspond to on the voltage trace? Now, slide I up and down, and watch how the arrows change direction as the V-nullcline passes by. How do these geometric observations relate to the balance of currents in the cell?

(1.5.7) It can also be instructive to repeat Exercise 1.5.6 on a finer scale to examine the sudden appearance of the limit cycle. Recall that the cycle appears around $I = 96$. Set $I = 90$, and temporarily reduce the slider range of I from 90 to 100. Nudge the slider to update the phase-plane image, then zoom in to a smaller box around the trajectory. (Click *(W)indow/zoom*, then *(Z)oom In*, and use the cursor to select the region of interest). The nullclines might not look smooth after zooming in. You can fix that by erasing everything *(e)*, and redrawing the nullclines and scaled direction field, but it will also fix itself when you move the I slider. Slide I up and down. How does the subtle geometric interaction of the nullclines and direction field contribute to the sudden appearance of the limit cycle? You may find it helpful to redraw the scaled vector field on a finer, 30×30, grid.

Stability of the equilibrium versus the limit cycle. Recall that the stability of an equilibrium is about the behavior of the system near the equilibrium. If nearby initial conditions are attracted to the equilibrium, it is stable. If they are generally repelled from the equilibrium, it is unstable. The same concept of stability applies to the limit cycle: if nearby initial conditions are attracted to the cycle, it is stable; if they are repelled, it is unstable.

(1.5.8) For a clean start, erase everything *(e)*, return the phase-plane window to default scale (*(W)indow/zoom, (D)efault*), and reset the I slider from 0 to 250. Choose a value of I, plot the nullclines *(n,n)* and test the stability of the equilibrium by checking what happens to nearby initial conditions. An easy way to do this is to choose *(I)nitital conditions* then *m(I)ce*. After clicking to activate the phase-plane window, you can choose lots of initial conditions with the mouse. When you are done, nudge the slider, or click *escape*, to liberate your mouse. Try it for a range of values of I to explore the stability of the equilibrium as it travels along the nullclines and the limit cycle appears and disappears. Is the equilibrium stable or unstable when there is a limit cycle? How about when there is no cycle? The case of a single action potential is like in Section 1.4. The equilibrium is stable, even tho some initial conditions take a large excursion before returning to rest.

(1.5.9) When there is a limit cycle, is it stable or unstable?

Exchange of stability. Roughly speaking, the equilibrium appears to be stable when there is no limit cycle, but unstable when there is a limit cycle. The limit cycle itself is stable, as if the equilibrium had passed its stability to the cycle. In fact, if you test initial conditions closely, right around the appearance and disappearance of the limit cycle, you will see the situation is a bit more subtle. We will return to that subtlety with the bifurcation diagram in Section 1.6.

The influence of instability. Unstable behavior is, by nature, very difficult to observe experimentally. For example, we have just seen that when the equilibrium is unstable in our simulations we observe tonic spiking instead. We might be tempted to argue that unstable behavior is irrelevant to biology. But invisible, unstable phenomena can play important roles in shaping the observable, stable behavior of a system. We will develop intuition for this fact in the next two exercises by exploring how the unstable equilibrium influences the voltage waveform when the cell is spiking.

(1.5.10) Reset the initial condition to $(V, W) = (-60, 0)$ (by clicking on it, or in the ICs window), and turn on the (unscaled) direction field (*(D)ir. field/flow, (D)irect field, return*). Recall that in the unscaled direction field, the length of the direction vector indicates the relative speed of motion around the phaseplane. Slide I up and down, and confirm that the arrows are very short near the equilibrium. Why is that? Use the definition of an equilibrium to explain. If you are not convinced, try zooming in closer to the equilibrium, or increasing the number of grid points.

(1.5.11) Set $I = 96$. Where is the equilibrium relative to the limit cycle? Activate the voltage trace window, and graph the waveform (*i,g*). Which part of the waveform corresponds to the stretch of the limit cycle closest to the equilibrium? For example, is it the depolarizing or hyperpolarizing phase of the action potential? Is it close to the peak or minimum voltage? The direction arrows are shortest close to the equilibrium, so the motion is slow. How is that reflected in the voltage waveform? Now, gradually increase I, so that the unstable equilibrium moves towards the middle of the limit cycle. What impact does this have on the voltage waveform and why does the spike frequency increase? Finally, increase I to a value just before the limit cycle disappears. Why does the spike frequency decrease again? And why does the waveform develop the "shoulders" seen in some cells?

Summarizing. As we increase I in this simulated current clamp experiment, there are two areas of qualitatively dramatic change: the onset and offset of tonic spiking, corresponding to the appearance and disappearance of a limit cycle in the phaseplane. There is an associated exchange of stability between the equilibrium and the limit cycle, but, even while unstable, the equilibrium continues to influence the waveform of the spikes. In the next section, we examine the *bifurcations* underlying the qualitative changes in behavior, and learn how to read the associated *bifurcation diagram*.

1.6 Reading a bifurcation diagram

We hope that the previous section convinced you that there is a value in studying both the stable and unstable behavior in a model. Sherman (2011) gives a nice analogy: the system is like a Shakespeare play, where some of the action is on-stage and observable, but influential events also happen off-stage, to be perceived only indirectly by their on-stage impact. Figure 1.6 shows the *bifurcation diagram* for our simulated current clamp experiment, succinctly summarizing information about all the stable and unstable equilibria and limit cycles. There is a lot of information packed into a bifurcation diagram, so we will spend some time unpacking it in this section. The *bifurcation parameter*, on the *x*-axis, is the parameter being controlled (applied current, in our case). The variable of interest (voltage) is plotted on the *y*-axis.

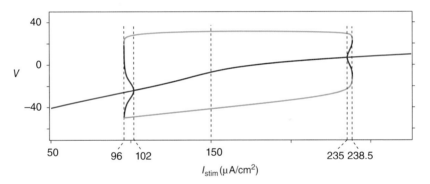

Figure 1.6 Bifurcation diagram for the Hopf parameter set. The diagram summarizes the behavior illustrated in Figure 1.5. Stimulus current, I, is the bifurcation parameter, and voltage, V, is the behavior variable plotted. For each value of the stimulus current, there is a corresponding phase plane, as shown in Figure 1.5. The equilibria and limit cycles from all the phase planes are charted on the bifurcation diagram, to show how they vary with stimulus current, and to highlight the bifurcations. The equilibrium voltage in each phase plane is plotted on the bifurcation diagram against the corresponding stimulus current; in red if the equilibrium is stable and in black if it is unstable. A limit cycle is represented by its peak and trough voltage levels; in green if the cycle is stable and in blue if it is unstable. In the simulated experiment in Section 1.5, repetitive firing begins where the branch of unstable limit cycles, born at the subcritical Hopf bifurcation ($I = 102$ μA), appears to fold back on itself to become stable, at the saddle-node bifurcation of limit cycles ($I = 96$ μA). Firing terminates in a similar mechanism. Note the regions of bistability around the onset and offset of spiking, where a stable equilibrium and stable limit cycle coexist.

(1.6.1) Locate the value $I = 150$ on the X-axis in Figure 1.6. There are three points on the bifurcation diagram at this value of I. What is the (approximate) value of the voltage at the black (middle) point? Use XPP to confirm that it is the voltage of the equilibrium (in the phaseplane) when $I = 150$. As we know, the location of the equilibrium changes as you slide I up and down. Check that the middle "branch" of the bifurcation diagram tracks the voltage of the equilibrium. The color coding tell us about the stability of the equilibrium. What does black mean? What does red mean?

(1.6.2) Now let us consider the the two green (upper and lower) voltage levels on the bifurcation diagram at $I = 150$. What do they represent? If it is not clear from the phaseplane, use the graph of voltage versus time to confirm that they correspond to the maximum and minimum voltage levels of the stable limit cycle corresponding to tonic spiking. As with the equilibrium, check that the green branches of the bifurcation diagram track the voltage extremes of the stable limit cycle (and action potentials) as you slide I up and down.

Unstable limit cycle. We are ready to examine the bifurcations underlying the sudden appearance and disappearance of stable limit cycles we observed in Section 1.5. To fix ideas, consider the region of the bifurcation diagram between $I = 235$ and $I = 238.5$, where the stable limit cycles disappear. The blue points in this region represent the maximum and minimum voltage levels of an *unstable* limit cycle. The unstable limit cycle is like an off-stage Shakespearean actor. We will see how it is "born" in a *Hopf bifurcation* at the equilibrium, and "dies" in a *saddle-node bifurcation of limit cycles* taking the stable limit cycle with it.

Hopf bifurcation. The bifurcation diagram shows us that at the exact value of I where the unstable equilibrium regains stability (turning from black to red on the diagram, around $I = 235$), a small unstable limit cycle is "born" around the equilibrium. The unstable nature of the equilibrium has been passed off to the new cycle. This creation of a limit cycle as an equilibrium changes stability is called a *Hopf bifurcation*. For a small range of subsequent values of I, the large stable limit cycle coexists with the small unstable limit cycle, so there is a stable equilibrium and *two* limit cycles: one stable and one unstable. Over the next few exercises, we will confirm this in XPP, and use a sneaky trick to plot the unstable limit cycle.

(1.6.3) According to the bifurcation diagram, the equilibrium regains stability at about $I = 235$, and we know from Section 1.5 the stable limit cycle disappears just before $I = 239$. So choose the intermediate value $I = 237$. Erase everything (e), plot the nullclines (n,n), and choose an initial condition like (−60,0) to see the stable limit cycle. Zoom in *((W)indow/zoom, (Z)oom In)* so that the limit cycle fills the view. Erase everything again *(e)*, redraw the nullclines *(n,n)*, and choose *(I)nitialconds, (L)ast* so that the last point computed at the end of the last trajectory is used as the initial condition for the next trajectory. Since the last point was very close to the stable limit cycle, this should yield a clean picture of the cycle.

(1.6.4) We will use XPP's graphics tools to "freeze" this clean picture of the stable limit cycle for $I = 237$. Click *(G)raphics stuff, (F)reeze*, and then *(F)reeze* again. At the color prompt, choose 7, for green, to be compatible with the bifurcation diagram. (The default color, 0, is black, 1–10 range thru shades of red, orange, yellow, green, blue and purple, in that order.) Choose "stable" for the name and key. Now, whenever you erase everything, if you click *(R)estore*, the frozen cycle will re-appear. (You can change the color and name, add a key, or unfreeze the cycle, using *(E)dit, (K)ey* and *(D)elete* respectively in the *(G)raphics stuff, (F)reeze* menu.)

(1.6.5) Click *i, i* to choose initial conditions with the mouse. Choose an initial condition inside and close to the stable limit cycle, to confirm that it is, indeed, stable. (Note that choosing the initial condition on one of the nullclines can help you keep track of where you started.) Now, choose another initial condition inside the stable limit cycle, but close to the equilibrium this time. If you are close enough, the trajectory will spiral in toward the equilibrium, confirming its stability. We have just shown that the system is *bistable*, meaning that the long-term behavior depends critically on the choice of initial condition. The unstable limit cycle acts as a threshold, also known as a *separatrix*, between the two modes of behavior. Try different initial conditions to get a sense of where the unstable limit cycle must be. (Remember to click the *escape* key to liberate your mouse when you are done.)

Plotting the unstable limit cycle. Here is the sneaky trick we will use: What would happen to a trajectory that spirals away from the unstable limit cycle and toward the stable equilibrium if we could run it *backward* in time? It would spiral *away* from the equilibrium and *toward* the limit cycle. "Backwards" time is surprisingly easy to implement for an autonomous system of differential equations; we just make the time step negative.

(1.6.6) In XPP, click *u* for *N(u)merics*, then *d* for the time step, *Dt*. The XPP command line will show the current value of *Dt*. Edit the command line (you can use the arrows on your keyboard) to put a negative sign in front of the value, and click the *return* key. Click the *escape* key to exit the numerics menu. Now, XPP will run time backward. Choose an initial condition that spiraled in to the equilibrium in the previous exercise, and watch the unstable limit cycle appear. For a clean picture of the unstable cycle, erase everything (*e*), redraw the nullclines (*n,n*), and choose the last point computed as the new initial condition (*i,l*). Freeze the unstable limit cycle (*g,f,f*) using color 9, for blue, and "unstable" for the name. Now, when you click *(R)estore*, both limit cycles should re-appear.

(1.6.7) Check that the voltage extremes of the two limit cycles agree with those given by the bifurcation diagram for $I = 237$ in Figure 1.6.

(1.6.8) While we are working with backward time, let us slide I to see the Hopf bifurcation in action. Change the I slider to range from 230 to 238. Click *n(U)merics, (T)otal* to change the total run time to 2500 in the XPP command line, to give trajectories more time to settle down in this delicate region. Warning: increasing the run time slows XPP down, so it is a good idea to change it back to 500 at the end of this section. Remember to click the *escape* key to exit from the numerics menu. Confirm that when $I = 230$, the equilibrium is unstable (i.e., stable in this backward time). Now, slowly increase I, to watch the birth of a limit cycle at the equilibrium, and the gradual growth of the limit cycle as I increases to 238. This limit cycle is stable in backwards time, so unstable in forward time. Use *Restore* to compare limit cycles for different values of I with the frozen limit cycles for $I = 237$.

(1.6.9) Exactly which part of the bifurcation diagram was Exercise 1.6.8 about? Take a moment to clearly describe the correspondence between the bifurcation diagram and your XPP results.

(1.6.10) Now, we will focus on the "fold" in the bifurcation diagram where the blue branch representing the unstable limit cycle meets the green branch representing the stable limit cycle. Continuing in backwards time mode, set the I slider to range from 237 to 238.35. Slide I up and watch the unstable limit cycle continue to grow as I increases. Freeze the unstable cycle for $I = 238.35$. Next we will compare it to the stable limit cycle for $I = 238.35$. Go back into the *n(U)umerics* menu, and make *Dt* positive so that time is running forwards again. (Remember to click on *escape* to exit the numerics menu.) Restore all the saved cycles, set $I = 237$, choose an initial condition on the stable limit cycle, and slowly slide I up to 238.35 again to watch the stable cycle shrink as I increases. Notice that the stable and unstable limit cycles are much closer together when $I = 238.35$ than they were when $I = 237$. it is not a coincidence that we chose the value $I = 238.35$ so carefully. If you try repeating this exercise for $I = 238.5$, you will find the limit cycles have disappeared.

Saddle-node bifurcation of limit cycles and the offset of tonic spiking. In the last exercise, we saw the two limit cycles converging to each other as I was increased, exactly as predicted by the bifurcation diagram. In the thin region between the pair of limit cycles, trajectories spiral outward.

Outside that region, trajectories spiral inward. The limit cycles separate the inward and outward cycling behavior. As the two limit cycles converge, the region between them shrinks to nothing, till the limit cycles coalesce and disappear, and all trajectories spiral inward. This convergence and disappearance of a pair of limit cycles is called a *saddle-node bifurcation of limit cycles*, and corresponds to the sudden offset of tonic spiking in the voltage trace. (The word *saddle* denotes the unstable limit cycle, while *node* denotes the stable limit cycle. The naming scheme seems strange, but originates from analogy with the *saddle-node bifurcation of equilibria* that we will see in Sections 1.7 and 1.9.)

Onset of tonic spiking. The sudden onset of tonic spiking in our simulated current clamp experiment of Section 1.5 is also associated with an unstable limit cycle that is born in a subcritical Hopf bifurcation and dies in a saddle-node bifurcation of limit cycles. But the sequence of events is slightly different. The birth of the unstable limit cycle as the equilibrium gains stability, and the converge and disappearance of the limit cycles, all happen as I is decreased rather than increased. In our simulated current clamp experiment, I was increased, so there was a spontaneous creation of a pair of limit cycles that appeared to come from nowhere, out of the "clear blue sky." This explains why a saddle-node bifurcation of limit cycles is sometimes called a *blue sky bifurcation*.

Subcritical versus supercritical Hopf bifurcations. The type of Hopf bifurcation exhibited by this system, where an unstable limit cycle is born, is called *subcritical*. There are also *supercritical Hopf bifurcations* in which a stable limit cycle is born as the equilibrium changes stability. Here, the word *critical* refers to the value of the bifurcation parameter where the equilibrium changes stability and the limit cycle is born. *Subcritical* and *supercritical* describe which side of that critical value the limit cycle is born into: as an unstable limit cycle surrounding the stable equilibrium (subcritical) or as a stable limit cycle surrounding the unstable equilibrium (supercritical).

In real applications, when a subcritical Hopf bifurcation occurs it is often paired with a saddle-node bifurcation of limit cycles (the large stable limit cycle maintains the large-scale stability of the system, so that trajectories do not grow without bound). In the bifurcation diagram, this manifests as the (blue) branch of unstable limit cycles, born at the Hopf bifurcation, appearing to "fold back" on itself, changing stability in the process. Thus, the saddle-node bifurcation of limit cycles is also called a *fold bifurcation of limit cycles*, and the pair of bifurcations is sometimes collectively referred to as a *backward Hopf bifurcation*.

Supercritical Hopf bifurcations are simpler to understand: the birth and growth of the limit cycle are observable (without resorting to backward time), and the oscillations grow gradually as the bifurcation parameter is varied, rather than appearing out of the blue. See, for example, the models of calcium driven oscillations in Chapter 3.

(1.6.11) Let us put it all together! Revisit the simulated current clamp experiment of Section 1.5, and explain how you can use the bifurcation diagram to predict the model cell's response to sustained current (the sequence of voltage traces and phase-plane portraits, and the associated values of I in Figure 1.5).

(1.6.12) Now, we will focus more closely on the appearance of tonic spiking, to investigate some consequences of bistability. Delete all the frozen trajectories (g,f,d) and return the phase plane to default size (w,d). Check the total run time is still 2500 (using $n(U)merics$, $(T)otal$, and the command line; remember to click the *escape* key to exit the numerics menu). Reset the initial condition to $(-60,0)$ to represent the cell at rest before any current is applied (using *IC's* button). Set the I slider to range from 90 to 105, and confirm that, with this initial condition, tonic spiking appears around $I = 96$, as in (Figure 1.5). Exactly which part of the bifurcation diagram does this represent? The point to notice is that from the initial condition $(-60,0)$, the trajectory "discovers" the stable limit cycle as soon as the blue sky bifurcation has occurred.

(1.6.13) What if the cell's history meant that it was starting at a different initial condition? For example, set the initial condition to $(V, W) = (-25, 0.15)$. Now, slide I again, from 90 to 105. When does the trajectory discover the stable limit cycle? You should find that it is different from the previous exercise. Why is that? Exactly which part of the bifurcation diagram does this represent? The initial condition $(-25, 0.15)$ was carefully chosen so that as I is increased, the cell stays quiescent, tracking the equilibrium voltage as long as the equilibrium point is stable, and happily oblivious of the "blue sky" bifurcation creating the pair of limit cycles. It is only when the equilibrium point loses stability at the Hopf bifurcation, around $I = 102$, that trajectories are forced to discover the large, stable limit cycle and the cell starts tonic spiking.

Bistability means history matters. For a parameter value where the system is bistable, such as $I = 98$, there are two *attractors* (in this case the stable equilibrium and the stable limit cycle). Each attractor has a *basin of attraction*, consisting of all the initial conditions it attracts. The basin of attraction of the stable limit cycle consists of all the initial conditions leading to tonic spiking, while the basin of attraction of the stable equilibrium consists of all the initial conditions leading to quiescence. The threshold, or *separatrix* between the two basins of attraction is the unstable limit cycle. Bistability means that we cannot predict the cell's behavior without knowing its recent history, since the history sets the initial condition. In Exercise 1.6.12, the initial condition represents a history of a cell at rest until a current step (from $I = 0$) is applied. In contrast, a cell *in vivo* may experience a slowly changing stimulus, more akin to a slow ramp of applied current, such as the slow modulation of calcium sensitive channels by slow accumulation of cytosolic calcium discussed in Chapters 3 and 4. If the stimulus current changes slowly enough, relative to the phase-plane dynamics, the cell can track the slowly changing stable equilibrium, resulting in a history that is better approximated by the initial condition of Exercise 1.6.13 than that of Exercise 1.6.12. These subtleties of multi-stability combined with time-scale separation are key to models of bursting.

Bifurcation and bursting. Now that we know how to read the bifurcation diagram, we can use it to predict the results of a fixed current injection, or of a slowly changing stimulus current. The bifurcation diagram predicts the sudden appearance and disappearance of large amplitude tonic spiking, including the subtleties of bistability associated with the cell's history. In Section 1.10, bursting behavior is modeled by adding a slowly changing variable, intrinsic to the cell, that drives the cell back and forth across bifurcations in a multistable regime, thereby "switching" tonic spiking on and off.

Plotting bifurcation diagrams. By now, you may be wondering how we (or the computer) establish the stability of the equilibrium or limit cycle with precision, and how we plot the bifurcation diagram. Section 1.11 is about how to determine stability. The bifurcation diagram was plotted using XPP's interface with the bifurcation software AUTO (indy.cs.concordia.ca/auto) in the *File* menu. Learning to use AUTO is exciting, but is beyond the scope of this tutorial. Our experience is that it works well to have an expert show you how to get started, then carefully follow the AUTO tips on Ermentrout's XPP help pages (Ermentrout, 2012) to build on that foundation.

Different bifurcations yield different spiking characteristics. In the next sections, we will see how manipulating the parameters of K-channel gating within the Morris–Lecar model yields two more bifurcation mechanisms for the onset of tonic spiking, each leading to different spiking characteristics. In the example we just worked through, tonic spiking was restricted to a narrow frequency range, as in Hodgkin's Class II, resonator, neurons (Hodgkin, 1948). The *SNIC bifurcation* in the next section yields tonic spiking with arbitrarily low frequency, depending on applied current, as in

Hodgkin's Class I, integrator, neurons. The *Homoclinic bifurcation* in Section 1.9 yields tonic spiking with a high baseline between the spikes. This collection of bifurcation mechanisms provides building blocks for modeling the rich diversity of cellular excitability, and biological oscillations more generally. See introductory textbooks on dynamical systems, such as Blanchard *et al.* (2011), Ellner and Guckenheimer (2006), Hirsch *et al.* (2012), and Strogatz (1994) for more introduction to bifurcations, and Bertram *et al.* (1995), Ermentrout and Terman (2010), Golubitsky *et al.* (2001), and Izhikevich (2007) for approaches to classifying bifurcations in the context of excitable systems.

1.7   Saddle node on an invariant circle (SNIC) bifurcation

Different cell types, ion channels, and conditions correspond to different ranges of parameter values. For example, recall that V_3 represents the half-activation voltage of the inhibitory conductance, and increasing V_4 decreases the slope of the conductance curve at half-activation. These gating parameters vary enormously between channel types and cells, and are easily shifted by mechanisms like phosphorylation, G-protein binding and steroid binding (Carrasquillo and Nerbonne, 2014; González *et al.*, 2012; King *et al.*, 2006; Lovell *et al.*, 2000, 2001; Pongs and Schwarz, 2010; Vacher and Trimmer 2011). Temperature can dramatically impact gating kinetics, captured in the model by ϕ (Hille, 2001), and the maximal conductances, $g_{Ca}, g_K,$ and g_L depend on the number and density of channels expressed, which vary widely between and within cells, as well as on single-channel conductance.

In this section, we will work with the SNIC parameter set of Table 1.1, which differs only in the voltage dependence of potassium-channel gating from the Hopf parameter set of the preceding sections. Our parameter choices are similar to choices often used in the literature, going back (in nondimensionalized form) to Rinzel and Ermentrout (1989) and to some extent to Morris and Lecar (1981). There is nothing extraordinary about the exact values, in the sense that nearby parameter values yield similar behavior. Sliders in XPP can be used to explore the *sensitivity* of the behavior to parameters (how much each parameter can change before a new bifurcation occurs).

(1.7.1) Set up XPP with a phase-plane window and a voltage trace window (as in Exercise 1.5.2), and change the total run time back to 500, if necessary (*u,t*). Select the SNIC parameter set using *(F)ile, (G)et par set.* Open the parameter window (using the *param* button at the top of the XPP window), enlarge it to see all the parameters, and check that they agree with the SNIC column of Table 1.1. Only the parameters V_3 and

V_4 have changed; perhaps representing a different K channel. What do the new parameters say about the voltage-dependent gating of the new channel compared to the old?

(1.7.2) Let us see what effect the new parameters have on the nullclines and equilibria of the system. Set up sliders for V_3 and V_4 so that each varies between the Hopf and SNIC values (Table 1.1), and plot the null-clines. Recall from Section 1.4 that the W nullcline is simply the graph of $W_\infty(V)$, the K-channel open probability at steady state as a function of V. Is this consistent with the way the nullcline changes as you slide V_3 and V_4? By contrast, the V nullcline does not change with V_3 and V_4. Look back at Equation (1.22) for the V nullcline to see why: V_3 and V_4 play no role in the equation.

(1.7.3) Set V_3 and V_4 at their SNIC values (12 and 17, respectively). When $I = 0$ the nullclines intersect three times, representing three equilibria. Click on some initial conditions close to each equilibrium (using i,i) to determine whether they are stable. Or quickly sample the behavior in the whole phase plane using the flow ($(D)ir.\ field/flow,\ (F)low$, with a 10×10 grid). Despite the new equilibria, the behavior is much the same as before. There is one stable equilibrium, giving a resting potential of approximately -60, and almost all initial conditions settle down to rest, either directly, or after the transient excursion of a single action potential.

(1.7.4) Activate the voltage trace window and simulate a sustained current injection experiment (as in Section 1.5), with the initial condition set at $(V, W) = (-60, 0)$ to represent a cell at rest before the current is applied. A good range for I is -25 to 150. The voltage response shows many similarities with the behavior in Section 1.5: as you increase I, rest gives way to tonic spiking, and eventually the spiking disappears in damped oscillations to plateau voltage. What are some differences from the behavior in Section 1.5? Check the onset of spiking carefully. Notice that there are no lone action potentials; the cell snaps straight from rest to tonic spiking. If you slide I delicately, you may be fooled into thinking you have found a lone action potential (around $I = 39.75$), but if you extend the t axis to 1000 ms and continue the run (click $(C)ontinue$ and choose run time 1000 in the command line), you find that it is really very low frequency tonic spiking. From there, the spike frequency increases rapidly with increasing I, so that small changes in I lead to dramatic frequency modulation.

(1.7.5) Now, watch the onset of spiking in the phase plane. What is going on? At $I = -25$ there is only one equilibrium. As you increase I, a pair of new equilibria are created when the V nullcline "pushes through" the W nullcline. So there are three equilibria by the time I reaches 0, as we know from Exercise 1.7.3. What happens to the middle equilibrium as you continue to increase I? It travels down the nullclines to coalesce and vanishes with the lower equilibrium when the V nullcline pushes through the W nullcline again. At exactly that moment, the stable limit cycle appears. This is not a coincidence.

(1.7.6) To understand how the stable limit cycle appears as the nullclines push through each other, it is helpful to focus on each of the two equilibria that coalesce and vanish together. Set $I = 27$, where there are three fairly evenly spaced equilibria. Zoom in closely on the lower equilibrium (click *(W)indow/zoom, (Z)oom in*, then use the cursor to select a very small box around the equilibrium). Erase *(e)* and redraw the nullclines *(n,n)* for accuracy at this scale, then plot the flow using *(D)ir field/flow, (F)low* and a 10×10 grid. If you zoomed in closely enough, it should look like Figure 1.7e. The equilibrium is asymptotically stable, meaning all nearby trajectories converge to it. There is also a pattern to the convergence. All the trajectories swoop around and approach the equilibrium along one of two directions, and those two directions line up along a single line. A stable equilibrium with this pattern of convergence along a line (rather than around a full spiral) is called a *stable node*. Nodes can be stable or unstable. An *unstable node* is like a stable node running in reverse time. See Section 1.11 for more detail about how we classify equilibria.

(1.7.7) Next, we will zoom in on the upper equilibrium. Return to the default phase-plane window size *(w,d)*, erase everything and redraw the nullclines. Zoom in on the upper equilibrium and plot the flow to get something like Figure 1.7g. These trajectories are truly spiraling, and get crowded, so we used a 6×6 grid for the figure. Click on some initial conditions to confirm that the equilibrium is unstable. An equilibrium with trajectories spiraling away like this is called an *unstable spiral*. An equilibrium with trajectories spiraling in is called a *stable spiral*.

(1.7.8) Now, let us zoom in on the middle equilibrium. Once again, return to the default phase-plane window size *(w,d)*, erase everything, and redraw the nullclines. Zoom in on the middle equilibrium, redraw the nullclines, and plot the flow to get something like Figure 1.7f. This time we used a 15×15 grid for the figure to emphasize the pattern. The tractories swoop toward the equilibrium from one direction, and away from the equilibrium in another direction. Click on some initial conditions to check which direction is "in" and which direction is "out." Pay particular attention to the diagonal line that separates trajectories swooping to the right from trajectories swooping to the left. A trajectory exactly on the diagonal line swoops neither left nor right, but instead converges directly to the equilibrium. This line is called the *stable manifold* of the equilibrium. There is another line separating trajectories coming from above versus below the equilibrium. A trajectory exactly on this line comes from neither above nor below. It comes directly from the equilibrium. In other words, in *backward* time, it converges directly to the equilibrium. This line is called the *unstable manifold* of the equilibrium. An equilibrium like this, with a stable manifold and an unstable manifold, is called a *saddle*. It is unstable, since most trajectories end up swooping away from it.

(1.7.9) Let us zoom back out again to see how these local pieces are globally connected. In particular, where do the trajectories on the unstable manifold of the saddle end up in forward time? It is hard to plot the exact trajectories, but choosing any initial conditions very close to the saddle, just to the right and just to the left, shows us what happens. The left branch of the unstable manifold converges directly to the stable node, while the right branch takes an excursion corresponding to a single action potential before settling down to the stable node (Figure 1.7a, top). Each branch of the unstable manifold consists of a *heteroclinic connection*, meaning a trajectory that connects two equilibria. Taken together, the two heteroclinic connections form a loop in phase plane. This loop is key to the SNIC bifurcation underlying the onset of tonic spiking in this section.

Invariant circle. The loop described in the previous exercise is the *invariant circle* of the *saddle node on an invariant circle bifurcation*. Here, the word *circle* is used loosely, to mean a closed loop, rather than a perfectly round circle. (In other words, it is used in the topological rather than geometric sense.) The word *invariant* refers to the fact that the circle is invariant under the flow, meaning that it is composed of trajectories of the flow.

Saddle-node bifurcation of equilibria. Each time the nullclines push past each other, a saddle and a node (either stable or unstable) coalesce and disappear in a *saddle-node bifurcation of equilibria*. This is often referred to, simply, as a *saddle-node bifurcation*, and is the *saddle node* of the *saddle node on an invariant circle bifurcation*. Viewed the other way around, each time the nullclines meet and push through each other, a pair of equilibria (one saddle and one node) are created in a saddle-node bifurcation. (The node may than evolve into a spiral as the equilibria separate, as in Exercise 1.7.7.) See Section 1.11 for more detail.

Saddle node on an invariant circle (SNIC) bifurcation. We are now ready to view the SNIC bifurcation as a saddle-node bifurcation of equilibria occurring along an invariant circle. On the short branch of the invariant circle in Exercise 1.7.9, between the two equilibria, the flow is clockwise. On the long branch, the flow is counterclockwise. As I is increased, the saddle and the stable node converge, and the short, clockwise branch of the invariant circle shrinks. At the moment of the saddle-node bifurcation, the clockwise branch of the invariant circle vanishes. What remains is a counterclock-wise invariant circle with a single equilibrium. As I is further increased, the equilibrium vanishes and the invariant circle becomes a stable limit cycle, inheriting the stability of the old node (Figure 1.7a, middle and bottom). Thus, at exactly the moment when the V nullcline pushes through the W nullcline, the cell starts tonic spiking.

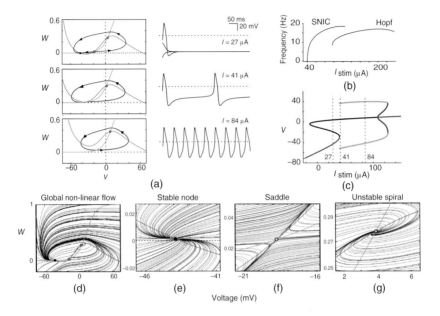

(a)   (b)   (c)   (d)   (e)   (f)   (g)

Figure 1.7   Sustained current injection with the SNIC parameter set. (a) Series of phase-plane trajectories and corresponding voltage traces obtained with the stimulus current amplitudes indicated. For $I = 27$ μA, there are three equilibria (at the nullcline intersections). The two branches of the unstable manifold of the (middle) saddle equilibrium follow different trajectories (one sub- and one super-threshold) to the stable node, forming a "circle." As I increases, the nullclines separate and the equilibria are lost from the circle, transforming it into a stable limit cycle. Firing begins at very low frequency when the limit cycle is first created, because the motion slows almost to a stop, in memory of the lost equilibria. As the nullclines separate further, firing frequency increases. (b) Firing frequency plotted against stimulus amplitude, for the SNIC and Hopf parameter sets. The two parameter sets differ only in the voltage dependence of K-channel gating, but the associated bifurcations yield behaviors exemplifying Hodgkin's excitability Classes I and II, respectively: firing frequency starts low and grades up smoothly with increasing current in the SNIC example, but is narrowly constrained in the Hopf example. (c) Bifurcation diagram, charting the equilibria and limit cycles from each phase plane, as in Figure 1.6. The SNIC bifurcation occurs just below $I = 41$ μA, where the large stable limit cycle is created at the moment the stable equilibrium is lost in a saddle-node bifurcation. The termination of firing follows the same bifurcation structure as in the Hopf example. (d) Flow in the phase plane when $I = 27$ μA, with enlargements. (e–f) Detailed flow structure close to each equilibrium.

(1.7.10) Figure 1.7c shows the bifurcation diagram for I ranging from −25 to 150. As usual, there is a lot of information packed into the diagram. Take some time to read it carefully. Which parts of the diagram correspond to the pairwise appearance and disappearance of equilibria? Which parts correspond to the stable node, saddle and unstable spiral? What color is the saddle, and why? Where is the SNIC bifurcation? Why does the end of the green branch representing the stable limit cycle line up with the fold in the middle branch? Finally, use the bifurcation diagram to explain the results of your simulated current injection experiment, including both the appearance and disappearance of tonic spiking.

(1.7.11) Why do the spikes first appear with such low frequency, as shown in Figure 1.7a and b? Hint: plot the (unscaled) direction field as you slide I through the SNIC bifurcation. Do you see the "ghost" effect of the vanished equilibria, slowing the motion on their stretch of the limit cycle? This ghost effect explains why the SNIC bifurcation yields Hodgkin's Class I, integrator neurons. Check the voltage trace again to confirm this is consistent with the waveform, and explain why the spike frequency increases as I increases.

Hodgkin's classification of neurons. In Figure 1.7b, spike frequency is plotted against applied current for the SNIC and Hopf parameter sets. Rinzel and Ermentrout (1989) describe how the associated bifurcations correspond to the characteristics of Hodgkin's Class I and Class II neurons (Hodgkin, 1948). In the SNIC bifurcation, tonic spiking appears with arbitrarily low frequency, as in Hodgkin's Class I, so the neuron has the capacity to be integrative, in the sense that the voltage response is graded with the strength of the stimulus. By contrast, in the saddle-node bifurcation of limit cycles (paired with the subcritical Hopf bifurcation), tonic spiking occurs over a very narrow frequency range, as in Hodgkin's Class II, so the neuron has the capacity to resonate with a specific stimulus frequency. See Izhikevich (2007) for a fuller characterization of classes of excitability.

1.8 Time-scale separation

Our final parameter set ("Homoclinic" in Table 1.1) differs from the SNIC parameter set only in the kinetics of K-channel gating. The parameter ϕ is increased in Equation (1.13), so that K channels respond more quickly to voltage change. In Section 1.9, we simulate a current clamp experiment and study the associated bifurcations for this parameter set. But first we explore the impact of changing the time scale of W, relative to that of V, on the overall dynamics of the system. Time-scale structure is a powerful point of contact between biology and mathematics. There is a vast range of time scales in biology, and the level of Time-scale separation between variables has important consequences for model behavior and analysis.

(1.8.1) Set up XPP with a phase-plane window and voltage trace window (as in Exercise 1.5.2). Adjust the phase-plane window (using *(V)iewaxes*) so that W ranges from -0.2 to 0.6. Set the initial condition to $(V, W) = (-60, 0)$, the total run time to 500 (using *u,t*), and I to 0. Choose either the SNIC or homoclinic parameter set (using *(F)ile, (G)et par set*), and check Table 1.1 to confirm that the only difference between these two parameter sets is the value of ϕ. Create a slider for ϕ that ranges between the two values, from 0.04 to 0.22. Plot the nullclines (*n,n*) and slide ϕ. Why are the nullclines unchanged? One way to explain it is by noticing that ϕ does not appear in either of the nullcline Equations (1.19) and (1.22). Now, explain it in terms of the the meaning of ϕ for K channels.

(1.8.2) Even though changing ϕ does not change the nullclines, it has a dramatic effect on the behavior of the system. Turn on the scaled direction field (using *d,s*) and slide ϕ. As ϕ increases, the arrows all get steeper. Why? First, let us think about it in terms of the equations. Recall from Section 1.4 that the slope of each arrow is given by its "rise/run," where the rise is the rate of change dW/dt in the W direction, and the run is the rate of change dV/dt in the V direction. Look back at Equations (1.12) and (1.13) for dV/dt and dW/dt. What role does ϕ play in each equation? How does this explain what happens to the slopes of the arrows as ϕ increases? Now explain it in terms of the meaning of ϕ.

(1.8.3) What impact do you predict the increase in ϕ will have on spike waveform and frequency?

(1.8.4) Let us test your prediction. Set I to 42 and ϕ to 0.04. Sketch the nullclines to confirm this is just after the SNIC bifurcation of Section 1.7. Plot the voltage trace, and with the voltage trace window active, gradually slide ϕ up to 0.22. Is this what you predicted? When ϕ is small, spike frequency is low: the model K channels open slowly, so the voltage reaches a high peak before the K current catches up. Similarly, the K current drives the voltage to a deep hyperpolarization before the channels have slowly closed. Higher values of ϕ represent K channels that open and close more quickly. Thus, the voltage peaks earlier, does not hyperpolarize so deeply, and the spike frequency increases. The high spike baseline is particularly striking. We will return to this feature in Section 1.10 when we extend the Morris–Lecar model to exhibit bursting.

(1.8.5) Now let us return to the phase plane and direction field to see what is going on. Plot the trajectory (*i, g*), and the scaled direction field (*d,s*). When $\phi = 0.04$, we recognize the large limit cycle resulting from the SNIC bifurcation in Section 1.7. Gradually increase ϕ, and notice how the direction field steepens, causing the limit cycle to narrow in the V

direction and elongate in the W direction. As you further increase ϕ, the limit cycle shrinks toward the equilibrium.

(1.8.6) Expand the ϕ slider to range from 0.01 to 0.5, to exaggerate the geometric phenomenon at play here. See Figure 1.8. As we change ϕ, the relative time scales of V and W change. When $\phi = 0.01$, V is much faster than W, the direction field is almost horizontal in most of the plane, and the flow is dominated by the fast change in V. It is only when dV/dt is close to 0, in the neighborhood of the V nullcline, that W, the slow variable, has much impact on the direction field and flow. As ϕ is increased to intermediate values, the V and W time scales become more similar, and the slopes in the direction field are more varied and less extreme. When ϕ reaches 0.5, W has become the fast variable, and the direction field is almost vertical in most of the plane.

Fast/slow dynamics. Notice how the shape of the limit cycle is tightly controlled by the folded shape of the V nullcline when V is the fast variable ($\phi = 0.01$) (see Figure 1.8a). On the "bottom" stretch of the limit cycle, the fast V dynamic "whisks" the trajectory to the right branch of the V nullcline. Now, the slow W dynamic comes into play. dW/dt is positive, albeit small, so the trajectory slowly climbs up the V nullcline, while the V dynamic ensures the trajectory "hugs" the nullcline tightly. At the nullcline's "knee", the fast V dynamic takes over again, whisking the trajectory

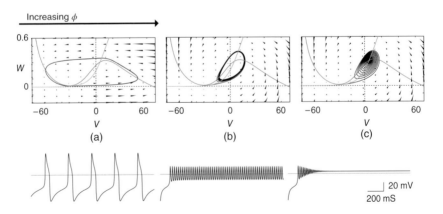

Figure 1.8   Changing time-scales. Only the rate constant of K-current activation, ϕ, is varied between the graphs, so the nullclines do not change. All other parameters are from the SNIC parameter set, as in Figure 1.7, with I held constant at 42 μA. Arrowheads represent the direction field. (a) $\phi = 0.01$, so W changes slowly relative to V. The direction field is primarily horizontal, and the large limit cycle (resulting from a SNIC bifurcation) hugs the V nullcline more tightly than in Figure 1.7, where $\phi = 0.04$. (b) $\phi = 0.22$. W changes on a similar time scale to V, and the cycle has a dramatically different shape, corresponding to low amplitude spikes with a high baseline. (c) $\phi = 0.23$. The cycle has disappeared altogether, so the spikes damp down to the attracting equilibrium.

over to the left branch of the nullcline, where dW/dt is negative, and so the cycle continues. This interaction between nullcline geometry and fast/slow separation of time scales has generated a rich body of mathematical research (see, for example (Jones, 1995) and (Zeeman, 1977)).

(1.8.7) Plot the voltage trace for $\phi = 0.01$ and describe how each of the fast and slow components of the limit cycle in the phase plane correspond to features of the voltage waveform. You can add extra detail by thinking about the location of the equilibrium, and the "ghost" of the SNIC bifurcation, relative to the limit cycle.

Time-scale separation and model reduction. Recognizing the separation of time scales and how they relate to your time scale of interest can be helpful for model simplification, as we will see throughout the book. For example, our model assumption that Ca channels activate instantly is a statement about the relative time scales of Ca-channel activation, K-channel activation, and action potentials in our model cell.

Time-scale separation and bursting. Separation of time scales also underlies many models of bursting. The basic idea is that a third variable with a time scale that is slow compared to both V and W, repeatedly tips the system across bifurcations from equilibrium to cycling and back. In Chapters 3 and 4, for example, calcium build up plays the role of the slow variable. If the third time scale is slow enough, the system tips between "hugging" the equilibrium and hugging the limit cycle, in much the same way as it hugs the two slow branches of the nullcline in Figure 1.8. In Section 1.10, we extend the Morris–Lecar model with a slow variable to illustrate the idea. To prepare for this, in Section 1.9, we study the homoclinic bifurcation mechanism that underlies the onset of high baseline spiking.

1.9 Homoclinic bifurcation

Figure 1.9a shows the bifurcation diagram when we set $\phi = 0.22$ (the "Homoclinic" parameter set in Table 1.1) and vary I to simulate a sustained current injection experiment. Comparing it with the previous two bifurcation diagrams, we see interesting similarities and differences. For example, there is a region of *tri-stability*, between $I = 37.2$ and $I = 39.6$, where two stable equilibria and a stable limit cycle co-exist. See Figure 1.9e–g for the case $I = 38$. You can use techniques from the previous sections to explore the phase plane and voltage traces, unpacking all the information in the bifurcation diagram. The following exercises focus on the differences from the SNIC example in the onset of spiking.

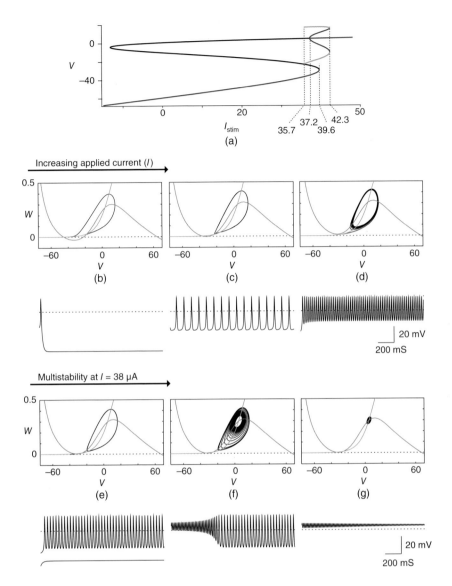

Figure 1.9   Sustained current injection with the Homoclinic parameter set. (a)
Bifurcation diagram, showing the homoclinic bifurcation at $I = 35.7$ μA, and
subsequent regions of bi- and tri-stabilities. (b–d) Phase-plane trajectories and nullclines
and corresponding voltage traces as applied current is increased through the bifurcation.
Notice the graded firing frequency response and the high spike baseline corresponding
to the limit cycle position. Viewed from (d) to (b), the stable limit cycle grows till it
collides with the saddle equilibrium to become a homoclinic loop and disappear in the
homoclinic bifurcation. (e–g) Tri-stability when $I = 38$ μA. There is a stable limit cycle
(e and f), with (e) a stable equilibrium outside and (f) a stable spiral equilibrium inside.

(1.9.1) Continuing from Section 1.8, check the total run time is still 500 (*u,t*, and remember to *escape* from the numerics menu). Select the Homo-clinic parameter set (*f, g*), and restrict the ϕ slider to range from 0.04 to 0.22 again. Set *I* at 42, plot the trajectory (with initial condition $(-60,0)$), and slide ϕ between the two extremes. Recall from Section 1.7 that when $\phi = 0.04$, the limit cycle is created by a SNIC bifurcation, so the limit cycle follows the shape of the SNIC invariant circle, enclosing the deli-cate region where the nullclines almost touch. As ϕ is increased, the limit cycle passes through that delicate region. This is our hint that when we fix ϕ at 0.22, and slide *I* in a simulated current injection experiment (as in Sections 1.5 and 1.7) we should expect to see a slightly different bifurcation mechanism for the onset of tonic spiking.

(1.9.2) Let us try it. Set $\phi = 0.22$, add a slider for *I* ranging from -25 to 50, and explore what happens in the phase-plane and voltage trace windows as you slide *I*.

(1.9.3) As *I* increases, the pairwise appearance and disappearance of equi-libria as the nullclines pass through each other should look familiar: it is exactly the same as in the SNIC bifurcation. Why? (For a hint, look back at Exercise 1.8.1. By contrast, the limit cycle and tonic spiking look quite different from those in the SNIC example.

(1.9.4) As with the SNIC bifurcation in Section 1.7, the stable equilibrium is lost when the stable node and the saddle coalesce and disappear, around $I = 40$. But this time the stable limit cycle appears far from the saddle-node bifurcation. What happened to the invariant circle of the SNIC example? To answer this, begin by setting $I = 27$, plot the flow (using *d, f* with a 10×10 grid), and compare it with the flow in Figure 1.7d. Describe some of the differences.

(1.9.5) Erase the flow (*e*), replot the nullclines (*n. n*), and choose an initial condition just to the right of the saddle equilibrium (*i, m*) to approxi-mate the right-hand branch of the unstable manifold of the saddle (see Exercises 1.7.8 and 1.7.9 to review stable and unstable manifolds). Notice how the unstable manifold returns fairly close to the saddle, from above, before heading over to the stable equilibrium, as shown in Figure 1.9b.

(1.9.6) Reset the *I* slider to range from 27 to 50, and gradually increase *I*. What happens to the unstable manifold of the saddle? Just before $I = 36$, it returns to become the stable manifold of the same saddle! See Figure 1.9c. A trajectory like this, that starts and ends at the same saddle, is called a *homoclinic loop*.

(1.9.7) Continue to increase *I*. The homoclinic loop disappears, giving birth to a stable limit cycle in its wake (Figure 1.9d). This is a *homoclinic bifurca-tion*. The unstable manifold of the saddle now spirals into the stable limit cycle. Set $I = 37$, and plot the entire flow again (*d, f* with a 10×10 grid) to see that the system is now bistable. There is a stable equilibrium around

$V = -35$, and the new stable limit cycle. Choose initial conditions in the phase plane (i, i) to plot the corresponding voltage traces (rest, and tonic spiking, respectively) for each stable state. (Remember you can turn sim-plot on (m,s) to plot the phase plane and voltage trace simultaneously.) Use the phase plane to explain why the spike baseline is so high, above the resting potential.

(1.9.8) It can be easier to understand the homoclinic bifurcation by con-sidering what happens to the stable limit cycle as I *decreases* through the bifurcation value $I \approx 35.7$. To explore this, zoom in (w,z) on the region of the phase plane containing the action (the equilibria and the limit cycle). Set the I slider to range from 34 to 41, and position it at $I = 41$. Choose an initial condition inside the stable limit cycle, and within the basin of attraction of the limit cycle, so it spirals out to the cycle. (Note, from the bifurcation diagram, that the equilibrium inside the limit cycle is also stable when $I = 41$, and there is an unstable limit cycle separating the basins of attraction of the stable limit cycle and the equilibrium. Try a few initial conditions inside the stable limit cycle to check this, and to find one that spirals out to the stable cycle.) Now, gradually decrease I, and watch what happens to the stable limit cycle and the equilibria.

Homoclinic bifurcation: a limit cycle collides with a saddle equilibrium. In Exercise 1.9.8, the stable limit cycle steadily grows as I is decreased. Around $I = 39.6$ the nullclines touch, and a saddle and stable node appear. As I continues to decrease, the stable limit cycle and saddle move inexorably towards each other. The *homoclinic bifurcation* is the moment of collision, when the limit cycle becomes a homoclinic loop, and vanishes. This viewpoint of bifurca-tions occurring when limit sets collide can help bring clarity to several of the bifurcations we have encountered where equilibria or limit cycles seem to appear out of "thin air."

Saddle-node bifurcation: a stable node and saddle collide. Every intersection of the nullclines is an equilibrium, and a saddle-node bifurcation occurs every time the nullclines push through each other. Depending on the direction that I is varied, a saddle-node bifurcation can be viewed as the creation of a saddle and node pair of equilibria where the nullclines first touch, or as the collision and disappearance of a saddle-node pair as the nullclines push past each other. In a bifurcation diagram, a saddle-node bifurcation appears as a fold in the branch of equilibria, as in Figures 1.7c and 1.9a. For this reason, it is also called a *fold bifurcation*.

SNIC bifurcation: a limit cycle collides with a degenerate equilibrium. In the SNIC bifurcation of Section 1.7, a saddle-node collision of equilibria occurs on the invariant circle as I is increased. Viewed from the other direction, as I is decreased, the limit cycle collides with an equilibrium at the moment of a saddle-node bifurcation. In other words, a homoclinic bifurcation occurs simultaneously with a saddle-node bifurcation. The equilibrium is called degenerate at that moment, because it is neither a saddle nor a node, but a hybrid of the two.

Saddle-node bifurcation of limit cycles: stable and unstable limit cycles collide. In Exercises 1.6.6–1.6.10, we saw an unstable cycle that was born at the equilibrium (in a Hopf bifurcation) grow inexorably till it collided with a stable limit cycle and the two cycles disappeared in a saddle-node bifurcation of limit cycles. In our bifurcation diagrams, a saddle-node bifurcation of limit cycles appears as a fold in the branch representing limit cycles, emphasizing the similarity with the saddle-node bifurcation of equilibria.

(1.9.9) Exactly where, on the bifurcation diagram (Figure 1.9a), is the homoclinic bifurcation? Why does the green branch representing the stable limit cycle end abruptly when it meets the black branch? What does that black branch represent? What does the fold in the black/red branch at $I = 39.6$ represent? What does the fold in the blue/green branch at $I = 42.3$ represent? (Hint: review Exercise 1.6.10).

(1.9.10) Use the same carefully chosen initial condition as in Exercise 1.9.8 to watch what happens to the voltage trace as you decrease I from 41, and the limit cycle approaches the saddle. The spike frequency decreases dramatically, as in the SNIC example and Hodgkin's Class I neurons. Why?

(1.9.11) Reset the initial condition to $(-60, 0)$, gradually increase I from 34, and watch what happens to the voltage trace again. Use the bifurcation diagram to explain why the tonic spikes appear with high frequency, instead of the low frequency we observed in the previous exercise.

Bifurcations switch spiking on and off. This completes our tour of parameter space for the Morris–Lecar model. It is by no means exhaustive. Indeed, we have only used three of an infinite choice of parameter sets. Nevertheless, we hope it has conveyed some of the richness of behavior of the model, and of the associated bifurcation mechanisms that switch spiking on and off with different characteristics of excitability. In the next section, we continue to follow Rinzel and Ermentrout (1989), using the Homoclinic parameter set to explore how a cycle of bifurcations, repeatedly switching spiking on and off again, can be used to model intrinsic bursting behavior.

1.10   Bursting

In this section, we extend the Morris–Lecar model to illustrate how bursting can arise as a slow passage, back and forth, across bifurcations from rest to spiking. For a range of stimulus currents, I, the homoclinic parameter set of the last section exhibits multiple stable modes of behavior, including rest and tonic spiking. Moreover, the different modes of behavior have voltage separation, in the sense that the spike baseline is above the resting potential. This creates an opportunity for the different behaviors to feed back and control the stimulus current via voltage, sweeping I back and forth across the bifurcations.

(1.10.1) To fix ideas, consider the homoclinic bifurcation diagram in Figure 1.9a, and suppose $I = 38$ (Figure 1.9e–g). Depending on the cell's history, it may be resting or spiking. If it is at rest, at the lower stable node, what happens if I gradually increases (in other words, if I is driven to the right on the bifurcation diagram)? We know from the diagram, and from our simulated current injection experiments, that the cell will track the stable node until it disappears in the saddle-node bifurcation. Then the cell will suddenly start spiking.

(1.10.2) Now, suppose the cell is spiking. What happens if I gradually *decreases* (i.e., is driven to the left on the bifurcation diagram)? We can read the diagram, or revisit Exercise 1.9.8 to answer this. The cell will continue to spike, tracking the limit cycle, until the cycle collides with the saddle and disappears. Then the cell will suddenly return to rest.

Voltage-dependent slowly varying current. From Exercises 1.10.1 and 1.10.2, we see that if I is driven to the right (increases) when the cell is at rest, but is driven to the left (decreases) when the cell is spiking, the cell will tip back and forth between rest and spiking, in a classic bursting fashion, as in Figures 1.1 (data) and 1.10 (model). In the model, the voltage separation between the resting and spiking states means that voltage feedback can be used to drive I in opposite directions during rest versus spiking. Let us translate this into a differential equation. The cell will burst if:

- the rate of change of I is positive when V is low (at resting levels), and
- the rate of change of I is negative when V is high (at spiking levels).

To clarify what we mean by "low" and "high" voltage levels, let V_b denote a voltage level between the resting and spiking levels. Check the bifurcation

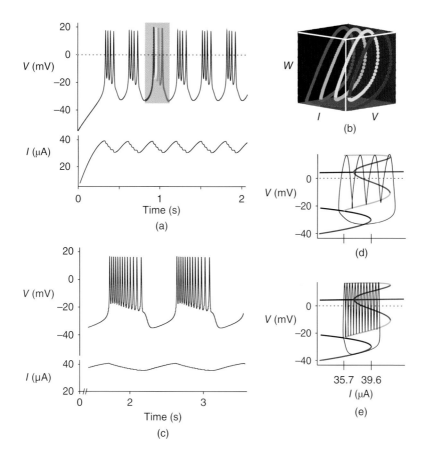

Figure 1.10   Bursting in the extended Morris–Lecar model. Starting with the homoclinic parameter set, internal voltage-dependent kinetics are included for the applied current, so that I slowly increases when $V < -20$ and slowly decreases when $V > -20$. (a) Burst firing, with rate constant $r = 0.005$ for I kinetics. Behavior of the added current is shown below the voltage trace. Gray highlight indicates the recurring cycle encompassing one burst. (b) The corresponding burst trajectory is a limit cycle in three-dimensional phase space. Each burst corresponds to a complete passage around the cycle. Individual spikes within the burst are colored as in A. The spike waveforms change slightly during a burst, but the burst as a whole follows the recurring cycle. (c) Longer bursts with more spikes are elicited when the added current, I, changes even more slowly ($r = 0.001$). (d and e) Details of the bifurcation diagram from Figure 1.9 onto which a two-dimensional projection of the three-dimensional burst cycles in (b) and (c), respectively, are superimposed. The projection is the view from directly "above" the cycle in (b), looking down on the I–V plane. During the interburst interval, $V < -20$ so I slowly increases, sweeping to the right on the bifurcation diagram. During this quiescent state, the cell tracks the low voltage stable equilibrium on the bifurcation diagram. When I passes 39.6 µA, the stable equilibrium disappears in a saddle-node bifurcation, and the cell, seeking an alternative stable state, jumps to the stable limit cycle and starts spiking. With the increase in voltage, I changes direction to decreasing, slowly sweeping to the left. The cell continues to spike, tracking the stable cycle until the cycle collides with the saddle and disappears in a homoclinic bifurcation when $I = 35.7$ µA. The cell is forced to seek the quiescent state again, the voltage drops, and the entire burst cycle repeats. The slower rate constant of I in (e) means there is less "momentum" (greater Time-scale separation), and the trajectory hugs the bifurcation diagram more closely.

diagram to confirm that we could, for example, choose $V_b = -25$ mV. Then, the cell will burst if

$$\frac{dI}{dt} > 0 \qquad \text{when} \qquad V < V_b, \quad \text{and} \qquad (1.23)$$

$$\frac{dI}{dt} < 0 \qquad \text{when} \qquad V > V_b \qquad (1.24)$$

(1.10.3) Confirm that, for positive values of r, conditions (1.23) and (1.24) are satisfied by the differential equation

$$\frac{dI}{dt} = r(V_b - V) \qquad (1.25)$$

We will examine the role of r in Equation (1.25) in the XPP exercises below.

Extended Morris–Lecar model. Recall that the Morris–Lecar model we have been exploring is defined (mathematically) by Equations (1.12)–(1.16), in which I is treated as an externally varied parameter. In the XPP program *BridgingTutorial-Burst.ode* (available online or from the authors), we extend the model with Equation (1.25), so that I is now treated as an intrinsic variable, with V, W, and I all feeding back on each other, either directly or indirectly. Equation (1.25) is somewhat abstract, in the sense that it was chosen for its simplicity, and is not modeling a specific physiological mechanism for slowly varying I. Physiological mechanisms that have an analogous effect on current would also promote bursting. See Chapters 3 and 4 for calcium-induced bursting, and Bertram *et al.* (1995), Ermentrout and Terman (2010), and Golubitsky *et al.* (2001), Izhikevich (2007) for surveys and classifications of bursting mechanisms.

Three-dimensional systems. The extended Morris–Lecar model is three dimensional, in the sense that it has three dependent variables (V, W, and I). Instead of a phase *plane*, there is a three-dimensional phase *space*. As with the phase plane, a set of initial conditions $V(0), W(0)$, and $I(0)$ corresponds to a point in phase space. Given the initial conditions, iteratively computing the future values of $V(t), W(t)$, and $I(t)$ may take a bit more computer time than for two variables, but is not conceptually different. The trajectory followed by $V(t), W(t)$, and $I(t)$ is a curve weaving around in three-dimensional phase space, instead of a two-dimensional plane. There *is* a conceptual difference here. Recall from Section 1.4 that trajectories cannot cross each other. In two dimensions, this has restrictive consequences. For example, a trajectory that starts inside a limit cycle can never get outside. Not so, in three dimensions! What does "inside" a limit cycle even mean in three dimensions? There is plenty of room for trajectories to weave around and around themselves and each other. Try "googling" *strange attractor*, and choosing *images*, to see some of the extraordinary and beautiful paths trajectories can take in three dimensions. The equations behind those images can be remarkably simple; see textbooks on dynamical systems and chaos, such as Blanchard *et al.*, (2011), Hirsch *et al.* (2012), and Strogatz (1994), to learn more.

(1.10.4) Returning to our extended Morris–Lecar model, look over the XPP program *BridgingTutorial-Burst.ode*. Find the parts of the code that correspond to:
- The new differential equation for I.
- The way that V feeds back into I.
- The way that I feeds back into V.
- The default initial conditions for V, W, and I.
- The new parameters r and V_b.
- The default parameter set being used.
- The total run time being used.
- The default window view that XPP will open to.

(1.10.5) Open XPP using *BridgingTutorial-Burst.ode*. It should open to a voltage trace window, with $r = 0.01$, $V_b = -20$, the homoclinic parameter set, and initial conditions $(V, W, I) = (-60, 0, 0)$. Run it (using *i,g*). You should see bursting behavior, similar, but not identical, to Figure 1.10a. Describe some of the differences from Figure 1.10a.

(1.10.6) Open a second window (using *m, c*), and plot the time course of I (using *Viewaxes*, or Xi versus t and the command line). Confirm that, as we planned, I increases when the cell is quiescent (at rest), and decreases when the cell is spiking. Why does I have a "sawtooth" shape? To answer this, look back at each of the terms in Equation (1.25), and the voltage trace.

(1.10.7) Use Equation (1.25) and the bifurcation diagram (Figure 1.9a) to explain why I and V steadily climb from their initial conditions until the bursting starts.

(1.10.8) Now, let us examine the role of r in Equation (1.25). What do you predict will happen if we decrease r? Create a slider for r, ranging from 0.001 to 0.01, and try it. Is it what you predicted? As you decrease r, I changes more slowly. So it takes longer for I to drive the cell from one bifurcation to the other, and back again. Thus, the burst frequency decreases. (Burst frequency means the number of entire bursts per time unit.) Near $r = 0.006$, it takes I so long to drive the cell through the spiking regime, that the cell suddenly increases to 4 spikes per burst, instead of 3.

(1.10.9) Why does the spike frequency decrease within each burst? And why does the spike baseline decrease within each burst? Hint: which bifurcation terminates the burst? Think about what is going on in the *V*-*W* phase plane.

(1.10.10) As you continue to decrease *r*, the bursts take longer, and the number of spikes per burst continues to increase. Why does it also take so much longer for the first burst to get started?

(1.10.11) Figure 1.10 shows several views of the bursting behavior at *r* = 0.005 and *r* = 0.001. When *r* = 0.005, the cell fires 4 spikes per burst (Figure 1.10a). Each spike represents a circuit around the slowly growing stable limit cycle in the slowly evolving *V*-*W* phase plane of Section 1.9, while each burst represents a circuit around the bifurcation diagram (Figure 1.10d). Let us isolate one burst. First, zoom into the voltage trace (*w,z*) to confirm that there is a complete burst between 900 ms and 1200 ms. We will select that burst. In the *n(U)merics* menu, set the *(T)otal* run time to be 1200 (use the command line, and remember to type *return*). Then set the *t(R)ansient* time to be 900. Click on *escape* to exit the numerics menu. Erase everything *(e)*, return the window to default size (*w, d*) and plot the single burst (*i, g*). Use *(V)iewaxes* to view the burst in lots of different ways. We have already seen *V* versus *t* and *I* versus *t*. What about *W* versus *t*? Or *V* versus *W*? Or *V* versus *I*? Or *W* versus *I*? In each case, make a prediction first. Good ranges for the axes are *V*: −40 to 30, *I*: 30 to 50, *W*: −0.2 to 1, and *t*: 900 to 1200.

(1.10.12) Let us view the burst in three dimensions. First we will view the time course of *V* and *W* changing together. Click *(V)iewaxes, (3)D*, and choose *t* for the *X*-axis, *V* for the *Y*-axis, and *W* for the *Z*-axis. You do not need to fill in the ranges, but be sure to fill in the last three boxes with the axis labels (*t, V*, and *W*). When you click *OK*, you may be presented with a blank screen. Fear not! Click *(W)indow/zoom, (F)it*, and your three-dimensional plot should appear. You can rotate the image by holding the mouse down and moving the cursor. Experiment with the rotation, to get "end on" views that look like your two-dimensional plots from the previous exercise, and "diagonal" views that show how the two dimensional plots (*projections*) relate to each other in three dimensions. (Use *(W)indow/zoom, (F)it* again if the image rotates out of view).

(1.10.13) Now, let us view the burst in *I, V, W* space, to reproduce Figure 1.10b. This is the *phase space* for the system; the three dimensional analogy of a two dimensional phase *plane*. It gives a beautiful view for understanding how the each burst corresponds to passage around a coiled, three-dimensional limit cycle. This limit cycle in phase space traces a circuit, tracking the stable equilibrium of the two-dimensional system during quiescence (as *I* increases), and the stable limit cycle of the two-dimensional system during spiking (as *I* decreases), thereby forming a loop as *I* slowly varies back and forth. Rotate this image to make sure that you see how to relate the full, three-dimensional loop to the two-dimensional projection of the loop in the V versus I plot. Note that you may need to change the order of V and W (and their axes labels) in *(V)iewaxes, (3)D* to get the views you want.

Visualizing bursting on the bifurcation diagram. Of the two-dimensional plots, V versus I is particularly informative, because V measures the behavior of the cell, and I is the bifurcation variable. Indeed, the V versus I plot has the same axes as the bifurcation diagram, so the two are often super-imposed, as in Figure 1.10d and e. There is some subtlety (slight of hand, even) to appreciate here. The bifurcation diagram is about the stable sets in the two-dimensional V, W phase plane *with I held constant*, for each value of I. The superimposed burst trajectory is about the path followed by V and W *when I is slowly varying*. If I slowed down all the way to a *stop*, the bifurcation diagram could tell us about the exact (deterministic) behavior of V and W for the value of I where we stopped. When I is varying, the bifurcation diagram tells us the approximate behavior of the trajectory. The slower I varies, the more closely the trajectory follows the bifurcation dia-gram. Compare Figure 1.10 parts D ($r = 0.005$) and E ($r = 0.001$). When I changes more slowly ($r = 0.001$), the burst trajectory "hugs" the stable branches of the diagram, and the bifurcations themselves, more closely.

1.11   Eigenvalues and stability

Throughout the tutorial, we have seen the importance of stability for understanding and predicting the behavior of a model. So far, we have used simulations to determine the stability properties of limit sets (equi-libria and limit cycles), we have worked with bifurcation diagrams that informed us of the stability properties, and we have noticed that changes in stability are associated with bifurcations. We close the tutorial by returning to the two-dimensional Morris–Lecar model, to describe how the stability properties of an equilibrium can be characterized by its *eigenvalues*. Recall that stability is about the behavior of trajectories close to the equilibrium. The essential idea of this section is *linearization* of the system close to the equilibrium. In other words, close to the equilibrium we approximate the nonlinear system with something linear (and, therefore, simpler), and deduce the stability properties from the approximation.

One-dimensional linear differential equation. We will start by developing intu-ition for one of the simplest, but most useful, differential equations out there:

$$\frac{dx}{dt} = kx \tag{1.26}$$

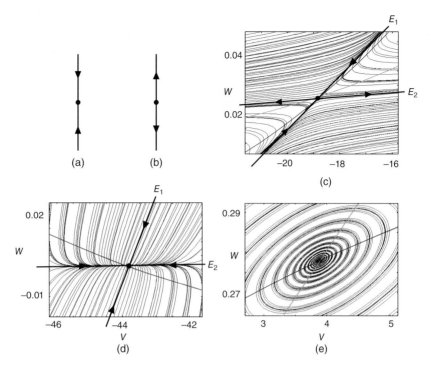

Figure 1.11   Eigenvalues and stability. (a and b) An equilibrium of a linear one-dimensional dynamical system has a single eigenvalue, indicating the direction and rate of flow (towards or away from the equilibrium). The eigenvalue is (a) negative when the equilibrium is stable and (b) positive when the equilibrium is unstable. (c–e) Magnified view, close to an equilibrium in a two-dimensional system. The equilibrium has two eigenvalues, organizing the direction of flow. (c) A saddle has one negative and one positive eigenvalue corresponding to flow towards and away from the saddle along eigendirections E_1 and E_2, respectively. (d) A stable node has two negative eigenvalues, $k_1 < k_2$, corresponding to flow along eigendirections E_1 and E_2, respectively. (e) A spiral equilibrium has complex eigenvalues (a complex conjugate pair). The equilibrium is unstable when the real part of the eigenvalues is positive, stable when the real part of the eigenvalues is negative. Parameter values given in the text.

Equation (1.26) is *one-dimensional*, because there is only one equation, and one variable x. There is also one parameter, k. Equation (1.26) is called *linear*, because the right-hand side, kx is a linear function of x. Recall that when we had two equations for two variables, V and W, we plotted the trajectories in a two-dimensional phase plane. When we extended the Morris–Lecar system to three equations, for the three variables V, W, and I, we plotted the trajectories in three-dimensional phase space. Equation (1.26) has one variable, so we plot the trajectories on a one-dimensional *phase line* as shown in Figure 1.11a and b.

(1.11.1)   We have not yet said what the variable x represents. For now, let us simply say x measures position on the phase line. Imagine yourself as an ant, living a one-dimensional life on the phase line. Suppose that x denotes your position, and Equation (1.26) determines your motion. Consider the case when $k = 2$.

- Which direction do you (the ant) walk from initial position $x = 3$?
- Which direction do you walk from initial position $x = -3$?
- Which direction do you walk from initial position $x = 0$?
- Which phase line shows your motion, Figure 1.11a or Figure 1.11b?

If $x > 0$, then $kx > 0$ (since $k = 2$), so $dx/dt > 0$, and you walk in a positive direction, further away from $x = 0$. Similarly, if $x < 0$, then $dx/dt < 0$, and you walk in a negative direction from your negative initial position. In other words, you walk further way from $x = 0$ again. If you start at exactly $x = 0$, then $dx/dt = 0$, so you do not move. In summary, when $k = 2$, $x = 0$ is an unstable (repelling) equilibrium, corresponding to Figure 1.11b.

(1.11.2) What if $k = -2$? There is an equilibrium at $x = 0$ again. Which direction do you walk from initial position $x = 3$ this time? And which direction from initial position $x = -3$? Confirm that, wherever you start, you head "home" to $x = 0$. So, when $k = -2$, $x = 0$ is a stable (attracting) equilibrium, corresponding to Figure 1.11a.

(1.11.3) What if $k = -1$? The phase line will look the same as for $k = -2$, but there is a difference. Do you head home to $x = 0$ faster when $k = -2$ or when $k = -1$?

(1.11.4) How do the cases $k = 1$ and $k = 2$ compare? In both cases, you are repelled from $x = 0$. Is the repulsion stronger when $k = 1$ or when $k = 2$?

The sign of k determines attraction versus repulsion. Summarizing, when k is positive in Equation (1.26), the equilibrium at $x = 0$ is repelling, and when k is negative, the equilibrium is attracting. The larger the magnitude of k, the stronger the attraction or repulsion. If we now think of x as representing displacement from the equilibrium at $x = 0$, then k characterizes the feedback of x onto itself. When $k < 0$, there is negative feedback, the displacement decays and we return to equilibrium. When $k > 0$, there is positive feedback and the displacement grows (exponentially). Equipped with this intuition for the one-dimensional flow of Equation (1.26) along a line, we now return to the two-dimensional Morris–Lecar model.

(1.11.5) Open XPP with *BridgingTutorial-MLecar.ode*, and choose the SNIC parameter set (f,g). Set $I = 27$ as in Exercises 1.7.6–1.7.9, and plot the global non-linear flow (using d, f, and a 10×10 grid), as in Figure 1.7d. We will focus on the saddle equilibrium first (Figure 1.7f). Recall that the saddle has a stable manifold and an unstable manifold, composed of trajectories. The two branches of the unstable manifold "emerge" directly from the saddle, and take different routes to the stable node (creating the invariant circle of the SNIC bifurcation). The two branches of the stable manifold head directly into the saddle. One branch emerges from the unstable spiral, the other comes from below. Close to the saddle, all other trajectories are guided towards the saddle by the stable manifold, swoop past, and are guided away again by the unstable manifold.

(1.11.6) Repeat Exercise 1.7.8, to zoom into a neighborhood of the saddle, as in Figures 1.7f and 1.11c. When you zoom in closely enough, the stable and unstable manifolds look like straight lines. Remind yourself which straight line is the stable manifold, and which is the unstable. If the flow does not happen to show the unstable manifold clearly (it depends where the grid of initial conditions falls), remember that you can plot a good approximation by choosing initial conditions with the mouse (i, i) just to the left and right of the saddle.

(1.11.7) Now repeat the process to zoom in even more closely, choosing a small box around the saddle within the already zoomed-in window. Replot the nullclines and flow. Do you see any difference? It should look like Figure 1.7c again, except the scale on the axes is finer. Do it again. And again. It still looks just like Figure 1.7c. If you keep zooming, you will find your computer's limits. But until that point, we are seeing fairly compelling evidence that no matter how closely we look, the flow close to the saddle is organized by the same two straight lines. These straight lines are called *eigendirections*. The eigendirections are *tangent* to the stable and unstable manifolds at the saddle point: the more closely we zoom in, the straighter the manifolds look, and the more closely they are approximated by the eigendirections. "Eigen" is a German word for "self." Why do you think it is used in this context? Flow on an eigendirection flows along itself. It is just flow along a straight line.

(1.11.8) Flow along a straight line is like flow in one dimension. In fact, it is a (mathematically proven) theorem that when we zoom in closely enough, the flow along an eigendirection is well approximated by $dx/dt = kx$ for the right choice of constant k. This theorem is key to how we quantify stability, so let us work with it. Imagine ignoring all of the phase plane except the attracting eigendirection (the line E_1 in Figure 1.11c). Along E_1, the flow is directed toward the saddle. Let x denote the distance from the saddle along the line E_1, positive x going up and to the right, negative x in the opposite direction. The saddle is at $x = 0$, so the flow is directed toward $x = 0$ from both sides. Is this reminding you of the ant in Exercises 1.11.1–1.11.4? What sign does k_1 have to be, for $dx/dt = k_1 x$ to give a good approximation to the flow on the attracting eigendirection? The number k_1 is called the *eigenvalue associated with the eigendirection E_1*.

(1.11.9) What role does the size of the eigenvalue play? Which would correspond to stronger attraction to the saddle along the attracting eigendirection, $k_1 = -2$ or $k_1 = -1/2$?

(1.11.10) Now, let us think about the repelling eigendirection (the line E_2 in Figure 1.11c), and let x denote distance from the equilibrium along E_2. What sign would k_2 have to be for $dx/dt = k_2 x$ to give a good approximation to the flow on the repelling eigendirection? In other words, what sign is the eigenvalue corresponding to the repelling eigendirection?

(1.11.11) What role does the size of the eigenvalue play in the repelling case? Which would correspond to stronger repulsion from the saddle, $k_2 = 2$ or $k_2 = 1/2$?

(1.11.12) Recall that changing ϕ changes the slopes in the direction field, but does not change the locations of the nulllclines or the equilibria. Change ϕ to 0.22 (as in the homoclinic example). Confirm that the flow around the saddle is organized by two eigendirections again, with one positive eigenvalue and one negative. How can you tell that k_1 is stronger relative to k_2 than it was for $\phi = 0.04$?

A saddle has eigenvalues of opposite signs. Let us review the overall saddle behavior again: trajectories are carried in toward the equilibrium by the eigendirection with a negative eigenvalue, and carried out again by the eigendirection with a positive eigenvalue. This is true for every saddle in the phase plane. Indeed, one way to define a saddle equilibrium is that it has one positive and one negative eigenvalue. Notice that one positive eigenvalue is enough to make an equilibrium unstable. Almost every trajectory is carried away by it.

(1.11.13) Let us apply the same way of thinking to the stable node. With $\phi = 0.22$ and $I = 27$, return to the default window size in XPP (using w, d), then zoom into the stable equilibrium. Once again, if you keep zooming in, you find the flow always looks the same. And once again, the flow is organized by two straight line eigendirections E_1 and E_2, as in Figure 1.11d. Explain how we know that the corresponding eigenvalues k_1 and k_2 are both negative.

(1.11.14) In the example of the previous exercise (Figure 1.11d), which eigenvalue has the larger magnitude, k_1 or k_2? In other words, is the attraction stronger along E_1 or E_2? This can be somewhat counter intuitive, so let us think carefully about it. The two eigendirections collaborate to guide trajectories toward the equilibrium, by guiding them toward each other. Attraction along E_1 guides trajectories toward E_2. Similarly, attraction along E_2 guides trajectories toward E_1. The fact that trajectories swoop first toward E_2 tells us the attraction *toward E_2* is stronger than the attraction *along* E_2. In other words, E_1 is the stronger eigendirection, and k_1 has the larger magnitude.

Nodes have eigenvalues of the same sign. A stable node has two negative eigenvalues, corresponding to a flow organized by two attracting eigendirections. An unstable node is like a stable node running in reverse time: it has two positive eigenvalues, corresponding to a flow organized by two repelling eigendirections.

(1.11.15) Now, let us focus on our third equilibrium, the unstable spiral. Continuing with $\phi = 0.22$ and $I = 27$, return to the default window. Zoom into the unstable spiral, redraw the nullclines, and plot the direction field with a 2×2 grid so the phase plane is not too densely filled. Zoom in again. The flow looks the same as you keep zooming in (see Figure 1.11e), but there are no eigendirections!

Spiral equilibria have complex eigenvalues. Spiraling flow is incompatible with straight lines. Nevertheless, there are still eigenvalues associated with spiraling into, or out of, an equilibrium, and the intuition we developed with straight lines can still help. The eigenvalues for a spiraling equilibrium are complex numbers, of the form $\alpha + i\beta$, where $i = \sqrt{-1}$. We call α the *real part* of the complex number, and β the *imaginary part*. Moreover, the eigenvalues for a spiral equilibrium are closely related: if $k_1 = \alpha + i\beta$, then $k_2 = \alpha - i\beta$ (that is, the eigenvalues form a *complex conjugate pair*). The real part of the eigenvalues matches our straight line intuition, and tells us about the attraction or repulsion of the equilibrium. If $\alpha < 0$, the equilibrium attracts, and the trajectories spiral inward. If $\alpha > 0$, the equilibrium repels, and the trajectories spiral outward. The imaginary part of the eigenvalues tells us about the rate of rotation around the equilibrium as the trajectory spirals in or out. If you have not thought about complex numbers recently (or ever), you can read about them on the web, or in an introductory textbook on differential equations, such as Blanchard *et al.* (2011). The essential message, for our immediate purposes, is that the real part of the eigenvalues tells us about the stability of the equilibrium.

(1.11.16) Equilibrium points are also called *singular points*. The *(S)ing pts* menu in XPP is worth exploring. Let us try it on the unstable spiral. Return to the default window, click on *(S)ing pts, (M)ouse*. A tiny window will open, instructing you to click where you guess there is a singular point. Click near the unstable spiral. A new tiny window will open asking whether to print eigenvalues. Choose *(Y)es*. Three things happen simultaneously:

- A square appears in the phase plane, marking the unstable spiral.

- The eigenvalues are printed in the XPP console window. Confirm that they are of the form $\alpha + i\beta$ and $\alpha - i\beta$ (approximately $0.016 \pm i0.036$).
- Another small window opens, titled "Equilibria." At the top of this window, we are told this equilibrium is *Unstable*. The middle of the window tells us the stability-relevant properties of the eigenvalues. For example, $c+ = 2$ tells us there are two complex eigenvalues with positive real part, so we know the equilibrium is an unstable spiral. Note that r stands for real eigenvalues (with imaginary part $\beta = 0$) and *im* stands for purely imaginary eigenvalues (with real part $\alpha = 0$). The bottom of the window shows the V, W coordinates of the equilibrium.

(1.11.17) We are currently using the homoclinic parameter set. Recall from the bifurcation diagram in Figure 1.9a that there is a Hopf bifurcation around $I = 37.2$. Before the bifurcation, the equilibrium is an unstable spiral (as in the previous exercise), so has eigenvalues with positive real part. After the bifurcation the equilibrium is a *stable* spiral, so the eigenvalues have negative real part. How does the transition from positive to negative real parts happen? To see how this works, set up a slider for I ranging from 27 to 40, and use the *(S)ing pts* menu to print the eigenvalues for different values of I as you cross the bifurcation. For example, try $I = 32$, $I = 35$, $I = 36$, $I = 37$, $I = 37.1$, $I = 37.2$, $I = 38$, $I = 39$, and $I = 40$. As you vary I through the Hopf bifurcation, the complex parts of the eigenvalues do not change much, but the real parts of the eigenvalues get smaller and smaller in magnitude until they pass through zero as they change from positive (unstable spiral) to negative (stable spiral).

At a Hopf bifurcation, the equilibrium has purely imaginary eigenvalues. In other words, the real part of the eigenvalues is zero. This is a powerful statement. Indeed, it is how we define the bifurcation. When the real part of the eigenvalues passes through zero, the equilibrium changes stability. If we can compute eigenvalues, we can locate the bifurcation.

Calculating eigenvalues. In this tutorial, we use XPP to compute eigenvalues. Most introductory texts in differential equations, dynamical systems or mathematical biology describe how to calculate eigenvalues directly from a model's differential equations. For example, see Blanchard *et al.* (2011), Edelstein-Keshet (2005), Ellner and Guckenheimer (2006), Hirsch *et al.* (2012), and Strogatz (1994). It is a two-step process. The first step is *linearization*: using calculus to find the best linear approximation to the non-linear system, close to the equilibrium of interest. In other words, formalizing our process of zooming-in to each equilibrium. The second step is to calculate the eigenvalues of the linearization, using matrix algebra. For two-dimensional systems, it is a fairly straightforward process, and eigenvalues can often be calculated by hand. For models with more variables, we are more likely to use the computer.

(1.11.18) Reset $I = 27$, and try the *(S)ing pts* menu on the saddle. Confirm that

- The saddle is marked with a triangle in the phase plane.
- The eigenvalues (shown in the console window) are real numbers with opposite signs, as expected.
- The "Equilibria" window tells us this is an unstable equilibrium with one positive real eigenvalue ($r+ = 1$), and one negative ($r- = 1$).

  Another tiny window opens for the saddle. XPP is offering to draw the *invariant sets*, meaning the stable and unstable manifolds of the saddle. Choose *(Y)es*. There are four branches to be drawn, and you need to click *escape* after each branch, to plot the next one. The unstable branches are drawn first, in "gold," taking their two different routes to the stable equilibrium. Next come the stable branches, one emerging from the unstable spiral, the other coming from below. (Note that, in truth, the four branches meet at the saddle, but in practice XPP plots them slightly offset.)

(1.11.19) What will XPP tell you about the stable node? Try it. As expected, the eigenvalues are both negative. Recall from Exercise 1.11.14 that we know the stronger eigenvalue corresponds to the "strong" eigendirection, E_1 (so $k_1 = -0.588$), and the weaker eigenvalue corresponds to the "weak," roughly horizontal eigendirection, E_2 (so $k_2 = -0.074$). A tiny window opens offering to draw the *strong sets*. Choose *(Y)es*. This time there are two branches to be drawn (and you need to click *escape* after each one). The strong set of a stable node is composed of trajectories that approach the stable node directly along the strong eigendirection. (All the other trajectories approach the node along the weak eigendirection.)

(1.11.20) Recall from the bifurcation diagram in Figure 1.9a that the saddle and stable node coalesce and disappear in a saddle-node bifurcation around $I = 39.6$. How does an equilibrium whose eigenvalues have opposite signs coalesce with an equilibrium with two negative eigenvalues? Print the eigenvalues for the two equilibria for different values of I to see how this works. (It will go more quickly if you decline the offer to draw invariant sets and strong sets.) For example, try $I = 37$, $I = 38$, $I = 39$, $I = 39.3$, and $I = 39.5$. It may help to zoom into the region where the two equilibria coalesce. As the equilibria converge, their eigenvalues also converge. In particular, the positive eigenvalue of the saddle and the weak eigenvalue of the stable node each converge to zero.

Locating bifurcations At the saddle-node bifurcation, the equilibrium has one negative eigenvalue and one zero eigenvalue. Once again, this is a powerful statement. If we can compute the eigenvalues, we can locate the bifurcation. These ideas recur throughout the book. You will see many discussions of real eigenvalues passing through zero, or complex eigenvalues crossing the imaginary axis (meaning that the real parts pass through zero). They signal bifurcations, where interesting or surprising qualitative changes in behavior can be expected. See a dynamical systems text, such as Hirsch *et al.* (2012), Izhikevich (2007), or Strogatz (1994) for more information, and for the analogous concept of *Liapunov exponents* for characterizing the stability of limit cycles.

1.12 Perspectives

The subject of computational neuroendocrinology is young, and full of captivating open questions with important medical consequences. To mention just a few: What is the role of the diversity and irregularity of firing patterns observed in secretory neuroendocrine cells? Do they enable interplay between unscheduled perturbations (e.g., stressors in the adrenal corticosteroid system) and endogenous oscillatory rhythms (e.g., on circhoral or circadian scales)? More generally, how are time and space scales crossed from firing patterns to tissue level secretory networks and thence to axis level feedback loops? And how does the beautiful structure of interwoven networks of different cell types in the anterior pituitary contribute to endocrine decision making? It is an exciting area of study, requiring collaboration among neuroscientists, endocrinologists, and mathematical scientists.

This tutorial was designed to help empower that collaboration. Through the lens of the Morris–Lecar model, we have introduced concepts of electrical excitability, mathematical modeling, and dynamical systems. We focused on excitability because neuroscientists have a strong intuition for it, and its graphic spikes and bursts provide an enticing launch pad for mathematical analysis. We worked in two dimensions, because the geometry of the phase plane provides an excellent point of contact for experimentalists and theoreticians, harnessing the visual intuition to help translate between the disciplines.

The modeling and dynamical systems techniques developed are extremely versatile, applying across the neuroendocrine system and in higher dimensions, as shown in the chapters that follow. At the cellular level, Bertram *et al.* model the diverse mechanisms of channel gating found in secretory pituitary cells, and describe the hybrid biological/computational system of the dynamic clamp. Sherman describes how the interaction between membrane potential and calcium dynamics can produce bursting; Sneyd *et al.* present a detailed model of bursting in GnRH cells and MacGregor and Leng introduce random processes into a dynamical model of firing to understand phasic spiking patterns in vasopressin neurons. Increasing scale to the tissue level, Hodson *et al.* analyze the network structure of cells in the anterior pituitary, and Leng and Feng apply dynamical systems methods to a network of oxytocin cells. Increasing scale again, to the level of whole endocrine axes, Terry *et al.* model feedforward and feedback systems of the stress axis, and Clement and Vidal model the dynamics of GnRH secretion in the female reproductive axis. Increasing scale to the planetary level, the dynamics of excitability are even finding important applications in climate science (Crucifix, 2012).

Acknowledgement

We are grateful to Bowdoin College (Faculty Leave Supplement and Porter Fellowship) and the National Science Foundation (DMS-0940243 and CCF-0832788) for their support of this work.

References

Bean BP (2007). The action potential in mammalian central neurons. *Nat Rev Neurosci.* **8**, 451–465.

Bertram R, Butte MJ, Kiemel T and Sherman A (1995). Topological and phenomenological classification of bursting oscillations. *Bull Math Biol.* **57**, 413–439.

Bertram R, Tabak J, Stojilkovic SS (2014), in press.

Blanchard P, Devaney RL and Hall GR (2011). *Differential Equations.* 4th ed. Brooks/Cole. [*Popular undergraduate text on differential equations and dynamical systems*].

Carrasquillo Y and Nerbonne JM (2014). Diverse regulatory mechanisms. *Neuroscientist* **20**, 104–111.

Coetzee WA, Amarillo Y, Chiu J, Chow A, Lau D, McCormack T, Morena H, Nadal MS, Ozaita A, Pountney D, Saganich M, Vega Saenz de Miera E and Rudy B (1999). Molecular diversity of K^+ channels. *Ann NY Acad Sci.* **868**, 233–285.

Crucifix M (2012). Oscillators and relaxation phenomena in Pleistocene climate theory *Phil Trans R Soc A* **370**, 1140–1165.

Dolphin AC (2009). Calcium channel diversity: multiple roles of calcium channel subunits. *Curr Opin Neurobiol.* **19**, 237–244.

Edelstein-Keshet L (2005). *Mathematical Models in Biology.* Classics in Applied Mathematics, SIAM.

Ellner SP and Guckenheimer J (2006). *Dynamic Models in Biology.* Princeton University Press. Supplementary materials available at http://press.princeton.edu/titles/8124.html.

Ermentrout GB, XPP (2012 or current version) available at http://www.math.pitt.edu/bard/xpp/xpp.html. [*Dynamical systems software package used in the exercises*].

Ermentrout GB and Terman DH (2010). *Mathematical Foundations of Neuroscience.* Springer.

Fall CP, Marland ES, Wagner JM and Tyson JJ (2005). *Computational Cell Biology.* Springer.

Fatt P and Katz B (1953). The electrical properties of crustacean muscle fibres. *J Physiol.* **120**, 171–204.

Fitzhugh R (1961). Impulses and physiological states in theoretical models of nerve membrane. *Biophys J.* **1**, 445–466.

Golubitsky M, Josic K and Kaper TJ (2001). An unfolding theory approach to bursting in fast-slow systems. In *Global Analysis of Dynamical Systems: Festschrift Dedicated to Floris Takens* (eds. Broer HW, Krauskopf B and Vegter G), Chapter 10, pp. 277–308. IOP Publishing Ltd.

González C, Baez-Nieto D, Valencia I, Oyarzún I, Rojas P, Naranjo D and Latorre R (2012). K^+ channels: function-structural overview. *Compr Physiol.* **2**, 2087–2149.

Hille B (2001). *Ion Channels of Excitable Membranes.* 3rd edn. Sinauer Associates, Inc. [*Basic electrophysiology and ion channel biology*].

Hirsch MW, Smale S and Devaney RL (2012). *Differential Equations, Dynamical Systems, and an Introduction to Chaos.* Academic Press.

Hodgkin AL (1948). The local electric changes associated with repetitive action in a non-medullated axon. *J Physiol.* **107**, 165–181.

Hodgkin AL and Huxley AF (1952). A quantitative description of membrane current and its application to conduction and excitation in nerve. *J Physiol.* **117**, 500–544.

Izhikevich EM (2007). *Dynamical Systems in Neuroscience: The Geometry of Excitability and Bursting.* MIT Press, Cambridge, MA. [*Popular introduction to modeling and dynamical systems in neuroscience*].

Jan LY and Jan YN (2012). Voltage-gated potassium channels and the diversity of electrical signalling. *J Physiol.* **590**, 2591–2599.

Jegla TJ, Zmasek CM, Batalov S and Nayak SK (2009). Evolution of the human ion channel set. *Com. Chem. High T. Scr.* **12**, 2–23.

Jones CKRT (1995). Geometric singular perturbation theory, In *Dynamical systems (Montecatini Terme, 1994) Lecture Notes in Mathematics, vol 1609.* (eds. Dold A and Takens G), pp. 44–118. Springer.

Keener J and Sneyd J (2008). *Mathematical Physiology: I: Cellular Physiology.* Springer.

Keynes RD, Rojas E, Taylor RE and Vergara J (1973). Calcium and potassium systems of a giant barnacle muscle fibre under membrane potential control. *J Physiol.* **229**, 409–455.

King JT, Lovell P, Rishniw M, Kotlikoff MI, Zeeman ML and McCobb DP (2006). $\beta2$ and $\beta4$ Subunits of BK channels confer differential sensitivity to acute modulation by Steroid hormones. *J Neurophysiol.* **95**, 2878–2888.

Koch C (1999). *Biophysics of Computation: Information Processing in Single Neurons.* Oxford University Press.

Liang Z, Chen L and McClafferty H (2011). Control of hypothalamic-pituitary-adrenal stress axis activity by the intermediate conductance calcium-activated potassium channel, SK4. *J Physiol.* **589**, 5965–5986.

Lipscombe D, Andrade A and Allen SE (2013). Alternative splicing: functional diversity among voltage-gated calcium channels and behavioral consequences. *Biochim Biophys Acta* **1828**, 1522–1529.

Lovell PV, James DG and McCobb DP (2000). Bovine versus rat adrenal chromaffin cells: big differences in BK potassium channel properties. *J Neurophysiol.* **83**, 3277–3286.

Lovell P V, King JT and McCobb DP (2004). Acute modulation of adrenal chromaffin cell BK channel gating and cell excitability by glucocorticoids. *J Neurophysiol.* **91**, 561–570.

Lovell PV and McCobb DP (2001). Pituitary control of BK potassium channel function and intrinsic firing properties of adrenal chromaffin cells. *J Neurosci.* **21**, 3429–3442.

Morris C and Lecar H (1981). Voltage oscillations in the barnacle giant muscle fiber. *Biophys J.* **35**, 193–213. [*Original description of the Morris–Lecar model*].

Nagumo J, Arimoto S, and Yoshizawa S (1962). An active pulse transmission line simulating nerve axon. *Proc IRE* **50**, 2061–2070.

Pongs O and Schwarz JR (2010). Ancillary subunits associated with voltage-dependent K+ channels. *Physiol Rev.* **90**, 755–796.

Rinzel J and Ermentrout GB (1989). Analysis of neural excitability and oscillations. In *Methods in Neuronal Modeling* (eds. Koch C and Segev I), pp. 251–291. MIT Press, Cambridge, MA. [*Seminal paper on bifurcations in the Morris–Lecar model on which this tutorial is based.*]

Sherman A (2011). Dynamical systems theory in physiology. *J Gen Physiol.* **138**, 13–19.

Stojilkovic SS, Tabak J and Bertram R (2010). Ion channels and signaling in the pituitary gland. *Endocr Rev.* **31**, 845–915.

Strogatz SH (1994). *Nonlinear Dynamics and Chaos: With Applications to Physics, Biology, Chemistry, and Engineering.* Perseus Books Publishing, LLC. [*Popular text on dynamical systems with applications across the sciences.*]

Tian L and Shipston MJ (2000). Characterization of hyperpolarization-activated cation currents in mouse anterior pituitary, AtT20 D16:16 corticotropes. *Endocrinology* **141**, 2930–2937.

Vacher H and Trimmer JS (2011). Diverse roles for auxiliary subunits in phosphorylation-dependent regulation of mammalian brain voltage-gated potassium channels. *Pflugers Arch.* **462**, 631–643.

Xu K, Terakawa S (1999). Fenestration nodes and the wide submyelinic space form the basis for the unusually fast impulse conduction of shrimp myelinated axons. *J Exp Biol.* **202**, 1979–1989.

Zakon HH (2012). Adaptive evolution of voltage-gated sodium channels: the first 800 million years. *Proc Natl Acad Sci – USA* **109** Suppl, 10619–10625.

Zeeman EC (1977). *Catastrophe Theory: Selected Papers, 1972–1977.* Addison-Wesley.

CHAPTER 2

Ion Channels and Electrical Activity in Pituitary Cells: A Modeling Perspective

Richard Bertram[1], Joël Tabak[1] and Stanko S. Stojilkovic[2]

[1] Department of Mathematics and Program in Neuroscience, Florida State University, Tallahassee, FL, USA
[2] Section on Cellular Signaling, National Institute of Child Health and Human Development, National Institutes of Health, Bethesda, MD, USA

2.1   Endocrine pituitary cells are electrically active

In 1975, Kidokoro showed that endocrine cells of the anterior pituitary were electrically excitable, producing action potentials like neurons do (Kidokoro, 1975). But why are pituitary cells excitable (Mollard and Schlegel, 1996)? Their role is to synthesize and secrete hormones in certain physiological conditions, with a time scale of minutes to hours (Stojilkovic *et al.*, 2010). Thus, there is no need for fast action potentials that can transmit information on a millisecond time scale. Kidokoro and colleagues quickly realized that pituitary action potentials, which are wider than neuronal action potentials, are largely mediated by the influx of Ca^{2+} ions, with Na^+ ions playing a minor role (Kidokoro, 1975). Such action potentials act as Ca^{2+} pulses to trigger Ca^{2+}-dependent hormone secretion and other cellular processes (Stojilkovic, 2006).

The many types of ion channels present in the pituitary cell membranes regulate electrical excitability and determine whether a cell is silent, generates action potentials or bursts (Stojilkovic *et al.*, 2010). Figure 2.1 shows several examples of spontaneous electrical activity in three types of endocrine pituitary cells. The recordings from somatotrophs and lactotrophs illustrate the fast bursting often seen in these cells. Occasionally, bursts consist of large spikes emanating from a depolarized plateau (top panel in Figure 2.1b). This is called *plateau bursting*. More often, the bursts have much smaller spikes (Figure 2.1a and lower three panels of Figure 2.1b). This is often called *pseudo-plateau bursting* (Stern *et al.*, 2008; Teka *et al.*, 2011). Gonadotrophs typically do not burst spontaneously,

Computational Neuroendocrinology, First Edition. Edited by Duncan J. MacGregor and Gareth Leng.
© 2016 John Wiley & Sons, Ltd. Published 2016 by John Wiley & Sons, Ltd.
Companion Website: www.wiley.com/go/Leng/Computational

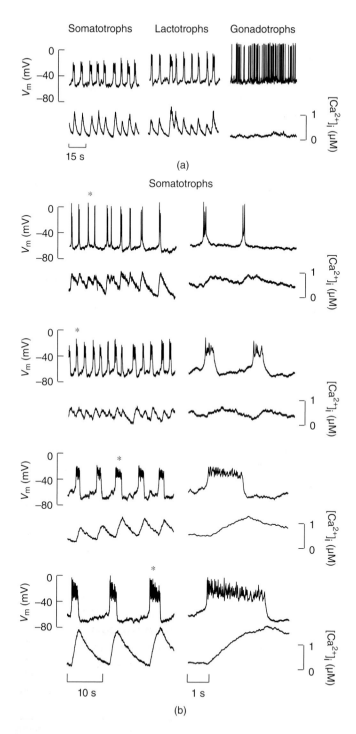

Figure 2.1 **Spontaneous activity in pituitary cells**. (a) Simultaneous measurements of membrane potential (V_m) and the intracellular Ca^{2+} concentration ($[Ca^{2+}]_i$) in pituitary somatotrophs, lactotrophs, and gonadotrophs. (b) Left: Variations in patterns of spontaneous electrical activity and associated $[Ca^{2+}]_i$ transients in somatotrophs from the same preparation. Right: Expanded time scales, showing selected bursts labeled with asterisks on left.

but instead produce action potentials with higher amplitude than those produced during bursting (Figure 2.1a). Although the gonadotroph action potentials are taller, they are also much narrower, so much less Ca^{2+} enters the cell with tonic action potentials than with bursts (Van Goor *et al.*, 2001a). This is clearly seen with measurements of intracellular Ca^{2+} concentration (Figure 2.1). Electrical excitability provides a versatile way to control pituitary output: hypothalamic and pituitary factors as well as steroid hormones can modulate Ca^{2+} influx in many ways by altering the electrical activity (Hodson *et al.*, 2012; Stojilkovic, 2012).

2.2   Endocrine pituitary cell types

The pituitary gland is composed of two embryonically, anatomically, and functionally distinct entities: the neurohypophysis or posterior pituitary and the *adenohypophysis,* composed of intermediate and anterior pituitary lobes. The adenohypophysis is populated with three groups of secretory (endocrine) cell types: pro-opiomelanocortin-producing cells, growth hormone (GH)/prolactin-producing cells, and heterodimeric glucoprotein-producing cells. All pituitary cell types are modulated by gonadal steroid hormones and agonists for ligand receptor channels and G protein-coupled receptors in a cell-specific manner.

The pro-opiomelanocortin gene is highly expressed in *melanotrophs* and *corticotrophs*. *Melanotrophs* are located in the intermediate lobe where they represent about 95% of endocrine cells. *Corticotrophs* are derived from the intermediate pituitary, but in adult animals these cells are scattered throughout the anterior lobe and make up 10%–15% of endocrine anterior pituitary endocrine cells. Both cell types are electrically excitable, but spontaneous action potentials are sufficient to trigger the release of pro-opiomelanocortin-derived peptides only in *melanotrophs*. *Melanotrophs* are regulated through the actions of dopamine, γ-aminobutyric acid (GABA), prostaglandin E2 and 5-hydroxytryptamine (Vazquez-Martinez *et al.*, 2003). *Corticotrophs* are primarily regulated through the action of corticotropin-releasing hormone, but also by urocortin 1–3 (a corticotropin-releasing hormone family of peptides) and arginine vasopressin (Aguilera *et al.*, 2004).

Lactotrophs account for 10%–25% of the endocrine cells located in the anterior lobe. Spontaneous electrical activity in these cells is sufficient to trigger prolactin secretion. The predominant hypothalamic influence is inhibitory and is mediated by dopamine (Freeman *et al.*, 2000). The sister cells, *somatotrophs*, represent up to 50% of all pituitary endocrine cells, and they are controlled by two hypothalamic neuropeptides: growth hormone-releasing hormone (GHRH), which stimulates GH release, and somatostatin, which inhibits GH release (DeAlmeida and Mayo, 2001; Patel *et al.*, 1996).

Gonadotrophs and *thyrotrophs* express the 92 amino acid α-glucoprotein hormone α-subunit, which is needed for the formation of follicle-stimulating hormone, luteinizing hormone, and thyroid-stimulating hormone with hormone-specific beta subunits. *Gonadotrophs* constitute about 10%–15% of the endocrine anterior pituitary cell population, while thyrotrophs constitute less than 10% of cells in the gland (Pazos-Moura *et al.*, 2003). The decapeptide gonadotropin-releasing hormone is the main agonist for *gonadotrophs* and is secreted in a pulsatile manner by neurons that are dispersed within the mediobasal hypothalamus preoptic areas (Stojilkovic *et al.*, 1994). Hypothalamic control of thyrotrophs is mediated by thyrotropin-releasing hormone, by numerous autocrine and paracrine factors.

2.3   Voltage-gated ion channels

Voltage-gated channels have been classified into two major subgroups: a superfamily of more than 140 members of *voltage-gated cation channels* that share structural similarity and a small family of structurally different *voltage-gated chloride channels*. Voltage-gated cation channels include Na^+, Ca^{2+}, and K^+ channels, as well as numerous less selective channels. The majority of voltage-gated channels contain voltage sensors, charged transmembrane helices that sense the electrical field in the membrane and which drive conformation changes, leading to opening and closing of the gates near the mouth of the pore (Yu *et al.*, 2005).

2.3.1   Voltage-gated sodium channels

Voltage-gated Na^+ (Na_v) channels are the primary molecules responsible for the generation of the rising phase of APs in excitable cells. The key electrophysiological features of these channels are: voltage-dependent activation, rapid inactivation, and selective Na^+ conductance. Tetrodotoxin (TTX) is a highly selective blocker of most types of voltage-gated Na^+ channels (Catterall *et al.*, 2005). Pituitary cells express functional channels that are composed of TTX-sensitive and TTX-resistant components (Stojilkovic *et al.*, 2012).

A mathematical model of the TTX-sensitive Na^+ current is the product of a conductance and a driving force. The conductance has an activation factor and an inactivation factor. The current through that conductance is given by Ohm's law as

$$I_{Na} = g_{Na} m_{Na} h_{Na} (V - V_{Na}) \tag{2.1}$$

where the *Nernst potential*, $V_{Na} = 50$ mV in our model, is such that the current is depolarizing. The maximal conductance g_{Na} varies from cell to cell, since it is determined in part by the number of Na_v channel proteins that are expressed in the plasma membrane. It is much larger in *gonadotrophs* than in *lactotrophs* and *somatotrophs* (Van Goor et al., 2001b). The *activation variable* (m_{Na}) and *inactivation variable* (h_{Na}) change over time according to the differential equations

$$\frac{dm_{Na}}{dt} = \frac{m_{Na,\infty}(V) - m_{Na}}{\tau_{m_{Na}}(V)} \tag{2.2}$$

$$\frac{dh_{Na}}{dt} = \frac{h_{Na,\infty}(V) - h_{Na}}{\tau_{h_{Na}}(V)} \tag{2.3}$$

These equations come from the application of the *law of mass action* to a channel with independent activation and inactivation gates, each of which can be in an open or a closed state. The variable m_{Na} represents the fraction of channels with an open activation gate, and h_{Na} is the fraction with an open inactivation gate. All voltage-dependent activation and inactivation variables satisfy equations of this form, and are thus said to satisfy first-order kinetics.

The steady-state activation and inactivation functions are Boltzmann functions, which have the form

$$x_\infty(V) = \frac{1}{1 + \exp\,[(v_x - V)/s_x]} \tag{2.4}$$

The parameter v_x sets the voltage at which the function is half-maximal (equal to $1/2$). The parameter s_x sets the slope of the function; smaller values give the curve a more step-like appearance. The sign of s_x is typically positive for an activation function (increasing with voltage) and negative for an inactivation function (decreasing with voltage). The v_x and s_x parameters are called *shape parameters* since they control the shape of the activation/inactivation function. The Na_v activation and inactivation functions are plotted in Figure 2.2. At the resting potential, the channel is deactivated ($m_{Na,\infty} \approx 0$), so the current does not contribute to the resting potential. In addition, the current is largely inactivated ($h_{Na,\infty} \approx 0.3$), so even if the cell becomes depolarized, the I_{Na} current will not contribute much to the membrane potential. For *lactotrophs* and *somatotrophs*, where the maximal conductance g_{Na} is also small, the current plays little role in the cell's electrical activity.

2.3.2 Voltage-gated calcium channels

Voltage-gated Ca^{2+} (Ca_v) channels are key sources of Ca^{2+} entry into the cytosol in excitable cells. Based on their biophysical profiles, Ca^{2+} channels are separated into two groups. The first group of channels is known as

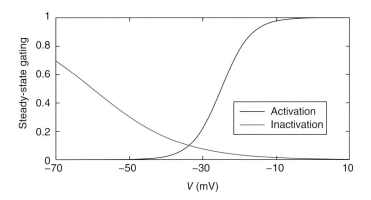

Figure 2.2   Gating properties of Na$_V$ channels. Steady-state activation function ($m_{\mathrm{Na},\infty}(V)$) and inactivation function ($h_{\mathrm{Na},\infty}(V)$) for the TTX-sensitive Na$^+$ current. Shape parameters are $v_{m,\,\mathrm{Na}} = -25$ mV, $s_{m,\,\mathrm{Na}} = 4$ mV, $v_{h,\,\mathrm{Na}} = -60$ mV, and $s_{h,\,\mathrm{Na}} = -12$ mV.

the *high-voltage activated* Ca^{2+} *channels*, because these require moderate to strong membrane depolarization to open. Among this group, biophysical and pharmacological studies have identified the *dihydropyridine*-sensitive L-type (Ca$_V$1.1, 1.2 and 1.3) and dihydropyridine-insensitive N-type (Ca$_V$2.1), P/Q-type (Ca$_V$2.2), and R-type (Ca$_V$2.3) channels, which are distinguished by their single-channel conductance, pharmacology, and metabolic regulation. The second group is known as the *low-voltage activated channels* (Ca$_V$3.1, 3.2, and 3.3), or T-type channels, because they require less depolarization for their activation and their subsequent inactivation and a strong membrane hyperpolarization to bring them out of their steady inactivation (Catterall, 2000). Both L- and T-type Ca$_V$ channels are expressed in pituitary cells (Stojilkovic *et al.*, 2012).

A model for current through L-type Ca$_V$ channels includes only channel activation, although inactivation can occur on a slow time scale of seconds. The current is modeled as

$$I_{\mathrm{CaL}} = g_{\mathrm{CaL}} m (V - V_{\mathrm{Ca}}) \qquad (2.5)$$

where the Ca^{2+} *Nernst potential* used in the model is $V_{\mathrm{Ca}} = 60$ mV. The *activation variable* m has first-order kinetics and the time constant τ_m is voltage dependent and small, with a value of a few milliseconds over a large voltage range. In practice, one often assumes that activation is instantaneous, and replaces the current with

$$I_{\mathrm{CaL}} = g_{\mathrm{CaL}} m_\infty(V)(V - V_{\mathrm{Ca}}) \qquad (2.6)$$

The advantage of using this *rapid equilibrium approximation* is that one differential equation, for m, is removed. The steady-state activation Boltzmann

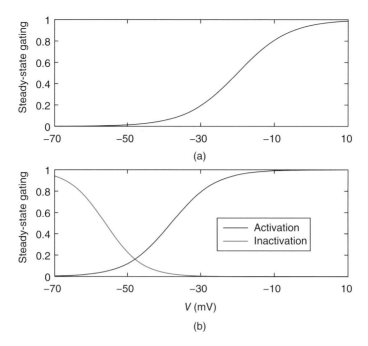

Figure 2.3 Gating properties of Ca$_V$ channels. (a) Steady-state activation function $(m_\infty(V))$ for the L-type Ca^{2+} current. Shape parameters are $v_m = -20$ mV and $s_m = 7$ mV. (b) Steady-state activation ($m_{T,\infty}(V)$, black) and inactivation ($h_{T,\infty}(V)$, red) functions for the T-type Ca^{2+} current. Shape parameters are $v_{mt} = -38$ mV, $s_{mt} = 6$ mV, $v_{ht} = -56$ mV, and $s_{ht} = -5$ mV.

function is shown in Figure 2.3a, with shape parameters given in the figure caption. Notice that this current is not activated at the resting potential, but begins to activate when the cell is depolarized to -40 mV or higher.

A model for the transient T-type Ca$_V$ current has both activation and inactivation factors. The activation is much faster than the inactivation, so we again use the *rapid equilibrium approximation* to remove the differential equation for the *activation variable*. The resulting expression is

$$I_{\mathrm{CaT}} = g_{\mathrm{CaT}} m_{T,\infty}(V) h_T (V - V_{\mathrm{Ca}}) \tag{2.7}$$

and the *inactivation variable* has first-order kinetics. The time constant τ_h would most accurately be described as a function of voltage, but the essential dynamics are not affected by treating it as a constant (10 ms), as we do here. Removing nonessential complexities facilitates the understanding of the system, and is an approach we typically take.

The steady-state activation and inactivation functions for the model T-type Ca$_V$ current are shown in Figure 2.3b. The activation curve is left-shifted compared with that for L-type Ca$_V$ channels. In fact, there is a window near the resting potential of the cell where this current is partially activated and not totally inactivated (between −60 and −40 mV in the model), so the current can depolarize the cell away from rest and toward the spike threshold.

2.3.3   Voltage-gated potassium channels

Voltage-gated K^+ (K_v) channels are widely expressed in excitable cells and play a critical role in membrane hyperpolarization during an action potential as well as in the propagation of action potentials. Electrophysiological studies have revealed that at least four functional classes of K^+ channels exist: fast or *rapidly activating delayed rectifier, slow delayed rectifier* (including M channels), A-type K^+ channels and the *ether-a-go-go-gene*-related (ERG) channels. The fast delayed rectifier is usually responsible for very short action potentials. Slow delayed rectifier channels are also involved in cell repolarization and, as indicated by their names, the gating kinetics of these channels is slow and the channels are noninactivating. A-type channels show rapid activation in the subthreshold range of membrane potential, fast inactivation and fast recovery from inactivation, and these channels contribute to the regulation of firing frequency in excitable cells (Hille, 2001). All four functional classes of K_v channels are expressed in endocrine pituitary cells (Stojilkovic *et al.*, 2010).

A model for the current through rapidly activating delayed rectifier K_v channels (M channels are not discussed further) accounts for voltage-dependent activation and no inactivation. The *rapid equilibrium* approximation is not used since the activation process is slow compared to Ca_v channel activation and this is crucial to the role of the current in action potential generation. The model current is

$$I_{K(dr)} = g_{K(dr)} n(V - V_K) \qquad (2.8)$$

where the *Nernst potential* is very negative ($V_K = -75$ mV in the model). The *activation variable* has first-order kinetics, and we use $\tau_n = 30$ ms. The steady-state activation function is shown in Figure 2.4a. Note that it is right shifted relative to the Ca_v channel activation functions. This and the slower activation rate slow down the negative feedback provided by this current; delayed negative feedback is an important element in the generation of an action potential.

Like the T-type Ca_v current, the A-type K^+ current has fast activation, slower inactivation, and a window for which the current is partially activated and not entirely inactivated at steady state. However, there are some important differences between those two currents. First, the A-type current is hyperpolarizing, while the T-type current is depolarizing. Second, the steady-state activation window is right shifted for A-type versus T-type,

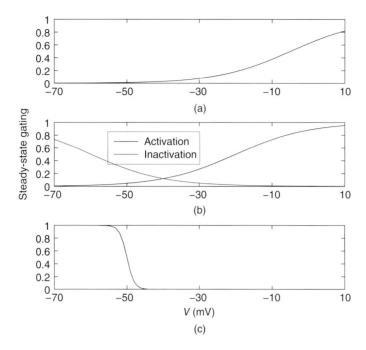

Figure 2.4   Gating properties of K_v channels. (a) Steady-state activation function $(n_\infty(V))$ for the delayed rectifier K^+ current. Shape parameters are $v_n = -5$ mV and $s_n = 10$ mV. (b) Steady-state activation $(a_\infty(V)$, black) and inactivation $(e_\infty(V)$, red) functions for the A-type K^+ current. Shape parameters are $v_a = -20$ mV, $s_a = 10$ mV, $v_e = -60$ mV, and $s_e = -10$ mV. (c) Steady-state activation function $(r_\infty(V))$ for the inward rectifying K^+ current. Shape parameters are $v_r = -50$ mV and $s_r = -1$ mV.

so that the current plays little role in setting the rest potential. Instead, it is important in modulating action potential frequency. The model for the current is

$$I_A = g_A a_\infty(V)e(V - V_K) \qquad (2.9)$$

where *rapid equilibrium* is used for the activation, and the *inactivation variable* has first-order kinetics with $\tau_e = 20$ ms. The activation and inactivation functions are shown in Figure 2.4b.

2.3.4   Inwardly rectifying potassium channels

Inwardly rectifying potassium (K_{ir}) channels produce an inward current under hyperpolarization, leading to K^+ influx, with little K^+ efflux under depolarization. Although the amplitude of the outward currents flowing through these channels is limited, they profoundly influence the resting membrane potential. There are 15 members of this family of channels that can be classified into three groups, based on their regulation patterns. Some of these channels are constitutively active at rest, leading to K^+

leaking from cells, whereas the activity of others is influenced by certain modulators, such as G proteins and nucleotides. The long cytoplasmic pore of these channels plays a critical role for inward rectification, and it provides the structural basis for the modulation of gating by G proteins and phosphatidylinositol 4,5 bisphosphate (Stanfield et al., 2002). The mRNA transcripts for numerous K_{ir} channels were identified in anterior pituitary cells. Functional studies have also indicated the presence of the constitutively active K_{ir}-like channels and *G protein-regulated* K_{ir} *channels* (Stojilkovic et al., 2010).

A model for the K_{ir} current is

$$I_{K_{ir}} = g_{K_{ir}} r_\infty(V)(V - V_K)$$ (2.10)

where *rapid equilibrium* is assumed for the activation. The activation function, shown in Figure 2.4c, drops rapidly from 1 (fully activated) to 0 (fully deactivated) near the rest potential.

2.4 Nonselective cation channels

The majority of transient receptor potential (TRP) channels are relatively nonselective cation-conducting channels. Six protein families comprise the mammalian TRP superfamily: the 'canonical' receptors (TRPCs), the vanilloid receptors, the melastatin receptors, the polysistins, the mucolpins, and the ankyril transmembrane protein 1 (Clapham et al., 2005). The mRNA transcripts for TRPC1, TRPC3, TRPC4, TRPC5, and TRPC7 have been identified in pituitary cells. The presence of these channels in endocrine pituitary cells was indicated pharmacologically, and they may contribute to the excitability of these cells (Tomic et al., 2011).

We model the current through nonselective cation channels as a constant-conductance current with a reversal potential between K^+ and Na^+. We use $V_{NS} = -20$ mV.

2.5 Ligand-gated ion channels

Many types of ion channels respond to chemical signals (ligands) rather than (or in addition to) changes in the membrane potential and they are called ligand-gated ion channels. The largest group of these channels is activated by neurotransmitters (Collingridge et al., 2009). Endocrine pituitary cells express these channels, including GABA-gated channels and ATP-gated P2X channels, and their role in the excitability of pituitary cells is discussed elsewhere (Stojilkovic et al., 2010). *Intracellular ligand-gated channels* have an intracellular ligand-binding domain and interact with intracellular messengers, such as Ca^{2+} and cyclic nucleotides. Pituitary cells express Ca^{2+}-activated K^+ channels (Van Goor *et al.*, 2001a,b) and hyperpolarization-activated cyclic nucleotide-gated channels (Kretschmannova *et al.*, 2012), both located at the plasma membrane. The main function of these channels is to convert Ca^{2+} and cyclic nucleotide signaling into electrical information. Other intracellular ligand-gated channels are located in intracellular membranes, such as the endoplasmic reticulum (ER). Pituitary cells express inositol trisphosphate (IP_3) receptor channels, which are selectively permeable to Ca^{2+}. In excitable cells, including pituitary cells, Ca^{2+} release from the ER has a profound effect on excitability (see Chapter 3).

2.5.1 Calcium-controlled potassium channels

Calcium-controlled potassium (K_{Ca}) channels are composed of two distinct families. One family includes three *small-conductance (SK) channels* (K_{Ca}2.1, 2.2 and 2.3) and the other includes one *intermediate-conductance (IK) channel* (K_{Ca}3.1). They are voltage-insensitive, and the rise in the intracellular Ca^{2+} concentration is critical for their activation. The other family consists of *high-conductance* K^+ *(BK) channels*. They are activated by voltage, and their open probability is modulated by Ca^{2+}. The BK channels, but not SK channels, form macromolecular complexes with Ca_V channels. This provides an effective mechanism for the control of the activity of these channels by Ca^{2+} influx through Ca_V channels (Wei *et al.*, 2005). Both SK and BK channels are present in endocrine pituitary cells (Van Goor *et al.*, 2001b).

A model for the SK- or IK-type current has a conductance that depends on the free Ca^{2+} concentration in the cytosol, rather than the voltage

$$I_{SK} = g_{SK}c_\infty(Ca)(V - V_K) \tag{2.11}$$

where Ca is the free cytosolic Ca^{2+} concentration. The activation is rapid, so the *rapid equilibrium* approximation is used, although the variable Ca changes slowly. The steady-state activation function is modeled as a second-order Hill function

$$c_\infty(Ca) = \frac{Ca^2}{Ca^2 + K_s^2} \tag{2.12}$$

where the value of Ca at which the function is half maximal is $K_s = 0.4$ μM. This is plotted in Figure 2.5a. At basal Ca levels (0.05 μM or less), there is little activation of the current. However, at the higher values of Ca which occur during bursting electrical activity (0.2 μM or more), the current is highly activated and can have a big impact on the cell's electrical activity.

Since BK-type K_{Ca} channels are co-localized with Ca^{2+} channels, they sense Ca^{2+} in nanodomains that form at the mouth of the open channel, and here the concentration is much higher than the bulk Ca^{2+} levels sensed

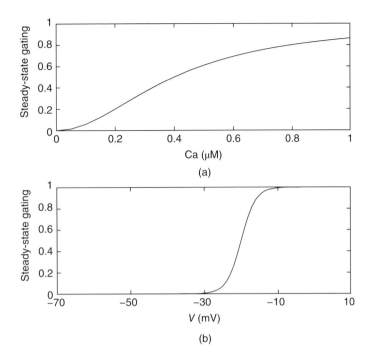

Figure 2.5   Gating properties of K_{Ca} channels. (a) Steady-state activation function $(c_\infty(Ca))$ for the SK-type or IK-type K^+ current. The shape parameter is $K_s = 0.4$ μM. (b) Steady-state activation function $(b_\infty(V))$ for the BK-type K_{Ca} current. The shape parameters are $v_b = -20$ mV and $s_b = 2$ mV.

by more distant channels. Since these nanodomains form only when the Ca^{2+} channels are open and dissipate quickly when the channels close, and since Ca^{2+} channel kinetics depend on the membrane potential, the BK conductance can be modeled as a purely voltage-dependent process (Sherman *et al.*, 1990; Simon and Llinas, 1985). The current is then

$$I_{BK} = g_{BK}b(V - V_K) \tag{2.13}$$

where the *activation variable b* has first-order kinetics with $\tau_b = 5$ ms. The steady-state activation function is described by a Boltzmann function, and is shown in Figure 2.5b. Since this function is quite steep, the current activates only during action potentials, and it plays a role in "shaping" action potentials and in the fast bursting pattern that is characteristic of *lactotrophs* and *somatotrophs*.

2.5.2 Hyperpolarization-activated cyclic nucleotide-gated (HCN) channels

HCN channels open upon hyperpolarization and close at positive potentials. The cyclic nucleotides cAMP and cGMP bind to the channel and

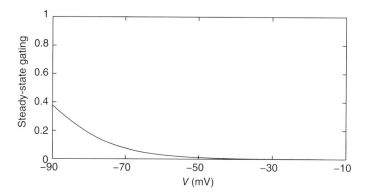

Figure 2.6 Gating properties of HCN channels. Steady-state activation function
$(h_\infty(V))$ for the h-current. The shape parameters are $v_h = -95$ mV and $s_h = -10$ mV.
Notice that the range of voltages shown here is different from that in previous figures,
since the current activates at very low voltages.

enhance its activity by shifting the activation curve of the channels to
more positive voltages. Activation of these channels leads to a slow
depolarization. HCN channels serve the following three principal functions
in excitable cells: (i) they contribute to the resting potential, (ii) they
generate or contribute to the pacemaker depolarization that controls the
rhythmic activity in spontaneously firing cells, and (iii) they compensate for inhibitory postsynaptic potentials (Robinson and Siegelbaum,
2003). Electrophysiological and pharmacological experiments confirmed
the presence of functional HCN channels in normal and immortalized
pituitary cells (Stojilkovic *et al.*, 2012).

Since HCN channels are nonselective, a model of the current through
the channels (called the h-current or I_h) uses a reversal potential ($V_{NS} =$
-20 mV) between that of K_v channels and that of Na_v channels:

$$I_h = g_h h(V - V_{NS}) \tag{2.14}$$

The steady-state activation function, shown in Figure 2.6, is very much like
that of the K_{ir} current, but is more left shifted. This current is only activated
at hyperpolarized voltages below the resting potential, unless the activation
curve is shifted rightward by the actions of cyclic nucleotides.

2.5.3 Inositol 1,4,5-trisphosphate (IP$_3$) receptor channels

These channels are composed of four similar subunits that are
noncovalently associated to form a four-leaf clover-like structure,
the center of which makes the Ca^{2+}-selective channel. Activation of
these Ca^{2+}-conducting channels is triggered by IP$_3$ and depends on the

intracellular Ca^{2+} concentration. There are three subtypes of IP_3 receptors, and further diversity of IP_3 receptor expression is created by alternative splicing. IP_3 receptors are commonly expressed in pituitary cells and are located on the ER membrane (Foskett *et al.*, 2007); they are activated in response to hormone activation of G-protein-coupled receptors (GPCRs) of the $G\alpha_q$ type, which is only briefly discussed in this chapter.

2.6 Spontaneous electrical activity and Ca^{2+} signalling

2.6.1 Channels contributing to the resting membrane potential

Experiments indicate that the K_{ir}-like channels contribute to the resting membrane potential in *lactotrophs, somatotrophs, corticotrophs,* and GH_3 cells (Stojilkovic, 2012). Recently, the contribution of TREK-1 (TWIK-related) channels to the resting membrane potential in *corticotrophs* was also suggested (Lee *et al.*, 2011). The finding that the resting membrane potential in endocrine pituitary cells is −50 to −60 mV suggests that, in addition to resting K^+ conductance, there is also a depolarizing conductance due to other ions. When extracellular Na^+ is substituted with large organic cations, the resting membrane potential rapidly reaches approximately −85 mV, suggesting that a Na^+-conducting channel has constitutive activity. The addition of TTX to inhibit all Na_V channels does not mimic the effect of the removal of bath Na^+. These and other data indicate that the constitutive activity of Na^+-conducting channels, termed background Na^+ channels (Sankaranarayanan and Simasko, 1996), contributes to the control of the resting membrane potential and may account for the pacemaking depolarization. Pharmacological experiments suggest that TRPC channels also contribute to the resting membrane potential (Tomic *et al.*, 2011).

2.6.2 Spontaneous spiking activity

Endocrine pituitary cells are spontaneously active independently of external stimuli. One form of spontaneous activity is a tonic spiking pattern. Here the action potentials are tall and narrow, with amplitudes of more than 60 mV (from initiation to peak), half-widths of less than 50 ms, and spiking frequencies of typically ~0.7 Hz. Despite being wider than neuronal action potentials, at these firing frequencies, pituitary action potentials generate a very limited increase in intracellular Ca^{2+}. Such a firing pattern is commonly observed in *gonadotrophs* (Figure 2.1a) and *thyrotrophs* and occasionally in other secretory cell types (Stojilkovic, 2006).

In most anterior pituitary cells, Ca_v channels give rise to action potentials in much the same way as Na_v channels in other excitable cells. The removal of extracellular Ca^{2+} and the addition of Ca_v channel blockers abolish electrical activity in the majority of endocrine pituitary cells without affecting the resting membrane potential, indicating that these channels are critical for spiking depolarization but not for the resting membrane potential (Stojilkovic *et al.*, 2010).

Spontaneous spiking can be achieved in a model cell that includes three elements: a depolarizing ionic current that is partially active at rest to bring the membrane potential above the spike threshold; a depolarizing current that is active at higher voltages and is regenerative, providing the positive feedback needed to produce the spike upstroke; and a hyperpolarizing current that activates more slowly, thereby providing the delayed negative feedback necessary for the action potential downstroke. This is demonstrated in Figure 2.7. In this simulation, the model contains the nonselective current I_{NS} (produced by a mix of background Na^+ and TRPC channels), an L-type Ca^{2+} current I_{CaL}, and a delayed rectifying K^+ current $I_{K(dr)}$. For the first 500 ms, the conductance of I_{CaL} is set to 0. The remaining

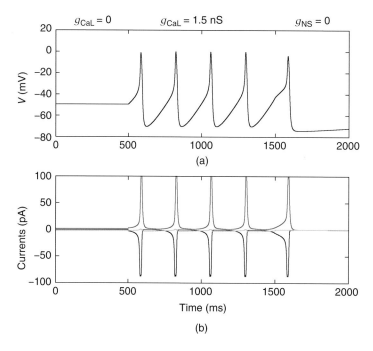

Figure 2.7 **Model cell simulation with three ionic currents:** I_{CaL}, $I_{K(dr)}$, and I_{NS}. (a) Voltage time course with I_{CaL} initially removed and then added at $t = 500$ ms. At $t = 1500$ ms, a nonselective current I_{NS} is removed. (b) Time-dependent changes in the ionic currents I_{CaL} (black), $I_{K(dr)}$ (red), and I_{NS} (green). Conductance values are $g_{CaL} = 1.5$ nS, $g_{K(dr)} = 10$ nS, and $g_{NS} = 0.06$ nS.

two currents combine to set the membrane potential near -50 mV. When g_{CaL} is increased to 1.5 nS, adding in the regenerative depolarizing current, the cell begins to fire action potentials. The three ionic currents are shown in the bottom panel. The current I_{CaL} is inward, and thus negative (black curve). The current $I_{K(dr)}$ is outward and positive (red curve). Both of these are very large compared with I_{NS}, which is inward when the voltage is low and outward when the voltage is high (green curve). Yet, this apparently insignificant current is actually crucial to the electrical activity, as we see when it is turned off at $t = 1500$ ms. Without this subthreshold current the membrane potential does not reach the spike threshold, so the model cell becomes quiescent and hyperpolarized. This demonstrates that even small ionic currents can be very important, particularly if they are active below the spike threshold.

2.6.3   Spontaneous bursting activity

The most common spontaneous pattern of activity in *lactotrophs* and *somatotrophs* is bursting, which consists of periodic depolarized potentials with superimposed small-amplitude spikes (Figure 2.1). The bursts have a much longer duration (several seconds) than gonadotroph action potentials, and the burst frequency is significantly lower (~ 0.3 Hz). The membrane potential rarely goes above -10 mV during a burst. The simplest explanation of why some cells exhibit a tonic spiking pattern, while others exhibit a bursting pattern could be that there is a cell-specific expression of channels. One channel type that has a greater expression level in *somatotrophs* and *lactotrophs* than in *gonadotrophs* is the BK type of K_{Ca} channels. These channels activate rapidly upon membrane depolarization, probably because they are co-localized with Ca_v channels. The BK current acts in conjunction with the delayed rectifying K^+ current to repolarize the cell membrane during the downstroke of an action potential. There is considerable evidence that BK channels are also a key element in the production of bursting, and that their greater expression in *somatotrophs/lactotrophs* is responsible for the different activity patterns of these cells versus *gonadotrophs*. The proximity of BK channels to Ca_v channels could be the major factor that determines the differential role of BK channels among endocrine pituitary cells. That is, K_{Ca} channels that are co-localized with Ca_v channels activate quickly and are gated by Ca^{2+} nanodomains, while those (either BK, IK, or SK types) relatively far from Ca_v channels activate more slowly by the accumulation of bulk free Ca^{2+} in the cytosol (Tsaneva-Atanasova *et al.*, 2007; Van Goor *et al.*, 2001a).

We use a model to illustrate the two spontaneous spiking patterns in Figure 2.8. For the first 3 s of simulation time, the spiking parameter set from Figure 2.7 is used. For the second half of the simulation, a parameter set is used that produces bursting. The main difference between

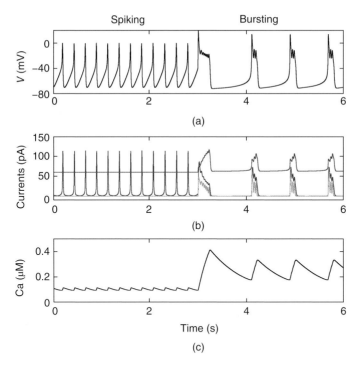

Figure 2.8 Spiking versus bursting. (a) Comparison of spontaneous spiking and bursting using the model cell with different parameter sets. The spiking parameter set is the same as that used in Figure 2.7, with the ionic currents I_{CaL}, $I_{K(dr)}$, and I_{NS}. The bursting parameter set includes two additional currents I_{SK} and I_{BK}. Parameter values for this set are $g_{CaL} = 2.5$ nS, $g_{K(dr)} = 3$ nS, $g_{NS} = 0.02$ nS, $g_{SK} = 2$ nS, $g_{BK} = 0.6$ nS, and $s_m = 10$ mV. (b) The three K$^+$ currents: $I_{K(dr)}$ (red), I_{BK} (brown), and I_{SK} (blue), which are translated up by 60 pA for clarity. (c) The free cytosolic Ca^{2+} concentration is much greater during bursting than during tonic spiking.

these parameter sets is the addition of SK and BK currents to the model. The bursting is clearly much slower, and the spikes emanating from the depolarized plateaus are much smaller than those produced during tonic spiking. The roles that the two K$_{Ca}$ currents play in the burst pattern are shown in the middle panel. The BK current (brown curve) activates quickly when the cell reaches the spike threshold, with a time course similar to $I_{K(dr)}$ (red curve). In contrast, the SK current (or equivalently, a BK current made up of channels located far from Ca$_v$ channels) builds up slowly during the burst (blue curve, translated up for clarity) and this buildup is ultimately responsible for the burst termination. Although the BK and delayed rectifying K$^+$ currents exhibit similar time courses, they have different contributions to bursting due to their different kinetics. BK channels promote bursting due to their rapid activation, while the delayed rectifying channels tend to inhibit bursting. If we increase the activation time constant of BK channels in the model, the BK current loses its burst promoting contribution and plays a role similar to that of the delayed rectifier (Tabak *et al.*, 2011, 2007; Van Goor *et al.*, 2001a).

Ca$_V$ channel activation is not only critical for firing of action potentials but also for intracellular Ca^{2+} and Ca^{2+}-controlled cellular processes, including hormone secretion. However, there is a major difference in Ca^{2+} influx in spiking and bursting cells. Ca$_V$ channels are open only briefly during a single action potential, and the elevated Ca^{2+} concentration is localized to nanodomains that form at the inner mouths of open Ca^{2+} channels. With the longer durations and smaller spike amplitudes during bursts, channels stay open longer and significant Ca^{2+} entry occurs, resulting in individual Ca^{2+} nanodomains overlapping and producing a global signal that can be easily resolved with fluorescent Ca^{2+} dyes. Simultaneous measurements of the membrane potential and cytosolic Ca^{2+} concentration showed that the bulk Ca^{2+} levels are low in spiking gonadotrophs (20–70 nM), while they are much higher (300–1200 nM) and clearly oscillatory in spontaneously bursting cells (Van Goor *et al.*, 2001a). Thus, the Ca^{2+} influx summed over time is much greater during bursting than during large-amplitude spiking. This is illustrated in the bottom panel of Figure 2.8. The variable shown here is the free bulk cytosolic Ca^{2+} concentration, which is computed from the differential equation

$$\frac{dCa}{dt} = -f(\alpha I_{Ca} + k_c Ca) \qquad (2.15)$$

where $f = 0.01$ is the fraction of cytosolic Ca^{2+} that is not bound to buffer, $\alpha = 0.0015$ μM fC^{-1} converts current to ion flux, $k_c = 0.12$ ms^{-1} is the pump rate of the plasma membrane Ca^{2+}-ATPases, and I_{Ca} is the sum of all Ca$_V$ currents (which in this case is just I_{CaL}). Calcium handling is described in more detail in Chapter 3.

2.6.4 Modulation of bursting by subthreshold channels

The model simulations of tonic spiking and bursting shown thus far have used only a few types of ionic currents, since only a few are needed for these behaviors. However, pituitary cells contain many channel types expressed at different levels. One advantage of a mathematical model is that it allows you to explore the different behaviors that your system can exhibit when components are added or subtracted. We have used this approach in Figures 2.7 and 2.8, and will use it further here to examine how three subthreshold currents, I_A, I_{CaT}, and I_{Kir} can influence the cytosolic Ca^{2+} level during bursting.

We examine first the impact of the A-type K$^+$ current (Toporikova *et al.*, 2008). Figure 2.9a shows the cytosolic Ca^{2+} concentration during 15 s of simulated bursting. For the first 5 s, there is no I_A, so the bursting and Ca^{2+}

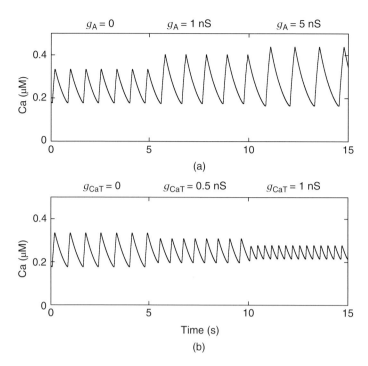

Figure 2.9   **The bursting model used in Figure 2.8 is augmented with different subthreshold currents**. (a) Addition of g_A slows down Ca^{2+} oscillations and increases the time-averaged mean Ca^{2+} level. (b) Addition of g_{CaT} speeds up Ca^{2+} oscillations and decreases the mean Ca^{2+} level.

oscillations are just as in Figure 2.8. For the next 5 s, the A-type conductance is increased to 1 nS, and for the last 5 s the conductance is increased further to 5 nS. These increases in conductance slow down the bursting, but make the duration of each burst active phase longer. The increased active phase duration results in an increase in the time-averaged Ca^{2+} level, but also an increase in the peak Ca^{2+} level, because Ca^{2+} accumulates during an active phase. Since hormone secretion may depend nonlinearly on the Ca^{2+} concentration, the increased peak could be more important than the increased mean level of Ca^{2+}. Figure 2.9b shows the effects of increasing the T-type Ca^{2+} conductance from 0 to 0.5 nS, to 1 nS. The first increase in conductance makes the bursts faster, with shorter active phases. This results in Ca^{2+} oscillations of smaller amplitude and a somewhat lower mean value. The second conductance increase converts the model cell to a tonic spiking state, further increasing frequency and further reducing the amplitude of the Ca^{2+} oscillations and the mean level of Ca^{2+}.

From these simulations (Figure 2.9), we see that the effects of subthreshold currents can be subtle and counterintuitive. Adding an A-type K^+ can slow down bursting, which is what one might expect from a hyperpolarizing current, but it also makes the oscillations larger, and increases the mean Ca^{2+} level, neither of which is expected *a priori* from the addition of a hyperpolarizing current. Addition of the low-threshold T-type Ca^{2+} current, a depolarizing current, speeds up bursting and slightly lowers the mean Ca^{2+} concentration. The reduction in mean Ca^{2+} is also counterintuitive. Finally, we saw in Figure 2.8 that the addition of two hyperpolarizing K^+ currents, I_{SK} and I_{BK}, can convert spiking to bursting and thereby increase the amplitude and mean level of Ca^{2+} oscillations, while the addition of a depolarizing T-type Ca^{2+} current does the opposite (Figure 2.9b). It appears, then, that ionic currents can have effects on the cell that are quite unexpected and hard to predict or understand without the aid of a model. Also, it is the mix and relative expression levels of channels that determine the electrical behavior and the resulting Ca^{2+} time course of the cell. For example, the expression level of T-type Ca^{2+} current is relatively high in *somatotrophs* (Van Goor *et al.*, 2001b). Taken alone, our simulations in Figure 2.9b suggest that this should bias the *somatotrophs* to a spontaneous tonic spiking pattern. However, they also have a higher level of the BK channel expression, which promotes bursting. This higher level of the BK channel expression likely explains why *somatotrophs* typically produce a spontaneous bursting pattern.

2.7 Modulation of spontaneous electrical activity by GPCRs

GPCRs are a very large and diverse superfamily of plasma membrane receptors that help define cellular responsiveness to extracellular signals. In excitable cells, this includes control of excitability and Ca^{2+} influx. GPCRs share a common structure of seven α-helix transmembrane domains with an extracellular N-terminus and an intracellular C-terminus, and are coupled to heterotrimeric *G proteins*, composed of α and $\beta\gamma$ subunits. Occupancy of receptors causes the dissociation of Gα-GTP from the G$\beta\gamma$-dimer, and these subunits function as transducers to relay information to different signaling pathways, which operate as amplifiers by producing intracellular messengers that carry information to intracellular sensors and effectors. Downstream effectors produce one or more actions, including membrane depolarization or hyperpolarization, activation and inactivation of voltage-gated channels and activation of Ca^{2+} release from the ER. Classically, *G proteins* are divided into four major families, based on their α-subunits: G_s, $G_{i/o}$, $G_{q/11}$, and $G_{12/13}$. GPCRs coupled to G_s stimulate and those coupled to $G_{i/o}$ inhibit adenylyl cyclases; the $G_{q/11}$-coupled receptors stimulate phospholipase C; and $G_{12/13}$ activates Rho proteins through Rho guanine-nucleotide exchange factors (Savarese and Fraser, 1992).

GPCRs modulate electrical activity directly through *G proteins* and indirectly through second messengers triggered by the activation of these receptors. Both pathways also contribute to the control of spontaneous electrical activity and Ca^{2+} signaling in endocrine pituitary cells. In this chapter, we focus our attention on the G_s and $G_{i/o}$ pathways, with only a short description of the G_q pathway. A key component of this latter pathway is the ER, which acts as an intracellular, high-capacity Ca^{2+} store. The handling of Ca^{2+} by the ER is discussed in Chapter 3.

2.7.1   Direct effects of G proteins on electrical activity

The $G_{i/o}$-coupled receptors are expressed in all endocrine pituitary cells. These are bound and activated by somatostatin in pituitary *somatotrophs*, where it inhibits electrical activity and the accompanied Ca^{2+} influx and GH secretion (Patel and Srikant, 1986). Dopamine acts as a principal inhibitory regulator of prolactin release by *lactotrophs* and of αMSH by *melanotrophs*; the dopamine D_2 subtype of receptors mediate the tonic inhibitory control of dopamine on hormone release by these cells (Missale *et al.*, 1998). Pituitary cells also express several other GPCRs linked to this signaling pathway, including receptors activated by adenosine, endothelins, GABA, melatonin, neuropeptide Y and 5-hydroxytryptamine (Stojilkovic *et al.*, 2010). Numerous observations indicate that the major inhibitory action of these receptors in pituitary cells is mediated directly by the *βγ*-dimers, rather than indirectly through cAMP or PKA, by altering the gating of inward rectifying K^+ channels and Ca_v channels.

The G-protein-regulated activation of K_{ir} channels has a well-established role in regulating electrical activity in pituitary cells. They are responsible for inhibition of activity and membrane hyperpolarization by somatostatin in *somatotrophs*, dopamine in *lactotrophs* and *melanotrophs*, and endothelins in *somatotrophs* and *lactotrophs*. The inhibitory actions of GABA via GABA$_B$ receptors are also mediated by K_{ir} channels (Stojilkovic *et al.*, 2010).

L-type Ca^{2+} channels are inhibited by a number of agents acting on receptors coupled to $G_{i/o}$. These include the inhibitory action of somatostatin on *somatotrophs* and AtT-20 cells, dopamine on *lactotrophs* and *melanotrophs*, neuropeptide Y on *melanotrophs*, and serotonin on *melanotrophs*. Serotonin also inhibits Q-type Ca^{2+} channels in *melanotrophs*. The activation of GABA$_B$ receptors also inhibits Ca^{2+} channels (Stojilkovic *et al.*, 2010).

2.7.2   Direct role of cAMP in electrical activity

cAMP is an intracellular messenger generated by adenylyl cyclase which regulates numerous cellular responses, including electrical activity and Ca^{2+} influx. There are nine plasma membrane isoforms of these enzymes, and the intrinsic activity of all adenylyl cyclase subtypes is upregulated by GPCRs linked to heterotrimeric G_s proteins through the α subunit (Willoughby and Cooper, 2007). GPCRs linked to the G_s-signaling pathways are operative in all endocrine pituitary cells. They are bound and activated by corticotropin-releasing hormone in *corticotrophs*, GHRH in *somatotrophs*, and vasoactive intestinal peptide and pituitary adenylyl cyclase-activating peptide (PACAP) in *somatotrophs*, *lactotrophs*, and *melanotrophs*. There is a great deal of data showing that the effect of G_s activation in pituitary cells is an increase of electrical activity, Ca^{2+} influx, and hormone secretion. What is not so clear is whether these actions are mediated through cAMP directly, indirectly through PKA activation, some combination of these, or by other signaling pathways (Stojilkovic *et al.*, 2012).

As mentioned earlier, HCN channels are expressed in endocrine pituitary cells and are gated directly by cAMP. Activation of the G_s pathway can, thus, leads to the cAMP-induced activation of HCN channels, increasing the depolarizing I_h current. The effects of this on the cell's electrical

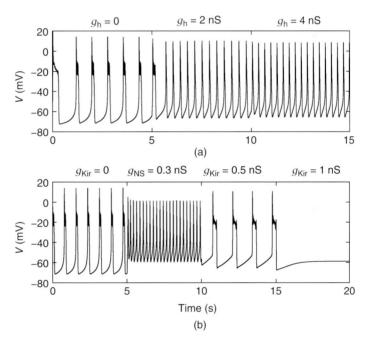

Figure 2.10   The bursting model used in Figure 2.8 is augmented with currents reflecting G-protein signaling. (a) $G\alpha_s$ signaling and the direct action of cAMP on HCN channels is simulated with the addition of an *h*-current. This converts bursting to spiking, and a larger value of g_h increases the spike frequency. (b) The G_s signaling pathway is simulated by the activation of a nonselective, depolarizing current, with g_{NS} increased from 0.02 to 0.3 nS. The $G_{i/o}$ signaling is simulated next by the activation of the K_{ir} current, with $g_{K_{ir}} = 0.5$ nS. This converts the spiking back to bursting. However, with too much K_{ir} conductance (g_{ir} increased to 1 nS), the electrical activity stops completely.

activity are simulated with the model in Figure 2.10a. In this simulation, a parameter set is chosen in which the model cell is initially bursting. After 5 s I_h is added, this converts the bursting pattern to tonic spiking. Further addition of the current increases the frequency of firing. Thus, in cells that are spontaneously bursting, such as many *lactotrophs* and *somatotrophs*, the activation of the G_s pathway can change the mode of activity to tonic spiking, whose frequency is modulated by the degree of activation of the pathway. While the amplitude of intracellular Ca^{2+} oscillations is lower when the cell is spiking, average intracellular Ca^{2+} increases with spike frequency, so the effect on hormone secretion is stimulatory once spike frequency is high enough.

2.7.3   Role of PKA in electrical activity

PKA is present in all eukaryotic cells and functions as the major mediator of the cAMP response. In the absence of cAMP, PKA is an inactive, asymmetric tetramer containing two regulatory and two catalytic subunits that bind to each other with high affinity. The binding of cAMP to the regulatory subunit decreases its affinity for the catalytic subunits by four orders of magnitude, leading to its dissociation into a dimer of regulatory subunits and two active monomeric catalytic subunits. The catalytic subunit phosphorylates numerous proteins, including plasma membrane channels (Taylor *et al.*, 1990).

PKA-dependent phosphorylation of K_{ir} channels silences them, leading to cell depolarization and enhanced excitability. It has been suggested that GHRH decreases the intrinsic activity of a K_{ir} channel in *somatotrophs* and *corticotrophs*, leading to enhanced excitability of these cells (Stojilkovic *et al.*, 2012).

The main effect of G_s-coupled receptors on the electrical activity in *somatotrophs* appears to be the facilitation of inward depolarizing currents, and the phosphorylation of several channels accounts for this effect. Both L- and T-type Ca^{2+} currents appear to be increased by GHRH in ovine *somatotrophs* and human adenoma GH cells. In rat *somatotrophs*, GHRH acts through PKA to activate TTX-insensitive Na_V channels. In *melanotrophs*, PACAP works through PKA to activate an inward nonselective cation current that depolarizes cells and stimulates Ca^{2+} influx. Recently, we provided evidence to support the hypothesis that TRPC channels could account for the inward nonselective cation current and that their phosphorylation by PKA facilitates Ca^{2+} influx in rat *somatotrophs* and other pituitary subtypes. Thus, the activation of G_s-coupled receptors can lead to the activation of numerous ion channels via the actions of PKA. These work together to increase the cell excitability and promote Ca^{2+} influx and Ca^{2+}-dependent hormone release (Stojilkovic *et al.*, 2012).

Pituitary cells receive many signals that are relayed through hormones and act on the cell's GPCRs. The cell's level and pattern of secretion are the output and reflect the integration of the various input signals, filtered through the steroid background that the cell is in. *In vivo*, then, it is most likely that several G-protein pathways are activated simultaneously, though at different levels. Also, some downstream actions are rapid, such as direct actions of $\beta\gamma$ subunits on K_{ir} and Ca_v channels, and some are slow, such as those involving PKA. An example of the integration process that a cell may go through is illustrated in Figure 2.10b. In this simulation, the influence of the different G-protein pathways is added sequentially. First, the G_s pathway is activated, and later the $G_{i/o}$ pathway is activated. (We neglect the time required for the downstream target to be activated by each G protein pathway.) The first, stimulatory, action is mediated in this example by activation of nonselective, depolarizing cation current (I_{NS}), and this converts the bursting pattern to continuous spiking. At time $t = 10\,s$, the $G_{i/o}$ pathway is activated, which activates K_{ir} current ($I_{K_{ir}}$). This current converts the spiking pattern back to a bursting pattern, thus increasing the mean Ca^{2+} level in the cell (not shown). However, if too much $I_{K_{ir}}$ is added, the model cell's electrical activity stops altogether, and the mean Ca^{2+} level of course declines. This demonstrates the complexity of the integration process that is performed by pituitary cells, and the utility of models in simulating and hopefully understanding this process.

2.7.4 Phospholipase C signaling pathway and electrical activity

The activation of GPCRs coupled to $G_{q/11}$ proteins leads to the activation of phospholypase C, causing phosphoinositide hydrolysis and the production of two intracellular messengers: IP_3 and diacylglycerol. IP_3 binds to its receptor channels and, along with Ca^{2+}, is required for their gating. Once activated, the IP_3 receptor functions as a Ca^{2+} channel, allowing Ca^{2+} to flow down its concentration gradient from the ER into the cytosol. The Ca^{2+} flux can be terminated by inactivating the receptor, which occurs through binding of Ca^{2+} to an inactivation site on each subunit on the cytoplasmic side of the receptor. The other signaling branch of $G\alpha_q$-coupled receptors follows the production of diacylglycerol, which together with Ca^{2+} activates protein kinase C, an enzyme that phosphorylates numerous channels and contributes to intracellular signaling by stimulation of phospholipase D and MAP kinase signaling pathways (Berridge and Irvine, 1989). In *gonadotrophs*, this signaling pathway is activated by gonadotropin-releasing hormone, which is the main agonist for these cells, as well as by endothelins, PACAP, substance P, arginine vasopressin and oxytocin. In *thyrotrophs*, the $G_{q/11}$ signaling pathway is activated by thyrotropin-releasing hormone, the main agonist for these cells, and endothelins. *Lactotrophs* express numerous Ca^{2+}-mobilizing receptors, activated by: acetylcholine, angiotensin II, ATP, endothelins, oxytocin, 5-hydroxytryptamine, substance P, thyrotropin-releasing hormone, and galanin. Mammalian *melanotrophs* express muscarinic receptors. In *corticotrophs*, the Ca^{2+}-mobilizing pathway is activated by arginine vasopressin, norepinephrine, and potentially by serotonin. *Somatotrophs* express Ca^{2+}-mobilizing ghrelin and endothelin receptors (Stojilkovic, 2012).

Models for Ca^{2+} handling by the ER, and the oscillations in cytosolic Ca^{2+} concentration, and consequently the membrane potential, which can be produced in pituitary cells, are discussed in Chapter 3. For additional information on the G_q pathway and its effects on the membrane potential and Ca^{2+} in pituitary cells, see the review Stojilkovic *et al.* (2010).

2.8   The dynamic clamp technique for studying the contributions of ion channels to electrical activity

Because there are so many inward and outward types of current, it is difficult to determine the contribution of each channel type to electrical activity patterns. This chapter shows that mathematical models are essential to develop understanding and intuition about the contribution of each channel type to electrical activity. Within a model we can manipulate any channel parameter, including kinetic parameters that are not accessible experimentally, and therefore identify which parameters control a given activity pattern. The drawback of models is that the results of a particular change in a channel parameter can have different effects depending on the other channels included in the model. Since pituitary cells are very heterogeneous, results obtained with a model may not be representative of many cells.

To manipulate key parameters of a channel and assess how they perturb the activity of real cells, we use the *dynamic clamp (DClamp) technique* (Robinson and Kawai, 1993; Sharp *et al.*, 1993) in which a model current is injected into a real cell. This requires the recording of the membrane potential V of the cell in current clamp mode (Figure 2.11). Using V, we can calculate what the current of interest should be using a mathematical model. If our computation is fast enough, we can then inject the computed current into the cell in real time. There are many systems available to perform DClamp; some systems run on the same Windows computers that are used to acquire electrophysiological data (Kemenes *et al.*, 2011; Milescu *et al.*, 2008). A dedicated computer is highly recommended, especially for modeling fast currents.

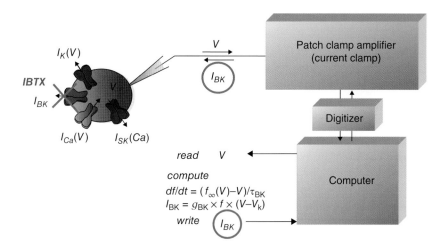

Figure 2.11   Dynamic clamp for injecting a model current in an intact cell. The cell's own BK current can be blocked pharmacologically with iberiotoxin (IBTX). In the current clamp, the recorded and digitized membrane potential (V) is used to calculate the BK current according to a mathematical model. This current is injected into the cell in real time. Modified with permission from Milescu *et al.* (2008). © 2008 The Biophysical society.

In the example illustrated in Figures 2.11 and 2.12, we wish to determine whether BK channels help produce bursting behavior. We begin by blocking the endogenous BK channels using a pharmacological blocker, which switches the cell's activity to spiking (Figure 2.12b). We then add back a model BK current via DClamp and the activity switches back to bursting (Figure 2.12c) (Tabak *et al.*, 2011). However, this burst-promoting effect of BK current occurs only when BK channel activation is fast enough (in this case, $\tau_{BK} = 10$ ms). When the BK activation time constant is increased to a level similar to that of the delayed rectifier ($\tau_{BK} = 20$ ms, Figure 2.12d), there is no burst-promoting effect. This was true for all cells examined.

While modeling had shown that BK activation needed to be fast to promote bursting, the experimental demonstration that this was true in most cells could not have been done without DClamp, because it is not otherwise possible to manipulate activation time constants in real time (Tomaiuolo *et al.*, 2012). Thus, DClamp provides a tool for bringing together the advantages of a model with the reality of an actual cell.

2.9   Perspectives

Endocrine pituitary cells have complex electrical signatures due to the interactions among many types of ion channels. The electrical activity plays a major role in the dynamics of the intracellular Ca^{2+} concentration,

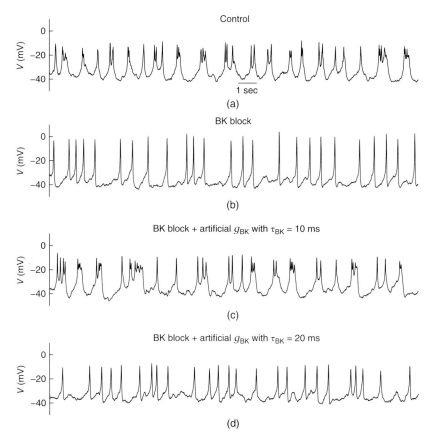

Figure 2.12 The burst-promoting role of BK channels depends on their activation kinetics. (a) Voltage recording from a GH_4 lacto-somatotroph cell. Under control conditions, this cell exhibits a mix of spiking and bursting. (b) Pharmacological block of BK channels switches the activity pattern to spiking. (c) Addition via *dynamic clamp* of an artificial BK conductance (g_{BK} = 0.5 nS) with fast activation (τ_{BK} = 10 ms) switches the electrical activity pattern back to bursting. (d) With slower kinetics (τ_{BK} = 20 ms), the addition of the artificial BK conductance cannot switch the activity back to bursting.

which in turn plays a major role in hormone secretion. Much is known about the individual ion channels underlying the electrical activity, but considerably less is known about how the channels interact in the different cell types. Mathematical modeling can and has played an important role in understanding how the channels contribute to the electrical activity of the cells. The *dynamic clamp* technique lies at the intersection of experimentation and modeling, and facilitates the testing of model predictions on actual cells.

Recommended reading

Essential references

Sharp AA, O'Neil MB, Abbott LF and Marder E (1993). The dynamic clamp: artificial conductances in biological neurons. *Trends Neurosci* **16**: 389–394. [*First use of dynamic clamp.*]

Stojilkovic SS (2006). Pituitary cell type-specific electrical activity, calcium signalling and secretion. *Biol Res* **39**: 403–423. [*Good description of pituitary cell activity.*]

Tabak J, Tomaiuolo M, Gonzalez-Iglesias AE, Milescu LS, Bertram R (2011). Fast-activating voltage- and calcium-dependent potassium (BK) conductance promotes bursting in pituitary cells: a dynamic clamp study. *J Neurosci* **31**: 16855–16863. [*First use of dynamic clamp in pituitary cells.*]

Van Goor F, Li YX and Stojilkovic SS (2001). Paradoxical role of large-conductance calcium-activated K^+ (BK) channels in controlling action potential-driven Ca^{2+} entry in anterior pituitary cells. *J Neurosci* **21**: 5902–5915. [*First explanation for why some pituitary cells burst and others do not.*]

Key reviews

Foskett JK, White C, Cheung KH and Mak DO (2007). Inositol trisphosphate receptor Ca^{2+} release channels. *Physiol Rev.* **87**: 593–658. [*A nice description of G-protein signalling.*]

Freeman ME, Kanyicska B, Lerant A and Nagy G (2000). Prolactin: structure, function, and regulation of secretion. *Physiol Rev.* **80**: 1523–1631. [*An extensive review of the biology of lactotrophs.*]

Hille B (2001). *Ion Channels of Excitable Cells.* Sinauer Associates, Inc., Sunderland, MA. [*An excellent text on ion channels.*]

Robinson RB and Siegelbaum SA (2003). Hyperpolarization-activated cation currents: from molecules to physiological function. *Annu Rev Physiol* **65**: 453–480. [*An extensive review of HCN channels.*]

Stojilkovic, S.S., Tabak, J. and Bertram, R. (2010). Ion channels and signalling in the pituitary gland. *Endocr Rev.* **31**: 845–915. [*A comprehensive review of ion channels and signalling in pituitary cells.*]

References

Aguilera G, Nikodemova M, Wynn PC and Catt KJ (2004). Corticotropin releasing hormone receptors: two decades later. *Peptides* **25**(3): 319–329.

Berridge MJ and Irvine RF (1989). Inositol phosphates and cell signalling. *Nature* **341**(6239): 197–205.

Catterall WA (2000). Structure and regulation of voltage-gated Ca^{2+} channels. *Annu Rev Cell Dev Biol.* **16**: 521–555.

Catterall WA, Goldin AL and Waxman SG (2005). International union of pharmacology. XLVII. Nomenclature and structure–function relationships of voltage-gated sodium channels. *Pharmacol Rev.* **57**(4): 397–409.

Clapham DE, Julius D, Montell C and Schultz G (2005). International union of pharmacology. XLIX. Nomenclature and structure–function relationships of transient receptor potential channels. *Pharmacol Rev.* **57**(4): 427–450.

Collingridge GL, Olsen RW, Peters J and Spedding M (2009). A nomenclature for ligand-gated ion channels. *Neuropharmacology* **56**(1): 2–5.

DeAlmeida VI and Mayo KE (2001). The growth hormone-releasing hormone receptor. *Vitam Horm.* **63**, 233–276.

Foskett JK, White C, Cheung KH and Mak DOD (2007). Inositol trisphosphate receptor Ca^{2+} release channels. *Physiol Rev.* **87**(2): 593–658.

Freeman ME, Kanyicska B, Lerant A and Nagy G (2000). Prolactin: structure, function, and regulation of secretion. *Physiol Rev.* **80**(4): 1523–1631.

Hille B (2001). *Ionic Channels of Excitable Membranes* 3rd edition edn. Sinauer Associates, Sunderland, MA.

Hodson DJ, Romanò N, Schaeffer M, Fontanaud P, Lafont C, Fiordelisio T and Mollard P (2012). Coordination of calcium signals by pituitary endocrine cells in situ. *Cell Calcium* **51**(3–4): 222–230.

Kemenes I, Marra V, Crossley M, Samu D, Staras K, Kemenes G and Nowotny T (2011). Dynamic clamp with StdpC software. *Nat Protoc.* **6**(3): 405–417.

Kidokoro Y (1975). Spontaneous calcium action potentials in a clonal pituitary cell line and their relationship to prolactin secretion. *Nature* **258**(5537): 741–742.

Kretschmannova K, Kucka M, Gonzalez-Iglesias AE and Stojilkovic SS (2012). The expression and role of hyperpolarization-activated and cyclic nucleotide-gated channels in endocrine anterior pituitary cells. *Mol Endocrinol.* **26**(1): 153–164.

Lee AK, Smart JL, Rubinstein M, Low MJ and Tse A (2011). Reciprocal regulation of TREK-1 channels by arachidonic acid and CRH in mouse corticotropes. *Endocrinology* **152**(5): 1901–1910.

Milescu LS, Yamanishi T, Ptak K, Mogri MZ and Smith JC (2008). Real-time kinetic modeling of voltage-gated ion channels using dynamic clamp. *Biophys J.* **95**(1): 66–87.

Missale C, Nash SR, Robinson SW, Jaber M and Caron MG (1998) Dopamine receptors: from structure to function. *Physiol Rev.* **78**(1): 189–225.

Mollard P and Schlegel W (1996) Why are endocrine pituitary cells excitable?. *Trends Endocrinol Metab.* **7**(10): 361–365.

Patel YC, Greenwood M, Panetta R, Hukovic N, Grigorakis S, Robertson LA and Srikant CB (1996) Molecular biology of somatostatin receptor subtypes. *Metab Clin Exp.* **45**(8 Suppl 1): 31–38.

Patel YC and Srikant CB (1986) Somatostatin mediation of adenohypophysial secretion. *Annu Rev Physiol.* **48**: 551–567.

Pazos-Moura CC, Ortiga-Carvalho TM and Gaspar de Moura E (2003). The autocrine/-paracrine regulation of thyrotropin secretion. *Thyroid* **13**(2): 167–175.

Robinson HP and Kawai N (1993) Injection of digitally synthesized synaptic conductance transients to measure the integrative properties of neurons. *J Neurosci Methods* **49**(3): 157–165.

Robinson RB and Siegelbaum SA (2003). Hyperpolarization-activated cation currents: from molecules to physiological function. *Annu Rev Physiol.* **65**: 453–480.

Sankaranarayanan S and Simasko SM (1996) A role for a background sodium current in spontaneous action potentials and secretion from rat lactotrophs. *Am J Physiol.* **271**(6 Pt 1): C1927–1934.

Savarese TM and Fraser CM (1992) In vitro mutagenesis and the search for structure–function relationships among g protein-coupled receptors. *Biochem J.* **283** (Pt 1): 1–19.

Sharp AA, O'Neil MB, Abbott LF and Marder E (1993) The dynamic clamp: artificial conductances in biological neurons. *Trends Neurosci.* **16**(10): 389–394.

Sherman A, Keizer J and Rinzel J (1990) Domain model for $Ca^{2(+)}$-inactivation of Ca^{2+} channels at low channel density. *Biophys J.* **58**(4): 985–995.

Simon SM and Llinas RR (1985) Compartmentalization of the submembrane calcium activity during calcium influx and its significance in transmitter release. *Biophys J.* **48**(3): 485–498.

Stanfield PR, Nakajima S and Nakajima Y (2002). Constitutively active and G-protein coupled inward rectifier K^+ channels: Kir2.0 and Kir3.0. *Rev Physiol Biochem Pharmacol.* **145**: 47–179.

Stern JV, Osinga HM, LeBeau A and Sherman A (2008). Resetting behavior in a model of bursting in secretory pituitary cells: distinguishing plateaus from pseudo-plateaus. *Bull Math Biol.* **70**(1): 68–88.

Stojilkovic SS (2006). Pituitary cell type-specific electrical activity, calcium signaling and secretion. *Biol Res.* **39**(3): 403–423.

Stojilkovic SS (2012). Molecular mechanisms of pituitary endocrine cell calcium handling. *Cell Calcium* **51**(3-4): 212–221.

Stojilkovic SS, Kretschmannova K, Tomić M and Stratakis CA (2012). Dependence of the excitability of pituitary cells on cyclic nucleotides. *J Neuroendocrinol.* **24**(9): 1183–1200.

Stojilkovic SS, Reinhart J and Catt KJ (1994) Gonadotropin-releasing hormone receptors: structure and signal transduction pathways. *Endocr Rev.* **15**(4): 462–499.

Stojilkovic SS, Tabak J and Bertram R (2010). Ion channels and signaling in the pituitary gland. *Endocr Rev.* **31**(6): 845–915.

Tabak J, Tomaiuolo M, Gonzalez-Iglesias AE, Milescu LS and Bertram R (2011). Fast-activating voltage- and calcium-dependent potassium (BK) conductance promotes bursting in pituitary cells: a dynamic clamp study. *J Neurosci.* **31**(46): 16855–16863.

Tabak J, Toporikova N, Freeman ME and Bertram R (2007). Low dose of dopamine may stimulate prolactin secretion by increasing fast potassium currents. *J Comput Neurosci* **22**(2): 211–222.

Taylor SS, Buechler JA and Yonemoto W (1990) cAMP-dependent protein kinase: framework for a diverse family of regulatory enzymes. *Annu Rev Biochem.* **59**: 971–1005.

Teka W, Tsaneva-Atanasova K, Bertram R and Tabak J (2011). From plateau to pseudo-plateau bursting: making the transition. *Bull Math Biol.* **73**(6): 1292–1311.

Tomaiuolo M, Bertram R, Leng G and Tabak J (2012). Models of electrical activity: calibration and prediction testing on the same cell. *Biophys J* **103**(9): 2021–2032.

Tomic M, Kucka M, Kretschmannova K, Li S, Nesterova M, Stratakis CA and Stojilkovic SS (2011). Role of nonselective cation channels in spontaneous and protein kinase A-stimulated calcium signaling in pituitary cells. *Am. J Physiol Endocrinol Metab.* **301**(2): E370–E379.

Toporikova N, Tabak J, Freeman ME and Bertram R (2008). A-type k(+) current can act as a trigger for bursting in the absence of a slow variable. *Neural Comput* **20**(2): 436–451.

Tsaneva-Atanasova K, Sherman A, van Goor F and Stojilkovic SS (2007). Mechanism of spontaneous and receptor-controlled electrical activity in pituitary somatotrophs: experiments and theory. *J Neurophysiol.* **98**(1): 131–144.

Van Goor F, Li YX and Stojilkovic SS (2001a). Paradoxical role of large-conductance calcium-activated K^+ (BK) channels in controlling action potential-driven Ca^{2+} entry in anterior pituitary cells. *J Neurosci.* **21**(16): 5902–5915.

Van Goor F, Zivadinovic D and Stojilkovic SS (2001b). Differential expression of ionic channels in rat anterior pituitary cells. *Mol Endocrinol.* **15**(7): 1222–1236.

Vazquez-Martinez R, Castaño JP, Tonon MC, Vaudry H, Gracia-Navarro F and Malagon MM (2003). Melanotrope secretory cycle is regulated by physiological inputs via the hypothalamus. *Am J Physiol Endocrinol Metab.* **285**(5): E1039–1046.

Wei AD, Gutman GA, Aldrich R, Chandy KG, Grissmer S and Wulff H (2005). International union of pharmacology. LII. Nomenclature and molecular relationships of calcium-activated potassium channels. *Pharmacol Rev.* **57**(4): 463–472.

Willoughby D and Cooper DMF (2007). Organization and Ca^{2+} regulation of adenylyl cyclases in cAMP microdomains. *Physiol Rev.* **87**(3): 965–1010.

Yu FH, Yarov-Yarovoy V, Gutman GA and Catterall WA (2005). Overview of molecular relationships in the voltage-gated ion channel superfamily. *Pharmacol Rev.* **57**(4): 387–395.

CHAPTER 3

Endoplasmic Reticulum- and Plasma-Membrane-Driven Calcium Oscillations

Arthur Sherman

Laboratory of Biological Modeling, NIDDK, National Institutes of Health, USA

3.1 Introduction

Calcium (Ca^{2+}) is of great importance throughout biology because it regulates many processes. In neuroendocrine cells, it plays a central role as the main trigger of hormone and peptide secretion. In the experimental literature, one often finds statements along the lines of "Agent X increases Ca^{2+} concentration ($[Ca^{2+}]_i$), which increases secretion". However, secretion is generally not controlled by a mere rise and fall of Ca^{2+} concentration, but rather by Ca^{2+} oscillations, and "Agent X" works by changing the pattern of those oscillations.

One of the key contributions of theorists has been to develop models that explain the mechanisms behind such oscillations and how they are regulated. Indeed, there are multiple mechanisms, so it is helpful to distinguish their origins and how they are regulated. In particular, we find oscillations that reflect variation in Ca^{2+} influx and arise from ion channels at the *plasma membrane* (PM), as well as oscillations that reflect release from internal stores and arise from ion channels in the membrane of the *endoplasmic reticulum* (ER). A particularly interesting scenario, where the analytical power of models really shines, is when both mechanisms are present in the same cell and interact with each other.

Our objectives are limited. We will consider simplified examples that illustrate the basic principles rather than aim to model in detail any particular system. An understanding of these principles will provide good preparation to tackle particular problems in the future. Our focus is cellular; other chapters will address systems level models that involve multiple cell types and organs. We also limit ourselves to temporal phenomena, modeling cells as spatially homogeneous. This is often adequate, sometimes not. Mathematically, this means that we only need to deal with ordinary differential equations (a single independent variable, time), rather than partial differential equations (time plus one or more spatial dimensions.) We also treat only deterministic systems, which leaves out the sometimes important effects of noise, but allows us to make good use of dynamical systems tools, such as phase planes and *bifurcation* diagrams (BDs).

3.2 Calcium balance equations

3.2.1 Derivation

The fundamental physical principle needed to model calcium dynamics in cells is the conservation of mass, which is determined by flux across boundaries. In physics, flux is the rate of flow of some quantity per unit area (http://en.wikipedia.org/wiki/Flux). As we will be dealing with small round cells with a fixed boundary, it is convenient to multiply implicitly by the cell surface area, giving just quantity per time, symbolized by J. Our goal is to calculate the changes in the cytoplasmic or intracellular Ca^{2+} concentration, $[Ca^{2+}]_i$, denoted here more simply as c, which means that we must divide by the cytosol volume to convert the rate of flux to the rate of change of concentration. The cytosol volume can be taken to be fixed, so that we can further simplify by absorbing the volume into the flux; we denote this scaled flux by j.

Cells can often (but not always) be well approximated with two compartments: one for the cytosol and one for the ER, as shown in Figure 3.1. The cytosolic Ca^{2+}, c, then satisfies the equation

$$\frac{dc}{dt} = f_i \left[j_{PM}^{in} - j_{PM}^{out} - \left(j_{ER}^{in} - j_{ER}^{out} \right) \right] \tag{3.1}$$

where we are using the volume-scaled fluxes.

The factor f_i accounts for the fact that most of the Ca^{2+} that enters a cell is buffered, that is, complexed with Ca^{2+}-binding proteins. Typically, only about 1% of the Ca^{2+} ions that enter remain free, which means that the rate of increase of the free Ca^{2+} concentration is only 1% of what it would be in the absence of buffering. This keeps the free concentration low and prevents runaway activation of the many reactions that are regulated by Ca^{2+}. This form of the equation is valid only because the buffering reactions are much faster than Ca^{2+} fluxes, so that it is safe to assume that free and bound Ca^{2+} are in the quasi-steady state. (A more complete derivation of this can be found in Sherman *et al.* (2002)).

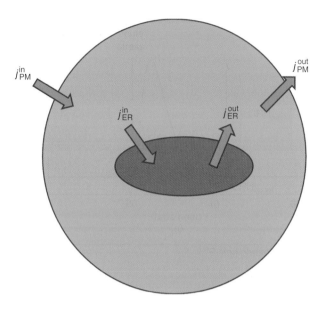

Figure 3.1   Calcium balance. j_{PM}^{in}, influx through plasma membrane; j_{PM}^{out}, efflux through plasma membrane; j_{ER}^{in}, influx through ER membrane; j_{ER}^{out}, efflux through ER membrane.

The equation for ER Ca^{2+}, c_{ER}, can be similarly written as

$$\frac{dc_{ER}}{dt} = f_{ER}\frac{\text{Vol}_i}{\text{Vol}_{ER}}\left(j_{ER}^{in} - j_{ER}^{out}\right) \tag{3.2}$$

Note that the ER gets its own fraction of free Ca^{2+}, which may differ from that in the cytosol. Also, because we absorbed the cytosolic volume into the fluxes, we have to multiply by the cytosolic-ER volume ratio to get the correct effect of the flux on c_{ER}. The ER volume is much smaller than that of the cytosol, so that the concentration change due to the flux will be much greater in the ER. However, the ER Ca^{2+} concentration is much greater, so the most typical case is small relative changes in the ER that result in large relative changes in the cytosol. We can make Equation (3.2) look much better, and reduce the number of parameters from 4 to 2, by multiplying the right-hand side by f_i/f_i:

$$\frac{dc_{ER}}{dt} = f_i\frac{f_{ER}}{f_i}\frac{\text{Vol}_i}{\text{Vol}_{ER}}\left(j_{ER}^{in} - j_{ER}^{out}\right) \text{ or}$$

$$\frac{dc_{ER}}{dt} = \frac{f_i}{\sigma}\left(j_{ER}^{in} - j_{ER}^{out}\right) \tag{3.3}$$

where

$$\sigma = \frac{f_i\text{Vol}_{ER}}{f_{ER}\text{Vol}_i}$$

3.2.2 Applications

We will flesh out the Ca^{2+} equations (3.1) and (3.3) and incorporate them into more complex models shortly, but pause here to show that even these simple equations can be used to draw nontrivial conclusions.

We choose the following expressions for the fluxes:

$$j_{PM}^{in} = -\alpha I_{Ca} \tag{3.4}$$

$$j_{PM}^{out} = k_{PMCA} c \tag{3.5}$$

$$j_{ER}^{in} = k_{SERCA} c \tag{3.6}$$

$$j_{ER}^{out} = P_{ER}(c_{ER} - c) \tag{3.7}$$

where PMCA is the "plasma-membrane calcium ATPase," which pumps Ca^{2+} out of the cell, and SERCA is the "sarco-endoplasmic reticulum calcium ATPase," which pumps Ca^{2+} into the ER. We assume that flux out of the ER is a passive, diffusive leak. Equations (3.4) and (3.5) correspond to Equation (2.15), Chapter 2, this volume, for bulk cytosolic Ca^{2+}, except that the plasma-membrane calcium current is for the moment constant, not voltage dependent. In general, the pump expressions are not linear, but rather saturating *Hill functions*, but these are not needed for the moment. There may also be multiple plasma-membrane Ca^{2+} currents (e.g., L-type and T-type currents, as described in Chapter 2, Equations (2.6) and (2.7)), multiple ER Ca^{2+} channels (e.g., *IP3* and *Ryanodine* receptors), and more than one Ca^{2+} efflux component (e.g., the Na^+–Ca^{2+} exchanger in addition to PMCA).

In Figure 3.2, the black curves show the effect of partial (50%) block of the SERCA pump, such as with *thapsigargin*, by cutting k_{SERCA} in half.

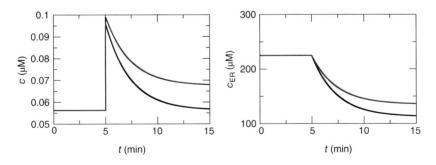

Figure 3.2 Illustration of the steady-state calcium theorem (Theorem 3.2.1) using the passive model, Equations (3.1) and (3.3), with fluxes as in Equations (3.4)–(3.7). c, cytosolic Ca^{2+}; c_{ER}, ER Ca^{2+}. Parameters: $\alpha = 4.5\ \mu M/pC$; $I_{Ca} = -1\ pA$, $I_{SOC} = -0.2\ pA$ (red), 0 (black); $k_{PMCA} = 8\ s^{-1}$; $k_{SERCA} = 0.4\ s^{-1}$, reduced to $0.2\ s^{-1}$ at $t = 5\ min$; $P_{ER} = 0.1\ s^{-1}$; $f_i = 0.01$; $\sigma = 0.04$.

For simplicity, we assume that the block becomes fully effective instantaneously at $t = 5$ min. Then, c rises to a peak and then recovers to baseline. One often hears or reads something like "thapsigargin was used to increase Ca^{2+}," but the simulation shows that such an increase is only transient because the Ca^{2+} released from the ER to the cytosol is pumped out of the cell, leaving the ER depleted (in proportion to the inhibition of SERCA) but the cytosol at its original level once equilibrium is re-established. It is simple to show that the rise in c must be transient: setting Equation (3.3) to steady state gives

$$j_{ER}^{in} = j_{ER}^{out}$$

and substituting this into Equation (3.1) and setting to the steady state implies that

$$j_{PM}^{in} = j_{ER}^{out}$$

Thus, the ER terms drop out of the c equation, and the steady-state value of c depends only on the parameters of j_{PM}^{in} and j_{PM}^{out}. We conclude that c cannot be affected by the change in k_{SERCA}. The same would be true if we had emptied the ER by increasing efflux, which could correspond to the activation of IP3 or Ryanodine receptors. This is in general enough that it is worth stating as a theorem that holds independent of our choices for the fluxes:

Theorem 3.2.1 The steady-state calcium theorem. *In a two-compartment Ca^{2+} model, the steady state of cytosolic Ca^{2+} is determined by the balance of plasma-membrane Ca^{2+} fluxes and can only be changed by changing a plasma-membrane ion current or pump.*

A maintained change in c is illustrated by the red curve in Figure 3.2. In that simulation, I_{Ca} is increased in magnitude at the same time that the PMCA is inhibited; this could correspond, for example, to a store-operated current (SOC) activated by the reduction in c_{ER} (Hogan *et al.*, 2010). The combination of the two effects results in an increase in c at the steady state. Conversely, if one observes a steady state increase in c when SERCA is inhibited in an experiment, one can be sure that a plasma-membrane ion current was affected (though not necessarily SOC).

The inability of c_{ER} to affect steady state c is not due to the depletion of the ER (indeed, we deliberately only depleted it partially in Figure 3.2 to emphasize this point), but to the fact that c_{ER} is constant. The reader may check this explicitly by solving for c in terms of c_{ER} in Equations (3.1) and (3.3) using the expressions in Equations (3.4)–(3.7).

We now illustrate that Theorem 3.2.1 does not hold when the system is not in steady state. In Figure 3.3, the black curves show the response to a train of square pulses of I_{Ca}; this represents roughly the effect of a train of action potentials. The red curves show the response when SERCA

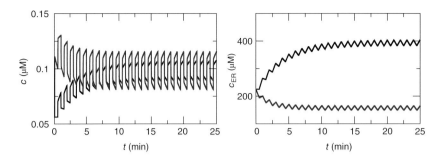

Figure 3.3   Depleting ER Ca^{2+} (c_{ER}) increases amplitude of cytosolic Ca^{2+} (c) response to pulses. Black: control, Red: SERCA (sarco-endoplasmic reticulum calcium ATPase) pump inhibited 50%. Equations and parameters as in Figure 3.2 but with I_{Ca} pulsed between -1 and -2 pA every 30 s.

is partially inhibited. The pulses of c are larger in amplitude. This happens because more of the Ca^{2+} that enters with each pulse stays in the cytosol instead of going into the ER. Theorem 3.2.1 does not apply because I_{Ca} fluctuates too rapidly for the system to reach steady state during each pulse.

Note that there are two time constants evident in Figure 3.3: with each pulse, c jumps up rapidly and then rises slowly. The rapid jumps reflect the fast intrinsic kinetics of c, whereas the slow rise reflects the slow kinetics of c_{ER}, which pushes c up slightly with each pulse as the ER fills. The slow kinetics of the ER are also manifest in the slow rise (*black*) and slow fall (*red*) of the envelope of c as the ER fills or empties. The mean trend of c, however, averaged over the rapid fluctuations, does approach approximately the same level irrespective of the fact whether the pump is inhibited or not. That is, Theorem 3.2.1 applies approximately to the averaged system.

3.3   ER-driven calcium oscillations

3.3.1   Closed cell

The model we have considered so far has a very limited repertoire because it is linear. There is a unique steady state, and the most the system can do is relax to that steady state exponentially or as a sum of exponentials. Put in other terms, the model has only negative feedback, embodied in the SERCA and PMCA pumps, which suppresses any fluctuation of c away from rest. There is a strong imperative to keep c stable, but some cells have evolved the ability to generate and profit from controlled large excursions away from rest. In order to obtain more dynamic responses, we need to make the model nonlinear, specifically to add positive feedback. We do this by postulating that c increases the flux out of the ER, often referred to as "calcium-induced calcium release" (CICR). Moreover, the negative feedback, which is needed to limit and terminate the excursions, has to develop slowly enough that it does not cancel out the rise in c too soon. We have already encountered examples of oscillations mediated by fast positive feedback combined with slow negative feedback in Chapter 1, McCobb and Zeeman, and Chapter 2, Bertram *et al.*, where they were the bases of action potentials. Indeed, the model we introduce here has much in common with those electrical oscillators, though it works via c rather than the membrane potential.

IP3 regulation of ER Ca^{2+}

A simple example of cytosolic Ca^{2+} oscillations is the model of Li and Rinzel (1994), which is a simplification of the model of DeYoung and Keizer (1992). This will serve as an exemplar of a wide class of models based on the IP3 receptor (IP3R), an internal receptor located on the ER membrane, which opens in response to the second messenger IP3. IP3 in turn is produced by the activation of a G-protein-coupled receptor (GPCR) on the plasma membrane that responds to an external signal, such as acetylcholine or GnRH; the GPCR is coupled to phospholipase C via G_q, which forms IP3 from phosphatidylinositol 4,5-bisphosphate (PIP2). The IP3R is moreover a ligand-gated Ca^{2+} channel; IP3 opens the channel and allows Ca^{2+} to flow down its concentration gradient from the ER to the cytosol. Thus, one way to introduce positive feedback is to assume that IP3 production is stimulated by rises in c. This was the basis of the earliest models for c oscillations (Meyer and Stryer, 1988; Swillens and Mercan, 1990). DeYoung and Keizer, in contrast, motivated by reports that c could oscillate even when IP3 is held fixed, proposed that c enhanced the activity of the IP3R directly. Both effects of c are known to exist, and there has been a long, yet unresolved debate about which is more important, or whether they each occur in different types of c oscillations. We will not enter that debate here, but simply use the hypothesis of DeYoung and Keizer as a learning tool.

Modeling the role of IP3

Bezprozvanny *et al.* (1991) showed that the steady state open probability of the IP3R was a bell-shaped function of c, which suggested that c in high concentrations inactivates the channel. DeYoung and Keizer proposed that this inactivation provides negative feedback beyond that of SERCA to terminate the Ca^{2+} spike, and that its time scale controls the period of the oscillation. They developed a model with eight states, for all the combinations of activating Ca^{2+}, activating IP3 and inactivating Ca^{2+}, bound or unbound.

Li and Rinzel (1994) simplified this in the following formula:

$$j_{ER}^{out} = (L + Pm_\infty(c; I)^3 h^3)(c_{ER} - c) \qquad (3.8)$$

where

$$m_\infty(c; I) = \frac{I}{K_I + I} \frac{c}{K_a + c}$$

I is the concentration of IP3, treated as a parameter; and h is the fraction of available IP3 receptors, that is, the fraction not inactivated by binding Ca^{2+}. h satisfies the differential equation

$$\frac{dh}{dt} = \frac{h_\infty(c) - h}{\tau_h(c)} \qquad (3.9)$$

where

$$h_\infty(c) = \frac{K_d}{K_d + c}, \quad \tau_h(c) = \frac{1}{A(c + K_d)}$$

Equations (3.8) and (3.9) together say that the IP3R open probability is for fixed h an increasing function of [IP3] and c, but decreases over time as receptors inactivate. This was deliberately formulated to highlight its similarity to the conductance of the voltage-dependent Na^+ channel, described in Chapter 2, Equation (2.1), which increases with the membrane potential V but inactivates over time.

We can now assemble the pieces to specify the *Li–Rinzel* model, taking Equations (3.1) and (3.3) with Equation (3.8) in place of Equation (3.7) and

$$j_{ER}^{in}(c) = \frac{V_e c^2}{K_e^2 + c^2}$$

in place of Equation (3.6) (not strictly necessary but customary and more accurate). The equations for c and c_{ER} then become

$$\frac{dc}{dt} = f_i \left\{ \left[L + P \left(\frac{I}{K_I + I} \frac{c}{K_a + c} h \right)^3 \right] (c_{ER} - c) - \frac{V_e c^2}{K_e^2 + c^2} \right\} \qquad (3.10)$$

$$\frac{dc_{ER}}{dt} = -\frac{f_i}{\sigma} \left\{ \left[L + P \left(\frac{I}{K_I + I} \frac{c}{K_a + c} h \right)^3 \right] (c_{ER} - c) - \frac{V_e c^2}{K_e^2 + c^2} \right\} \qquad (3.11)$$

Finally, we add Equation (3.9) for receptor inactivation.

This system with three dependent variables (c, c_{ER}, and h) can be simplified by assuming that the cell is closed, that is, that the fluxes across the plasma membrane, j_{PM}^{in} and j_{PM}^{out} are 0. This serves two purposes. First, it emphasizes that the oscillations only require flux in and out of the ER. Second, it reduces the number of equations to 2. The total Ca^{2+} content of the cell is

$$C_T = \sigma c_{ER} + c \qquad (3.12)$$

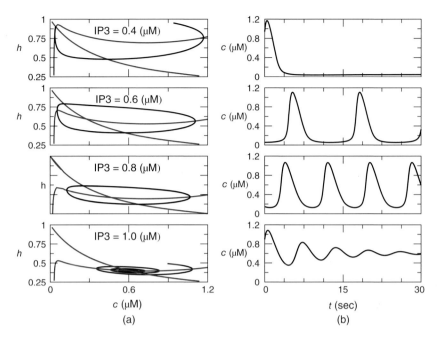

Figure 3.4   Phase planes (a) and timecourses (b) for the closed-cell Li–Rinzel model, Equations (3.9)–(3.11). h, fraction of IP3 receptors that are available to be opened (i.e. are not inactivated). Oscillations exist for an intermediate range of IP3 concentrations and, within that range, frequency increases with IP3. Parameters: I as specified in the panels; $f_i = 0.01$; $L = 0.0925$ μM/s; $P = 6660$ 1/s; $K_i = 1.0$ μM; $K_a = 0.4$ μM; $V_e = 100$ μM/s; $K_e = 0.3$ μM; $A = 0.5$ 1/μMs; $K_d = 0.4$ μM; $\sigma = 0.185$.

where σ takes into account the differences in ER and cytosolic volume and buffering. This quantity is constant when the cell is closed: its time derivative is 0, as can be verified by multiplying Equation (3.3) by σ and adding to Equation (3.1). This reduction to two equations now allows us to use phase planes, shown in Figure 3.4, to understand the behaviors. (The concept and usage of phase planes are explained in Chapter 1, McCobb and Zeeman.)

We solve the model equations for c and h (but can recover c_{ER} from Equation (3.12) should the need arise; see Figure 3.6). The left column shows the phase planes for three values of [IP3], and the right column shows the corresponding timecourses. The h nullcline (*blue*) is obtained by setting the right-hand side of Equation (3.9) to 0 and solving for h as a function of c. It decreases monotonically, reflecting the increase of inactivation with c (see Equation (3.9)).

The c nullcline (*red*) is obtained by setting the right-hand side of Equation (3.1) to 0. Conceptually, we want to solve for c as a function of h, but that equation can have up to three solutions for some values of h, so it is easier to solve for h as a function of c. The c nullcline is, thus, defined by

$$h = \left[\frac{1}{P} \left(\frac{j_{ER}^{in}(c)}{(c_{ER} - c)} - L \right) \right]^{\frac{1}{3}} \frac{1}{m_\infty(c; I)}$$

$$\approx \left[\frac{j_{ER}^{in}(c)}{P c_{ER}} \right]^{\frac{1}{3}} \frac{1}{m_\infty(c; I)}$$

where we have neglected the small terms c and L in the second line (the latter is valid as long as c is not too small). The resulting curve has a distorted N shape, increasing for small c, then decreasing, and then increasing again. The left branch of the c nullcline has a steep slope because $m_\infty \to 0$ as $c \to 0$. The N shape results from the competition between activation, m_∞, of the receptor, which increases c, and SERCA, j_{ER}^{in}, which refills the ER. The general trend is for h to increase due to SERCA, but in the range where the IP3R is strongly activated, h turns down. This is typical for *activator–inhibitor systems*, where the positive feedback mechanism creates a kink in the activator variable nullcline and thereby creating instability and oscillations. In Hodgkin–Huxley-type systems, the activation of the Na^+ current plays the same role. In that context, it creates a dip in the current–voltage relation, which translates to a negative resistance and gives away its role as the source of dynamism.

The intersection of the two nullclines is the steady state, and in each row there is only one. Increasing IP3 pulls down the c nullcline because m_∞ is an increasing function of I and moves the steady state along the c nullcline. In the top row, IP3 = 0.4 µM, the steady state is on the rising left branch of the c nullcline, and is therefore stable. The trajectory (*black*) swings around from the upper right to end at the steady state, producing a single transient spike and then steady c, as shown in the right panel. In this state, the system is not oscillatory but is said to be excitable, meaning that a suitable perturbation away from the rest state is amplified into a spike rather than returning immediately to rest.

For IP3 = 1.0 µM, the steady state is on the rising right branch of the c nullcline and is again stable, but the approach to rest is a damped oscillation. In order to get sustained oscillations, the steady state must be destabilized, which is guaranteed if it lies on the falling middle branch of the c nullcline. This is the case for IP3 = 0.6 µM, shown in the middle panels. The trajectory now takes the form of a closed curve (a limit cycle, see Chapter 1, McCobb and Zeeman) that orbits around the steady state.

The phase plane also explains a characteristic feature of the oscillation, namely that the spikes are narrow and the interspike intervals are long. This happens because the trajectory is closer to the unstable steady state during the interspike portion, and the flow is therefore slow. The period decreases markedly as IP3 is increased within the oscillatory range because the steady state moves to the right, away from the low c values traversed during the interspike period (compare IP3 = 0.6 μM to IP3 = 0.8 μM in Figure 3.4). Thus, it is not difficult for models like this to capture the frequency encoding observed experimentally as the IP3-generating stimulus is varied (Goldbeter *et al.*, 1990).

If we stack a series of phase planes like those in Figure 3.4 and plot the values of c (the steady states as well as the minima and maxima of the periodic orbits when those are present), we get Figure 3.5. A similar picture would be obtained if h were plotted against IP3, so we omit the third dimension. The line shows the steady states, *solid* and *black* for stable, *dashed* and *red* for unstable. The *green* dotted line shows the average c during spiking, and the filled circles the amplitude of the oscillations, which exist for a range of values of IP3, or between lower and upper thresholds. Those thresholds are labeled "HB" for Hopf bifurcation, which indicates the particular way in which the steady state goes unstable (see Chapter 1, McCobb and Zeeman). The existence of upper and lower thresholds, dividing the system behaviors into off, oscillating and fully on, is a ubiquitous feature of activator–inhibitor systems.

The peak c of the oscillation is in most cases higher than the steady c level when I is above the upper threshold, but the average is lower. The model

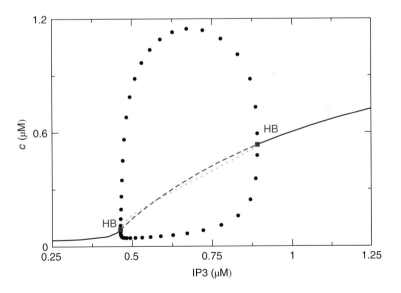

Figure 3.5   Bifurcation diagram for the closed-cell Li–Rinzel model. Oscillations in cytosolic Ca^{2+} (c) exist for an intermediate range of IP3, demarcated by Hopf bifurcations (HB). Black: stable; *lines*: steady states; *filled circles*: min and max of oscillation; red: unstable steady states; *green*: average cytosolic Ca^{2+} during oscillations. Equations and parameters as in Figure 3.4

thus suggests that if one could measure c experimentally but not IP3, then the average would be a better indicator of the IP3 level (or "activity") than the peak.

3.3.2 Open cell

Suppose now that the cell is open. Now during each Ca^{2+} spike, some of the Ca^{2+} will be pumped out of the cell rather than back into the ER. Unless there is some Ca^{2+} influx to balance the efflux, the ER would eventually empty out and oscillations would cease. We restore the plasma-membrane fluxes, setting j_{PM}^{in} to a constant and introducing a saturating PMCA pump:

$$j_{PM}^{out}(c) = \frac{V_p c^2}{K_p^2 + c^2}$$

The equations for c and c_{ER} are now

$$\frac{dc}{dt} = f_i \left\{ \left[L + P \left(\frac{I}{K_I + I} \frac{c}{K_a + c} h \right)^3 \right] (c_{ER} - c) - \frac{V_e c^2}{K_e^2 + c^2} \right.$$
$$\left. + \left(j_{PM}^{in} - \frac{V_p c^2}{K_p^2 + c^2} \right) \right\} \tag{3.13}$$

$$\frac{dc_{ER}}{dt} = -\frac{f_i}{\sigma} \left\{ \left[L + P \left(\frac{I}{K_I + I} \frac{c}{K_a + c} h \right)^3 \right] (c_{ER} - c) - \frac{V_e c^2}{K_e^2 + c^2} \right\} \tag{3.14}$$

This model (Equations (3.9), (3.13), (3.14)) is used to illustrate the role of Ca^{2+} influx in Figure 3.6. Note that each spike causes only a small reduction in c_{ER} in this model, so that oscillations persist for quite a few spikes. This is consistent with experiments showing continued spiking in pituitary gonadotrophs in 0 Ca^{2+} medium (Li *et al.*, 1994). In other

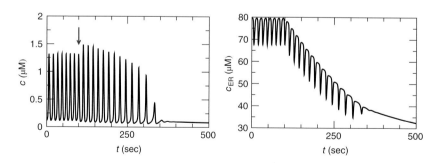

Figure 3.6 In the open-cell Li–Rinzel model (Equations (3.9), (3.13), (3.14)), Ca^{2+} influx is needed to sustain oscillations. Parameters as in Figure 3.4 except: $I = 0.3$ μM; $V_e = 50$ μM/s; $K_e = 0.2$ μM; $K_d = 0.2$ μM; $\sigma = 0.1$. We also add the plasma-membrane parameters: $V_p = 5$ μM/s; $K_p = 0.3$ μM; and j_{PM}^{in}, which is initially 2.5 μM/s and at $t = 100$ s (*red arrow*) reduced to 0.

models, the depletion of the ER is much deeper and removal of external Ca^{2+} terminates spiking abruptly (Friel, 1995; Friel and Tsien, 1992). The Li–Rinzel model can act in this mode as well (see Li and Rinzel (1994), Figure 5c). In such models, the ER sets frequency of spiking, not IP3R inactivation. This figure shows an effect of the PM on the ER, and is complementary to Figure 3.2, which showed an effect of the ER on the plasma membrane. For fixed IP3, the open-cell model, in fact, has upper and lower thresholds and a BD with respect to j_{PM}^{in} (not shown) similar to that of the closed-cell model with respect to IP3 (Figure 3.5). In the next section, we explore bi-directional interaction with a more fleshed-out plasma-membrane component.

3.4 Combining ER and PM oscillators

The first models for ER-driven Ca^{2+} oscillations were developed for nonexcitable cells (Goldbeter *et al.*, 1990), but the same processes often occur in electrically excitable cells. The combination of these two pathways can increase the dynamic repertoire of cells considerably.

3.4.1 Bursting driven by the ER

Our first goal in this section is to simulate *bursting* like that seen in pituitary gonadotrophs (Li *et al.*, 1994), which is driven by periodic Ca^{2+} releases from the ER, by adding a PM oscillator (electrical subsystem). We will use the following simplified Hodgkin–Huxley-type model (Tsaneva-Atanasova *et al.*, 2010):

$$C_m \frac{dV}{dt} = -I_{Ca}(V) - I_{K(V)}(V, n) - I_{K(Ca)}(V, c) \tag{3.15}$$

$$= -\bar{g}_{Ca} m_{\infty}(V)^2 (V - V_{Ca}) - \bar{g}_{K(V)} n (V - V_K) - g_{K(Ca)}(c)(V - V_K) \tag{3.16}$$

$$\frac{dn}{dt} = \frac{n_{\infty}(V) - n}{\tau_n} \tag{3.17}$$

where

$$m_{\infty}(V) = \frac{1}{1 + \exp(-(V - V_m)/K_m)} \, n_{\infty}(V) = \frac{1}{1 + \exp(-(V - V_n)/K_n)} \tag{3.18}$$

and

$$g_{K(Ca)}(c) = \bar{g}_{K(Ca)} \frac{c^4}{K_{m,kca}^4 + c^4} \tag{3.19}$$

The last corresponds to the SK conductance in Chapter 2.

Note that we have ignored the Na^+ current found in gonadotrophs, but just have the Ca^{2+} current do double duty to produce both tall, brief action potentials and c entry.

The equations are incomplete because we have to specify c, which comes from the open-cell Li–Rinzel model. Finally, in that model, we replace the constant j^{in}_{PM} used in Figure 3.6 with

$$j^{in}_{PM} = -\alpha I_{Ca}(V) \tag{3.20}$$

where α converts units of current to units of flux, as described in Chapter 2, Eq. 2.15. The ER and PM components communicate via the shared variable c. The models are now more complicated, so the parameters are in Table 3.1.

Figure 3.7 shows the solution of Equations (3.15)–(3.20). The oscillations differ from those in Chapter 2, where calcium oscillations were driven by electrical oscillations, either spiking or bursting: here the bursting electrical oscillations are driven by periodic releases of Ca^{2+} from the ER. The signature of this scenario is that c peaks between the bursts of V rather than during the bursts, as in Chapter 2. This reflects the finding that by itself the electrical component of the system can only produce spikes, not bursts. The silent periods are produced by the releases of Ca^{2+}, which activate the K(Ca) current. The role of the electrical subsystem is to produce

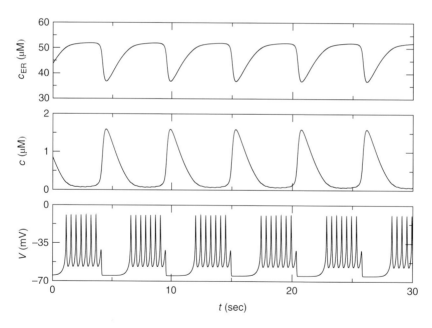

Figure 3.7   Bursting in combined endoplasmic reticulum–plasma membrane (ER-PM) model (Equations (3.9), (3.13)–(3.20)). The PM would spike continuously on its own but is interrupted by periodic releases of Ca^{2+} from the ER, as seen in pituitary gonadotrophs (Li *et al.*, 1994). The rise in cytoplasmic Ca^{2+} (c) thus occurs between the bursts of action potentials. Parameters are shown in Table 3.1.

Ca^{2+} influx to refill the ER after each Ca^{2+} release; the action potentials are so fast compared to the time scale of the ER that they look like a constant influx.

3.4.2 Regulation of Ca^{2+} entry by the ER via K(Ca) channels

We now use the same model to illustrate a more subtle scenario of ER-PM communication via K(Ca) following Li et al., 1997. In order to clarify the governing principles, we set IP3 to 0 to eliminate ER-driven rhythmicity, so that the only efflux from the ER is the passive leak L in Equation (3.10).

Figure 3.8 begins with the system in a state of periodic spiking (leftmost V panel) and nearly constant c and c_{ER}. At $t = 60$ s, the leak L is halved, filling the ER nearly exponentially to a new steady level that is twice as high. This lowers c, reduces g_{KCa} and increases spike frequency (second V panel). Thus, the ER signals the PM to increase the rate of Ca^{2+} entry needed to increase c_{ER}. As the ER reaches its new steady level after about 5 min, the spike rate returns to its baseline level (third V panel). At $t = 360$ s, the process is reversed: L is doubled, returning it to its initial value. This

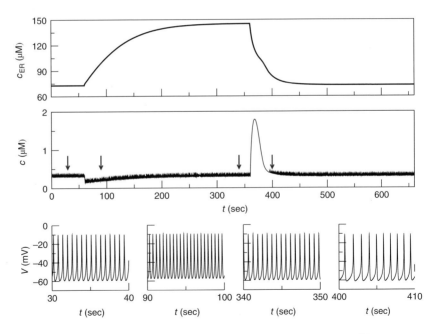

Figure 3.8   ER regulates firing frequency by sourcing or sinking Ca^{2+}. Equations as in Figure 3.7, but $I = 0$ to disable ER rhythmicity and L initially set to 6.25 μM/s to provide constant efflux from the ER. L is halved at $t = 60$ s and restored at $t = 360$ s. See Table 3.1 for other parameter changes. Bottom: V traces from indicated time segments beginning at the *red arrows* in the middle panel.

elicits a large spike of c, which inhibits spiking (not shown). Spiking then resumes at a reduced rate (fourth V panel) and finally recovers to baseline as c recovers.

Considerations like this may apply *in vivo*, where gonadotrophs are under the control of GnRH secreted by GnRH neurons in the hypothalamus in addition to their own intrinsic dynamics. Oscillations in GnRH would result in oscillations in IP3 in the gonadotrophs and lead to cycles of ER filling and emptying.

The general principle illustrated here is that when the ER communicates with the PM via $g_{K(Ca)}$, it increases the AP frequency when it fills and reduces the AP frequency when it empties. When the ER level is constant, it has no effect on the AP frequency. This is a corollary of Theorem 3.2.1. Although this result holds strictly only when the ER is nonoscillatory, it holds approximately for a bursting cell like that in Figure 3.7 (Li *et al.*, 1997).

In contrast, if the PM had a SOC channel, the ER level could control spike frequency even when it was unchanging. Moreover, whereas K(Ca) can refill the store only after the increased leak is relieved, SOC can refill it in the face of a maintained leak.

3.4.3   Bursting driven by the PM

In the previous subsection, we considered bursting driven by the ER. Now we revisit bursting driven by the PM, similar to that discussed in Chapter 2, from the point of view of the bifurcations involved. First, we disable ER-driven rhythmicity by setting the IP3 concentration, ER leak rate and SERCA pump rate to 0 (parameters L, I, and V_e in Equation (3.10)); passive ER dynamics will be added back later to complete the picture. We retain the PM equations (3.15)–(3.19), making parameter adjustments to illustrate several canonical patterns.

Plateau bursting

Figure 3.9a shows an example of "plateau" bursting, so-called because it is characterized by alternating active phases of spikes from an elevated plateau and silent phases. Because the timecourse resembles a square wave (though with spikes superimposed on the upper state), this is also called "square-wave bursting." The only substantive difference from the parameter set used in Figure 3.8 is that the time constant of the voltage-dependent K⁺ (K(V)) channel has been decreased from 60 to 30 ms; the other changes are cosmetic. Speeding up K(V) reduces the amplitude of the spikes because the K⁺ channels can react more rapidly to the changes in V triggered by the Ca²⁺ channels and limit the size of the fluctuations. Similar to Figure 3.8, there is no active ER in Figure 3.9, but now the elevation of the spike minima to about −45 mV allows for sustained Ca²⁺ entry and much greater

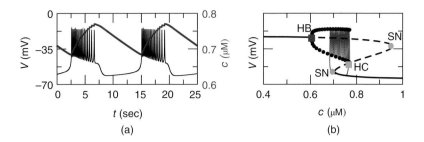

Figure 3.9   Plateau or square-wave bursting. Equations as in Figure 3.7 but with ER removed; parameters in Table 3.1. Timecourses of V and cytosolic Ca^{2+} (c) in (a). In contrast to Figure 3.7, c rises *during* the bursts of APs, not between them. Bifurcation diagram with superimposed trajectory shown in *blue* in (b). HB = Hopf bifurcation; SN = saddle-node bifurcation; HC = homoclinic bifurcation.

rises in c. The slow, nearly exponential rise in c terminates the spiking and allows c to recover, in contrast to the active ER dynamics in Figure 3.7.

A good way to understand the dynamics is to recognize that c varies much more slowly than V and n, which is evident by comparing the rapid spikes of V with the sluggish changes in c in the left panel. Thus, the PM subsystem (Equations (3.15) and (3.17)), heretofore distinguished by its cellular location and function, can be distinguished dynamically as the fast V–n subsystem, of the full fast–slow, V–n–c system. This allows us to treat c as a *parameter* of the fast subsystem and study the behaviors of the latter as c is varied.

Figure 3.9b shows the BD in *black* of the V–n subsystem of the PM oscillator with c as the bifurcation parameter. The V–c trajectory is superimposed in *blue*. The *solid black lines* show the steady states, and the *black circles* show the minima and maxima of the fast spike oscillations, as in Figure 3.5. As c increases, V tends to decrease because of the inhibition through the K(Ca) channels, but there is a switchback that produces a range of c values in which there are three steady states, only the bottom one of which is stable.

The turning points of the Z-shaped steady-state curve are defined by saddle–node bifurcations (SN), where one eigenvalue changes sign. Thus, the bottom branch is stable because it has two negative eigenvalues, the middle branch consists of saddle points that have one positive and one negative eigenvalue, and the upper branch has two positive eigenvalues.

In addition, the upper branch changes stability via a Hopf bifurcation (HB), which demarcates the lower threshold for spiking, much as for the Ca^{2+} spikes in Figure 3.5. The upper threshold for spiking is not, however, a second HB as in the Li–Rinzel model, but a more complex object called a "homoclinic orbit," labeled HC.

Note that the HC occurs when the spike minimum touches the middle branch of saddle points. It can be appreciated that something important should happen, as the orbit cannot pass through a steady state. Instead, the orbits progressively deform as c increases until a curve is formed that begins and ends at one of the saddle points. Because it begins and ends at a steady state, this is a brief spike with an infinitely long interspike interval, or, in other words, an oscillation with infinite period. Its function here is to mark the highest level of c for which spike oscillations exist. See Chapter 1 and Rinzel and Ermentrout (1998) for further discussion of homoclinic orbits.

To summarize what we have so far, for fixed c, there are four behavior regimes for this model: to the left of HB, there is only a depolarized steady state; between HB and the left SN, there is only a spiking state; between SN and HC, there is bistability between a spiking state and a low-V steady state; and to the right of HC there is only a low-V steady state.

In order to have bursting, however, c must vary, albeit slowly. That is, c provides the slow negative feedback that terminates each episode of spiking and fades away to permit the next episode. This is the same role played by IP3R inhibition, h, in the Li–Rinzel model.

We can make the analogy more apparent by setting n to steady state, reducing the V–n–c system to a V–c system, with V playing the role of fast activation and c playing the role of slow inhibition. This is illustrated in Figure 3.10a, which shows the V–n phase plane, with the V nullcline in *red*, the c nullcline in *green* and the trajectory in *black*. Relative to Figure 3.4, the activator and inhibitor axes are flipped. Note that c has switched allegiance, now playing on the inhibitor side. As in the Li–Rinzel case, the system changes from silent to oscillating to fully on as the steady state moves from the bottom branch of the activator (fast) nullcline to the middle branch to the upper branch.

In Figure 3.10b, we pretend that the third dimension of the system, n, is absent and think of the BD in Figure 3.9 as the V–c phase plane. This

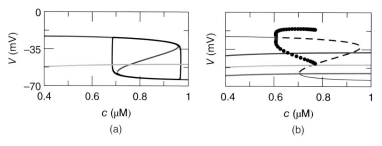

(a) (b)

Figure 3.10 (a) V–c phase plane for the model of Figure 3.9 but with $V_p = 7.5 \, \mu M \, s^{-1}$ and n set to n_∞ (equivalently, $\tau_n = 0$) to reduce the dimension to two and eliminate spiking. V nullclline, *red*; c nullcline, *green*; trajectory, *black*. (b) Bifurcation diagram from Figure 3.9 with c nullclines added. Intersection of c nullcline with Z-curve, controlled by PMCA pump rate V_p, determines whether behavior is silent ($V_p = 2.5$, *magenta*), bursting ($V_p = 7.5$, *green*), or continuously spiking ($V_p = 30$, *blue*).

is a good approximation, and gives the right conceptual picture, because c is much slower than V and n. In the full three-variable system, shifting the c nullcline again switches the system behavior, in this case from silent (*magenta*) to bursting (*green*) to continuously spiking (*blue*).

The square-wave bursting described above is reminiscent of the electrical activity seen in pancreatic β cells, as first modeled by Chay and Keizer (1983). They proposed that the shift of the c nullcline described above, mediated by the ATP-dependent PMCA pump, accounts for the experimentally observed transitions induced by changes in glucose concentration and which drive the corresponding increases in insulin secretion. The models have become more complex and involved, with molecular actors, notably the ATP-dependent K$^+$ channel, which were not known at the time, but the dynamic structure and its modulation by glucose remain essentially the same more than 30 years on (Sherman, 2011).

One limitation of the *Chay-Keizer model* was that the slow oscillations were not quite slow enough (the observed periods vary from tens of seconds to more than a minute). A more serious problem is that when the timecourse of c was measured a few years later, it was not a sawtooth, but closer to a square wave.

Figure 3.11 shows that both these problems can be fixed by adding back the ER. The only differences between Figures 3.11 and 3.9 are the nonzero values for the ER leak and SERCA pump rate, which are responsible for the roughly three fold increase in the period. The period varies inversely with the leak and directly with the pump rate, as first shown by Chay (1997). This is a plausible explanation for the effect of acetylcholine to increase burst frequency in β cells by stimulating IP3 production and partially emptying the ER (Bertram and Sherman, 2004). The physiologically important increase in insulin secretion that accompanies this depends on the activation of SOC, which layers a gross depolarization onto the frequency increase.

When a burst begins, c rises rapidly, due to its own intrinsic dynamics, and equilibrates with c_{ER}. Its slow rise during the remainder of the active phase is due to the slow rise in c_{ER}. The process unwinds in reverse at the end of the active phase. This is the same situation as described earlier in Figure 3.3. The slow rise of c in time corresponds to the accumulation of spikes near the homoclinic bifurcation (Figure 3.11, *upper right panel*). During that time, the c nullcline intersects the set of spike orbits (as shown in Figure 3.10b, blue nullcline). If c_{ER} remained fixed, the cell would spike forever, but c_{ER} slowly rises, which moves the nullcline slowly to the right and drags the trajectory across the homoclinic. It then falls to the bottom branch of the Z-curve and the silent phase begins.

Slow and fast phases of c rise are seen in experimental recordings from β cells, and the slow tail can be eliminated by blocking the SERCA pump,

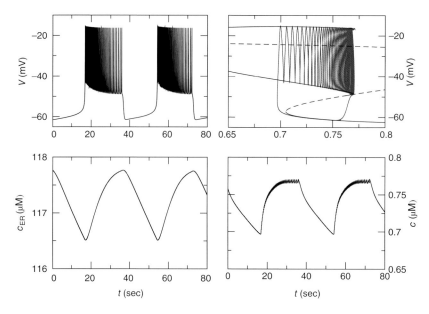

Figure 3.11 Switching on ER fluxes in the square-wave burster of Figure 3.9 increases the period dramatically. Note change in time base. Parameters in Table 3.1. c (*lower right*) now has fast and slow components from its intrinsic kinetics and the ER, respectively. The bifurcation diagram (*upper right*) is calculated with respect to c with c_{ER} fixed at its average value during bursting. The accumulation of spikes at the end of the periodic branch is responsible for the increased period.

lending credence to the model (Gilon *et al.*, 1999). Note that the period of the oscillations could have been increased by reducing the buffering ratio f_i, but this would not have corrected the sawtooth timecourse of c.

Although they look rather different, Figures 3.8 and 3.11 actually exemplify the same fundamental feature of ER-PM communication via K(Ca): in both cases, the ER steals Ca^{2+} from the K(Ca) channels and fills at the expense of c. In the former case, spike frequency is increased, and in the latter case, the active phase of the bursts is prolonged, and, either way, Ca^{2+} influx is increased.

Pseudo-plateau bursting

Next we consider a variant of plateau bursting that is more typical of pituitary cells, particularly somatotrophs and lactotrophs. A model example is shown in Figure 3.12a. At first glance, this does not seem very different from the square-wave example, Figure 3.9: both exhibit spikes from a depolarized plateau alternating with silent periods. The most apparent difference is that the spikes are smaller, and might be called "spikelets," but this could just be a quantitative difference, not a qualitative one.

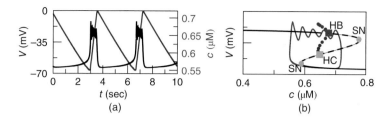

Figure 3.12 **(a) Pseudo-plateau bursting reminiscent of electrical activity in somatotrophs and lactotrophs**. Equations as in Figure 3.9; parameters in Table 3.1. (b) Bifurcation diagram. In contrast to the bifurcation diagram in Figure 3.9, the periodic orbits emanating from the Hopf bifurcation (HB) are unstable (max and min denoted by *filled red circles*).

The BD, Figure 3.12b, however is rather different. The HB now occurs between the two knees and is *subcritical*, meaning that the branch of periodic orbits bends back over the region of stable steady states. In such a case, the orbits are always unstable, though if the branch reverses back (here, that would be to the right), the orbits become stable. In this case that does not happen. Instead, the unstable branch of orbits terminates in a homoclinic orbit before it has a chance to turn around.

Consequently, there are *no stable periodic orbits* for any value of c in this model, yet there are spikes. How is this possible? The answer is that the spikes are transients. For this reason, this form of bursting is sometimes called *pseudo-plateau* bursting. We have enhanced the spikes by increasing the Ca^{2+} buffering factor f_i by a factor of 4 from the square-wave case, so that c sweeps the trajectory across the upper branch too rapidly for the spikes to squeeze down onto the stable upper branch. Nonetheless, the spikes do diminish in amplitude as they progress to the right, but only until they cross the HB, when they start to expand again.

If we looked in the V–n plane, perpendicular to the plane of the diagram, we would see them spiraling lazily toward the stable steady state to the left of the HB and then spiraling lazily away. In fact, the movement away from the unstable steady state is so slow that several spikes can be seen to the right of the HB, like Road Runner hanging in the air after running off a cliff until he realizes there is no solid ground beneath his feet. So, in order to get spikes that resemble those seen in pituitary plateau bursters, the rate of attraction of the stable steady states and the repulsion from the unstable ones have to be weak compared to the rate at which c increases.

The parameter change from the square-wave case that is mainly responsible for the above combination of properties is a shift in the activation curve of the Ca^{2+} channel to the left. The dynamic consequence is that more inhibition by K(Ca), and hence higher c, is needed to destabilize the upper steady state. This moves the HB to a point between the knees of the Z-curve. Because the HB is where the steady state changes from attracting to repelling, the upper state is weakly attracting near the bifurcation. Increasing f_i did not affect those rates because it appears only in the c equation, but helped by increasing the speed of c (and recall that it is the relative rates that matter).

In addition, we slightly increased the time constant of the V-dependent K^+ channel, τ_n to ensure that the periodic branch would end in a homoclinic before restabilizing. It has been shown that, if the system is sitting in the right part of parameter space, a single parameter change is sufficient (Osinga et al., 2012), and in Teka et al. (2011) it was shown that it can be done either by shifting the Ca^{2+} channel activation to the left or shifting the K^+ channel activation to the right. Additional changes to the slow c equation to prettify the spikes do not figure in this accounting, only changes to the V–n fast subsystem. All this can be summarized by saying that, at a sufficiently abstract level, β cells and pituitary bursters lie along a one-dimensional continuum of dynamical systems.

We do not mean to imply that pancreatic and pituitary bursters only differ in a single-ion channel property. These cells do many other things besides burst, and their developmental origins are different. It might, however, indicate that cells are sampling the space of dynamical behaviors in the way proposed here. This is all well and good; but is there any evidence that the BDs look like the ones we have drawn?

For β cells there is: Cook et al. (1981) showed that β cells could be reset from the active phase to the silent phase or vice versa by brief current pulses or external ion concentration changes. This is strong evidence for bistability between a low-V steady state and a small amplitude spiking oscillation, as predicted by the BD in Figure 3.9.

The corresponding experiment has not yet been done for pituitary cells, but the diagram in Figure 3.12 makes a clear prediction (Stern et al., 2008): resetting downward from active to silent should be possible as in the square-wave case. Resetting upward from silent to active should be much more difficult because there is no set of stable periodic orbits to be attracted to. For c to the left of the HB, there is an attracting steady state, but the examination of the V–n phase plane reveals that the basin of attraction is small – precise timing and duration of the stimulus would be required. This is a good example of a nonobvious prediction that can be made by looking at a system from an abstract dynamical systems point of view rather than the more straightforward biophysical point of view.

Losing bursting by increasing spike amplitude ...

A set of experiments on somatotrophs that *has* been done lends itself to a simple explanation using bifurcations. Van Goor et al. (2001) showed that blocking BK channels in somatotrophs could eliminate bursting and

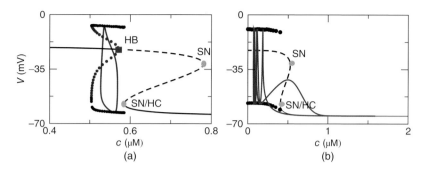

Figure 3.13   **(a) Bifurcation diagram for model of Figure 3.12 but with "BK" channel blocked to convert pseudo-plateau bursting to spiking, as seen in pituitary somatotrophs (Van Goor** *et al.***, 2001)**. Parameters in Table 3.1. The homoclinic bifurcation (HC) in that diagram has shifted leftward compared to diagram in Figure 3.12 and has merged with the saddle-node bifurcation (SN) at the left knee. (b) Bifurcation for electrical subsystem corresponding to Figure 3.7. The HB has shifted left so far that is has coalesced with a mirror-image HB at negative c and disappeared, leaving large-amplitude spiking that continues down to $c = 0$.

induce large amplitude spiking. This was discussed in terms of channel biophysics in Chapter 2, where the BK K(Ca) channel was modeled as a fast V-dependent K^+ channel. This is a reasonable approximation under the assumption that BK channels are located very close to Ca^{2+} channels and are gated by Ca^{2+} in a small domain that is in equilibrium with the single-channel Ca^{2+} flux.

We can view the V-dependent K^+ current in our simple three-variable model as a composite of BK and the slower delayed-rectifier channel. If we accept this for the sake of argument, then blocking BK would increase the effective time constant of our composite current. Figure 3.13a shows the BD of the "somatotroph" model with τ_n increased from 40 to 120 ms, along with a cosmetic decrease in the PMCA pump rate. The superimposed V–c trajectory in *blue* does indeed show a large amplitude spiking solution instead of bursting.

The BD shows why this happens: increasing the amplitude of the periodic branch tends to move the HC to the left, until it merges with the lower SN. Once this happens, there is no longer any overlap between spiking and the low-V steady state. For any fixed value of c, the system can either be silent or spiking but not both. Thus bursting of the sort in Figures 3.9 and 3.12, which depends on such co-existence, is no longer possible.

... and gaining it back by ER-PM cooperation

Bursting is, however, possible if another variable is added to the system that carries c left and right across the lower knee. In fact, we have seen such a case already. In Figure 3.7, the ER subsystem was active and included the variable h for the inactivation of the IP3R. In Figure 3.13b, we show the V–n BD with the trajectory from Figure 3.7 superimposed in *blue*. The spikes of c generated by the ER provide a drive, external to the PM subsystem, that carries the trajectory between the silent and spiking portions of the diagram.

The BDs in Figure 3.13, with branches of large amplitude spikes that terminate in a homoclinic orbit at a knee, are ubiquitous in neural models, much more common than the small amplitude spiking in Figures 3.9 and 3.12.

Such diagrams do not permit large increases in c due to spiking in the soma, but this is not a problem for neurons, which only need to send action potentials down the axon to the nerve terminal. There they trigger Ca^{2+} entry locally to drive peptide or neurotransmitter release. In small, round endocrine cells that lack axons, electrical activity and hormone release must take place in the same compartment, and plateau bursting is a way to achieve this.

An example of particular interest for this book is the GnRH model of Duan *et al.* (2011), a version of which is discussed in Chapter 4 of Sneyd *et al.* The BD of that model is very close to those shown in Figure 3.13. As such, the PM subsystem is not capable of bursting by itself – on the slow time scale it is excitable, not oscillatory (only fast oscillations, no slow oscillations). That model is also equipped with an excitable ER. It cannot generate c oscillations like those in Figure 3.7 but can throw a spike of c when Ca^{2+} entry is sufficient to trigger CICR. These two excitable subsystems can then combine in a ping-pong fashion to produce sustained oscillations.

3.5 The road goes ever on

This is the part where we have to acknowledge that the story we have told is incomplete and, in many respects, likely incorrect. For example, we have modeled the uptake and release of Ca^{2+} from the ER (in the absence of stimulation) as a balance between distinct leak and SERCA mechanisms. There is evidence, however, that SERCA is bi-directional and that the "leak" is really the pump running backward (MacLennan *et al.*, 1997). An appealing feature of this model is that as the ER fills, the pump is inhibited by the increased c_{ER}, so that at equilibrium there is no influx or efflux. This is more efficient than having large opposite fluxes, which requires constant consumption of ATP.

Also, we have discussed only the Li–Rinzel and DeYoung–Keizer models for the IP3R, in which Ca^{2+} and IP3 binding are parallel and independent. An alternative model that drops both of those assumptions and can account for more details of observed IP3R activity can be found in Sneyd and Dufour (2002).

We have moreover assumed that IP3 concentration is constant, and that the negative feedback during c oscillations is due to the inactivation of the IP3R. It is likely that in at least some cells, IP3 itself oscillates (Swillens and Mercan, 1990), particularly those with oscillations that are too slow to be governed by the relatively fast inactivation of receptors. A few studies have tried to distinguish these cases (Dupont *et al.*, 2003) (hepatocytes), (Sneyd *et al.*, 2006) (pancreatic acinar cells), but there have not been many conclusive results to date.

We have also neglected the other main ER Ca^{2+} release channel, the Ryanodine receptor, which mediates CICR in many cell types for positive feedback. Though these receptors display some degree of inactivation, this is not thought to play a role in oscillations. Negative feedback is more likely to come from depletion of the ER. An early model based on this idea is that of Friel and colleagues (Friel, 1995; Friel and Tsien, 1992). A distinguishing characteristic of such models is that the removal of extracellular Ca^{2+} rapidly terminates c oscillations as even one spike is sufficient to empty the ER (contrast with Figure 3.6).

As stated at the outset, we have only considered well-mixed cells in which Ca^{2+} gradients and diffusion are neglected. This is not justified for very large cells, such as cardiac myocytes and Xenopus oocytes, which exhibit dramatic Ca^{2+} wave propagation patterns. It is also not valid for small subregions of cells, notably the microdomains near both PM and ER Ca^{2+} channels, where Ca^{2+} concentrations can transiently be orders of magnitude larger than those in the bulk cytosol (Berridge, 2006). This means that models of, for example, IP3Rs, that assume that the receptor sees only bulk Ca^{2+} are not correct. See Smith (2002) for a worked out case of refitting DeYoung–Keizer using domain Ca^{2+} concentrations. Domain Ca^{2+} has been used to model the Ca^{2+}-dependent inactivation of Ca^{2+} channels (Sherman *et al.*, 1990), and, in this book, domain Ca^{2+} has been invoked in modeling the gating of BK K(Ca) channels (Chapter 2). Domains are also important for properly modeling Ca^{2+}-dependent exocytosis of hormones and neurotransmitter (Chen *et al.*, 2008; Pedersen and Sherman, 2009).

For more comprehensive surveys of the large literature in this area, we refer the reader to Falcke (2004) and Keener and Sneyd (2009).

We have made extensive use of fast–slow decomposition to analyze a variety of model parameter regimes with fast V and n and slow c. If the reader feels that this is not completely satisfactory for the case of pseudo-plateau bursting (Figure 3.12), this feeling is justified. In order to get the model to produce spike patterns like those seen in pituitary bursters, we had to make c considerably faster, which is at odds with the basic assumption that c can be treated as a parameter. It is also not possible to rigorously approximate the bursting system by a two-dimensional relaxation oscillator, as we did for the square-wave case (Figure 3.10a) because there is no attracting set of limit cycles. A recent alternative method of analysis classifies V as fast, but n and c as slow, and studies the two-dimensional slow subsystem (Vo *et al.*, 2010).

Certain phenomena, such as the transition from bursting to continuous spiking, require dropping fast–slow dissection entirely (Tsaneva-Atanasova *et al.*, 2010, Ermentrout and Terman, 2010). Embracing the three dimensionality of the system is in particular necessary to explain the chaotic oscillations that both square-wave and pseudo-plateau oscillations exhibit in certain parameter regimes, as chaos is not possible in two-dimensional systems.

3.6 Conclusions

The three main themes of this chapter have been ER-PM interactions, the ubiquity of activator–inhibitor kinetics and an emphasis on dynamical features rather than biophysical mechanisms. We close with general comments on the latter two.

We have used the simplest models possible and have also been guided by a metaphor based on the "Transformers" line of toys, which can change from truck to animal to robot (http://en.wikipedia.org/wiki/Transformers_(toy_line)). Thus, we have made step-wise parameter changes to produce models for "gonadotroph", "somatotroph" and "beta-cell". The resulting models are consequently not robust, incomplete in the behaviors they can exhibit and not the best model of any particular cell type. The trade-off is that they capture some key features and demonstrate the unity that lies behind the apparent diversity of cell attributes and behaviors. This approach also revealed a number of instances in which things that look similar are actually different, and things that look different are actually similar, which may not be apparent if one only does simulations of timecourses. For more examples of this with regard to bursting, see Bertram *et al.* (1995).

The didactic stress on canonical dynamic scenarios has resulted in models that ignore recent progress in understanding the biophysics and are in some sense likely incorrect, as discussed in the previous section. Hopefully, however, the models are wrong in a productive way, like the frictionless, inclined plane of elementary physics, and not the phlogiston theory of combustion. The study of physics arguably should begin with the inclined plane, not full-scale simulation of a Boeing 787. Often, more complex models can be decomposed into subsystems that operate on different time scales and hence can be analyzed semi-independently (Tyson *et al.*,

2003). Those subsystems may be two dimensional, or approximatable by two-dimensional systems, so that the phase plane methods relied on in this chapter can be applied. See, for example, Goel and Sherman (2009).

It has been argued that using models to estimate parameters may be futile once the model becomes sufficiently complex (say, 10 or more variables) because at least one of those parameters will exhibit high sensitivity and ruin the fit for the whole set (Gutenkunst *et al.*, 2007). Since any model that tries to achieve biophysical fidelity is likely to exceed this threshold of complexity, it is unlikely that models can be ruled in or out by measuring all the components. An alternative is to fit the overall behavior and use that to generate predictions that can distinguish competing hypotheses. A clear understanding of the bifurcation structure of a model and the patterns it permits is indispensable in this context.

An extreme version of such a programme is to use "normal forms," minimal models involving only polynomials. Such models have been shown to be capable of producing and rigorously classifying all the forms of bursting described here as well as many others (Osinga *et al.*, 2012).

We do not mean to suggest that specificity and biophysical verisimilitude are not also important goals. Sometimes one really needs to know such details, such as which flavour of the BK or K(V) channel is involved in a given behavior, because it could be modulated by a hormone or neurotransmitter or is a potential drug target. A limitation of simplified models is that the parameters are generally composites of multiple biophysical parameters, so it is difficult to infer what ranges of values the latter must have to generate a given pattern. Therefore, a balanced approach that uses both simplified and detailed models is needed for full understanding.

Activator–inhibitor dynamics are ubiquitous among biological models, but one may wonder whether this is due to our lack of imagination or is a genuine feature of biological systems. In favor of the latter interpretation, we note that life depends on both positive feedback and negative feedback. Without negative feedback, systems are unstable, and without positive feedback, they are inert. Dynamism requires further that the negative feedback be slower than the positive feedback. Given these elements, N-shaped nullclines will emerge and result in useful properties such as bistability and oscillations. We thus suggest that the subsets of phenomena discussed in this chapter are a microcosm of biology. As experimental techniques improve to permit observation of dynamic changes in time (and space) of general genetic and biochemical processes in cells as readily as we now track c and membrane potential, the phenomena and methods described here will become pertinent in more and more fields of investigation.

Table 3.1 Parameters for combined ER-PM model.

Name	Figure 3.7	Figure 3.8	Figure 3.9	Figure 3.11	Figure 3.12	Figure 3.13	Units
Channels							
C_m	1.0	1.0	1.0	1.0	1.0	1.0	$\mu F/cm^2$
$\bar{g}_{Ca}$	300	300	300	300	300	300	$\mu S/cm^2$
V_m	−22.5	−22.5	−22.5	−22.5	−25.5	−25.5	mV
K_m	12.0	12.0	12.0	12.0	12.0	12.0	mV
V_{Ca}	0.0	0.0	0.0	0.0	0.0	0.0	mV
$\bar{g}_{K(V)}$	720	720	720	720	720	720	$\mu S/cm^2$
V_n	0	0	0	0	0	0	mV
K_n	8.0	8.0	8.0	8.0	8.0	8.0	mV
$\bar{g}_{K(Ca)}$	500	500	60	60	200	200	$\mu S/cm^2$
$K_{m,kca}$	1.25	1.25	1.25	1.25	1.25	1.25	μM
V_K	−65	−65	−65	−65	−65	−65	mV
τ_n	0.06	0.06	0.03	0.03	0.04	0.12	s
Calcium handling							
f_i	0.002	0.002	0.001	0.001	0.004	0.004	–
α	0.05	0.2	0.05	0.05	0.05	0.05	$\mu M\ cm^2/nC$
σ	0.1	0.1	0.1	0.1	0.1	0.1	–
K_p	0.3	0.3	0.3	0.3	0.3	0.3	μM
V_p	25	100	15	15	45	20	$\mu M/s$
K_e	0.2	0.2	0.2	0.2	0.2	0.2	μM
V_e	625	625	0	2500	0	0	$\mu M/s$
L	0	6.25	0	20	0	0	$\mu M/s$
IP3R							
I	0.5	0	0	0	0	0	μM
P	20000	–	–	–	–	–	1/s
K_I	1.0	–	–	–	–	–	μM
K_d	0.4	–	–	–	–	–	μM
K_a	0.4	–	–	–	–	–	μM
A	2.0	–	–	–	–	–	$1/(\mu M\ s)$

Acknowledgments

This work was supported by the Intramural Research Program of the National Institute of Diabetes and Digestive and Kidney Diseases, National Institutes of Health, USA. Les Satin, Richard Bertram, Joe McKenna and the editors gave helpful suggestions about the presentation.

References

Berridge MJ (2006). Calcium microdomains: organization and function. *Cell Calcium* **40**(5–6): 405–412.

Bertram R, Butte MJ, Kiemel T and Sherman A (1995). Topological and phenomenological classification of bursting oscillations. *Bull Math Biol.* **57**(3): 413–439.

Bertram R and Sherman A (2004). A calcium-based phantom bursting model for pancreatic islets. *Bull Math Biol.* **66**(5): 1313–1344.

Bezprozvanny I, Watras J and Ehrlich BE (1991). Bell-shaped calcium-response curves of Ins(1,4,5)P3- and calcium-gated channels from endoplasmic reticulum of cerebellum. *Nature* **351**(6329): 751–754. *This paper showed that the steady-state open probability of the IP3R was a bell-shaped function of* Ca^{2+}, *which was the critical datum for the Deyoung–Keizer model.*

Chay TR (1997). Effects of extracellular calcium on electrical bursting and intracellular and luminal calcium oscillations in insulin secreting pancreatic beta-cells. *Biophys. J.* **73**(3): 1673–1688.

Chay TR and Keizer J (1983). Minimal model for membrane oscillations in the pancreatic beta-cell. *Biophys J.* **42**(2): 181–190. [*The first model for bursting in β cells and a foundational example for the mathematical analysis of bursting.*]

Chen YD, Wang S and Sherman A (2008). Identifying the targets of the amplifying pathway for insulin secretion in pancreatic beta-cells by kinetic modeling of granule exocytosis. *Biophys J.* **95**(5): 2226–2241.

Cook DL, Porte Jr. D and Crill WE (1981). Voltage dependence of rhythmic plateau potentials of pancreatic islet cells. *Am J Physiol.* **240**(3): E290–E296.

DeYoung GW and Keizer J (1992). A single-pool inositol 1,4,5-trisphosphate-receptor-based model for agonist-stimulated oscillations in Ca^{2+} concentration. *Proc Natl Acad Sci U.S.A.* **89**(20): 9895–9899. [*The first model for ER-driven* Ca^{2+} *oscillations based on* Ca^{2+} *feedback on IP3R*].

Duan W, Lee K, Herbison AE and Sneyd J (2011). A mathematical model of adult GnRH neurons in mouse brain and its bifurcation analysis. *J Theor Biol.* **276**(1): 22–34.

Dupont G, Koukoui O, Clair C, Erneux C, Swillens S and Combettes L (2003). Ca^{2+} oscillations in hepatocytes do not require the modulation of InsP3 3-kinase activity by Ca^{2+}. *FEBS Lett.* **534**(1–3): 101–105.

Ermentrout GB and Terman DH (2010). *Mathematical Foundations of Neuroscience.* Springer, New York, NY. [*A more mathematical approach to some of the dynamical systems ideas used in this chapter.*]

Falcke M (2004). Reading the patterns in living cells – the physics of Ca^{2+} signaling. *Adv Phys.* **53**: 255–440.

Friel DD (1995). Ca_i^{2+} oscillations in sympathetic neurons: an experimental test of a theoretical model. *Biophys. J.* **68**(5): 1752–1766.

Friel DD and Tsien RW (1992). Phase-dependent contributions from Ca^{2+} entry and Ca^{2+} release to caffeine-induced [Ca^{2+}] oscillations in bullfrog sympathetic neurons. *Neuron* **8**(6): 1109–1125.

Gilon P, Arredouani A, Gailly P, Gromada J and Henquin JC (1999). Uptake and release of Ca^{2+} by the endoplasmic reticulum contribute to the oscillations of the cytosolic Ca^{2+} concentration triggered by Ca^{2+} influx in the electrically excitable pancreatic B-cell. *J Biol Chem.* **274**(29): 20197–20205.

Goel P and Sherman A (2009). The geometry of bursting in the dual oscillator model of pancreatic β-cells. *SIAM J Appl Dyn Syst.* **8**(4): 1664–1693.

Goldbeter A, Dupont G and Berridge MJ (1990). Minimal model for signal-induced Ca^{2+} oscillations and for their frequency encoding through protein phosphorylation. *Proc Natl Acad Sci U.S.A.* **87**(4): 1461–1465. [*One of the first models for ER-driven* Ca^{2+} *oscillations that helped launch the field.*]

Gutenkunst RN, Waterfall JJ, Casey FP, Brown KS, Myers CR and Sethna JP (2007). Universally sloppy parameter sensitivities in systems biology models. *PLoS Comput Biol.* **3**(10): 1871–1878.

Hogan PG, Lewis RS and Rao A (2010). Molecular basis of calcium signaling in lymphocytes: STIM and ORAI. *Annu Rev Immunol.* **28**: 491–533.

Keener J and Sneyd J (2009). *Mathematical Physiology, I: Cellular Physiology*, 2nd edition. Springer, New York, NY. [*A good source book for models of* Ca^{2+} *oscillations in many different cell types, as well as other physiological models.*]

Li YX and Rinzel J (1994). Equations for InsP3 receptor-mediated $[Ca^{2+}]_i$ oscillations derived from a detailed kinetic model: a Hodgkin–Huxley like formalism. *J Theor Biol.* **166**(4): 461–473. [*A simplified version of the Deyoung–Keizer model, used for examples in this chapter.*]

Li YX, Rinzel J, Keizer J and Stojilkovic SS (1994). Calcium oscillations in pituitary gonadotrophs: comparison of experiment and theory. *Proc Natl Acad Sci U.S.A.* **91**(1): 58–62.

Li YX, Stojilkovic SS, Keizer J and Rinzel J (1997). Sensing and refilling calcium stores in an excitable cell. *Biophys J.* **72**(3): 1080–1091.

MacLennan DH, Rice WJ and Green NM (1997). The mechanism of Ca^{2+} transport by sarco(endo)plasmic reticulum Ca^{2+}-atpases. *J Biol Chem.* **272**(46), 28815–28818.

Meyer T and Stryer L (1988). Molecular model for receptor-stimulated calcium spiking. *Proc Natl Acad Sci U.S.A.* **85**(14): 5051–5055.

Osinga HM, Sherman A and Tsaneva-Atanasova K (2012). Cross-currents between biology and mathematics: The codimension of pseudo-plateau bursting. *Discrete Contin Dyn Syst Ser A* **32**(8): 2853–2877. (ENG).

Pedersen MG and Sherman A (2009). Newcomer insulin secretory granules as a highly calcium-sensitive pool. *Proc Natl Acad Sci U.S.A.* **106**(18): 7432–7436.

Rinzel J and Ermentrout B (1998). Analysis of neural excitability and oscillations In *Methods in Neuronal Modeling* (eds. Koch C and Segev I). The MIT Press, Cambridge, MA, pp. 251–291. [*A more mathematical treatment of the dynamical systems ideas used in this chapter.*]

Sherman A (2011). Dynamical systems theory in physiology. *J Gen Physiol.* **138**(1): 13–19. [*An elementary discussion of the utility of bifurcation diagrams for a physiology audience.*]

Sherman A, Keizer J and Rinzel J (1990). Domain model for Ca^{2+}-inactivation of Ca^{2+} channels at low channel density. *Biophys J.* **58**(4): 985–995.

Sherman A, Li YX, and Keizer J (2002). Whole cell models. In *Computational Cell Biology* (eds. Fall C, Marland E, Wagner J and Tyson J). Springer, New York, NY, pp. 101–139.

Smith GD (2002). An extended DeYoung-Keizer-like IP_3R model that accounts for domain Ca^{2+}-mediated inactivation In *Recent Research Developments in Biophysical Chemistry* (eds. Condat CA and Baruzzi A) Research Signpost Trivandrum, India.

Sneyd J and Dufour JF (2002). A dynamic model of the type-2 inositol trisphosphate receptor. *Proc Natl Acad Sci U.S.A.* **99**(4): 2398–2403.

Sneyd J, Tsaneva-Atanasova K, Reznikov V, Bai Y, Sanderson MJ and Yule DI (2006). A method for determining the dependence of calcium oscillations on inositol trisphosphate oscillations. *Proc Natl Acad Sci U.S.A.* **103**(6): 1675–1680.

Stern JV, Osinga HM, LeBeau A and Sherman A (2008). Resetting behavior in a model of bursting in secretory pituitary cells: distinguishing plateaus from pseudo-plateaus. *Bull Math Biol.* **70**(1): 68–88.

Swillens S and Mercan D (1990). Computer simulation of a cytosolic calcium oscillator. *Biochem J.* **271**(3): 835–838.

Teka W, Tsaneva-Atanasova K, Bertram R and Tabak J (2011). From plateau to pseudo-plateau bursting: making the transition. *Bull Math Biol.* **73**(6): 1292–1311.

Tsaneva-Atanasova K, Osinga HM, Riess T and Sherman A (2010). Full system bifurcation analysis of endocrine bursting models. *J Theor Biol.* **264**(4): 1133–1146.

Tyson JJ, Chen KC and Novak B (2003). Sniffers, buzzers, toggles and blinkers: dynamics of regulatory and signaling pathways in the cell. *Curr Opin Cell Biol.* **15**(2): 221–231.

Van Goor F, Li YX and Stojilkovic SS (2001). Paradoxical role of large-conductance calcium-activated K$^+$ (BK) channels in controlling action potential-driven Ca^{2+} entry in anterior pituitary cells. *J Neurosci.* **21**(16): 5902–5915.

Vo T, Bertram R, Tabak J and Wechselberger M (2010). Mixed mode oscillations as a mechanism for pseudo-plateau bursting. *J Comput Neurosci.* **28**(3): 443–458.

CHAPTER 4

A Mathematical Model of Gonadotropin-Releasing Hormone Neurons

James Sneyd[1], Wen Duan[1], and Allan Herbison[2]

[1] Department of Mathematics, University of Auckland, New Zealand
[2] Department of Physiology, University of Otago, New Zealand

4.1 Introduction

Gonadotropin-releasing hormone (GnRH) neurons exhibit complex patterns of electrical spiking. Action potentials occur in groups, often called *bursts*, and each burst is closely correlated with an increase in the concentration of intracellular Ca^{2+}. Each burst is separated by a quiet interval with no action potentials, of length ranging from a few seconds to a few tens of seconds. Although it is unclear exactly what is the physiological function of these patterns of electrical bursting, it is highly likely that they play a role in the regulation of the release of GnRH from the nerve terminal in the median eminence of the hypothalamus. GnRH in turn controls the release from the anterior pituitary of luteinizing hormone and follicle-stimulating hormone, which are crucial for sexual development and fertility. Thus, there is ample motivation for the study of the mechanisms underlying the patterns of electrical spiking seen in GnRH neurons.

Because of the highly complex dynamical phenomena observed in GnRH neurons (and, indeed, many other types of neurons), mathematical models have an important role to play. It is difficult, if not impossible, to attain a detailed understanding of the mechanisms underlying electrical bursting, and other kinds of complex oscillations, using qualitative models alone. Qualitative models (i.e., nonmathematical explanations of the behavior) are important for suggesting underlying structures and possible mechanisms, but, to test whether or not such mechanisms actually work, and to make specific predictions, a mathematical model is necessary.

Neuroendocrine neurons have, in general, some features of particular interest to modelers. The complex electrical bursting behavior is

Computational Neuroendocrinology, First Edition. Edited by Duncan J. MacGregor and Gareth Leng.
© 2016 John Wiley & Sons, Ltd. Published 2016 by John Wiley & Sons, Ltd.
Companion Website: www.wiley.com/go/Leng/Computational

necessarily a combination of at least two different oscillatory processes – one oscillatory process giving the fast electrical spiking, and the other, slower, process, causing the transitions from bursting to nonbursting regions. Although this must be true in general, it has not proven to be an easy task to determine exactly what each of these mechanisms is.

The fast spiking is reasonably well understood in many cell types, being the result of the modulation by the voltage of ionic conductances (usually, Na$^+$ and K$^+$ conductances) in the plasma membrane. Models of such fast spiking are usually based, more or less explicitly, on the model of Hodgkin and Huxley (1952). The precise nature of the conductances change, as do the parameter values, but the underlying model structure remains essentially the same.

However, the nature of the slow process (or processes) that causes the transitions between silent and active phases remains elusive, and is almost certainly different in each cell type. Some models use the intrinsic oscillatory dynamics of intracellular Ca^{2+} as the additional slow process (Chay and Keizer, 1983). Others use mechanisms based on metabolism or mitochondrial transport (Bertram *et al.*, 2004, 2007a,b).

Ultimately, it is not an easy task to determine the exact combination of oscillatory processes that causes bursting oscillations in any particular cell type. Mostly, models strive to present possible hypotheses which can then be tested, leading to the refinement of the models and additional tests. As this cycle of experiment and theory progresses through multiple models, we hope to get closer to an understanding of what is actually happening in the cell.

Here, we present a model of electrical bursting in GnRH neurons, a model that has already assisted us in understanding some of the basic mechanisms that control the length of the burst, and the length of the interburst interval.

4.1.1 Experimental data

The experimental results on which our model is based are described in detail by Lee *et al.* (2010). Here, we present only a very brief description. Intracellular calcium concentration and membrane potential were measured simultaneously in GnRH neurons in brain slices from GnRH-Pericam transgenic mice. Three different subpopulations of GnRH neurons were found. In one subpopulation (about 41%), there were no spontaneous action potentials, although action potentials could be stimulated by depolarization with KCl. In the second, small, subpopulation (3%), the action potentials were continuous, but not associated with a transient rise in [Ca^{2+}], while in the third subpopulation (56%), bursts of electrical spikes were accompanied by [Ca^{2+}] transients. It is this third subpopulation only that we consider here.

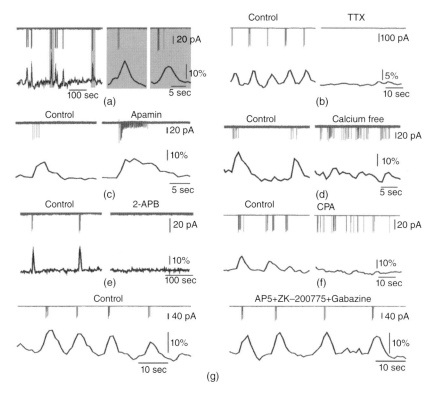

Figure 4.1   Recorded behavior of live GnRH neurons in the acutely prepared mouse brain slice, adapted from Lee *et al.* (2010). In each panel, the upper traces are the action currents, and the lower traces are the intracellular $[Ca^{2+}]$ transients. (a) Spontaneous short bursts are associated with long duration (about 10 s) $[Ca^{2+}]$ transients. (b) A blocker of voltage-gated Na^+ channel, tetrodotoxin (TTX, 0.5 μM). (c) A blocker of $[Ca^{2+}]$-dependent K^+ channels, apamin (300 nM). (d) Extracellular zero $[Ca^{2+}]$ solution. (e) A blocker of inositol trisphosphate receptors, 2-aminoethoxydiphenyl borate (2-APB, 100 μM). (f) An inhibitor of sarco/endoplasmic reticulum Ca^{2+} ATPase, cyclopiazonic acid (CPA, 30 μM). (g) Ionotropic glutamate and $GABA_A$ receptor blockers (AP-5 20 μM + ZK − 20077510 μM + Gabazine 10 μM).

For a bursting GnRH neuron, there is a clear correlation between the bursts of action potentials (or, more precisely, action current (AC) spikes) and the corresponding $[Ca^{2+}]$ transients (Figure 4.1a). The interburst interval varies from about 10 s to about 60 s, and the number of AC spikes within a burst is mostly between 2 and 10. The $[Ca^{2+}]$ transients are synchronized with the short bursts (Figure 4.1a). Importantly, the peak of the $[Ca^{2+}]$ transient occurs a few seconds after the burst has ended.

Although there is a clear evidence of stochasticity, both in the intraburst spiking pattern and in the interburst interval, here we shall focus our attention on deterministic mechanisms for controlling the bursting pattern. This allows for a simpler analysis of the model, while preserving the majority of the important dynamic features of the bursting, such as the interspike interval.

To investigate the mechanisms underlying this bursting behavior, pharmacological manipulations were used to perturb potential $[Ca^{2+}]$, influx mechanisms, and other ionic currents. Tetrodotoxin (TTX; a Na^+ channel blocker) depresses both AC spikes and $[Ca^{2+}]$ transients (Figure 4.1b). This suggests that the activation of the voltage-dependent Na^+ channel is needed for the initiation of an AC spike, with $[Ca^{2+}]$ transients following. Apamin, a blocker of Ca^{2+}-activated K^+ channels (SK channels), highly increases the number of spikes within each burst, but has little effect on the $[Ca^{2+}]$ transients (Figure 4.1c). In the absence of extracellular Ca^{2+}, $[Ca^{2+}]$ transients are almost eliminated while the bursting pattern is disorganized (Figure 4.1d).

Interestingly, blockers of the inositol trisphosphate (IP_3) receptor (IPR), such as 2-APB or Xestospongin, also eliminate both AC bursting and $[Ca^{2+}]$ transients (Figure 4.1e). The IPR is a Ca^{2+} channel located on the membrane of the endoplasmic reticulum (ER) that is activated by the second messenger IP_3. $[Ca^{2+}]$ has a biphasic effect on the IPR; at low $[Ca^{2+}]$, the steady-state open probability of the IPR increases with $[Ca^{2+}]$, but at high $[Ca^{2+}]$, the reverse is true. Thus, the IPR mediates a phenomenon known as Ca^{2+}-induced Ca^{2+} release. When $[Ca^{2+}]$ is low, a small increase in $[Ca^{2+}]$ increases the open probability of the IPR, which then releases additional Ca^{2+} from the ER, leading to a large Ca^{2+} transient. When $[Ca^{2+}]$ is high enough, the IPR shuts off, and the Ca^{2+} transient returns to baseline.

When the intracellular Ca^{2+} store is emptied by inhibiting the sarco/endoplasmic reticulum Ca^{2+} ATPase pumps (SERCA pumps) with cyclopiazonic acid (CPA), $[Ca^{2+}]$ transients are strongly depressed, while the pattern of short bursts is again disorganized (Figure 4.1f).

Since 2-APB blocks the IPR, it prevents Ca^{2+}-induced Ca^{2+} release and so eliminates the Ca^{2+} transients. At first glance, the fact that 2-APB also eliminates electrical spiking would seem to indicate that it is the Ca^{2+} transient which initiates the action potential spiking, not vice versa, as suggested by the response to TTX. This is a discrepancy we shall be considering in more detail later.

The AC spikes and $[Ca^{2+}]$ transients continue even after blocking ionotropic glutamate and $GABA_A$ receptors with a combination of receptor blockers (AP5, ZK-200775 and gabazine for NMDA, AMPA, and $GABA_A$ receptors, respectively, Figure 4.1g), from which we conclude that GnRH neurons have an intrinsic capacity to generate bursting, that is, the bursts are not generated by synaptic input from elsewhere. Although we know that neither GABA nor glutamate input is necessary to drive bursting in GnRH neurons (Lee *et al.*, 2012) – and, indeed, the blockage of

GABA/glutamate signaling has little effect on the burst properties – one has to be careful with this assumption, as it is possible that other afferent inputs play a regulatory role. However, our data indicate that, although afferent input may have a role to play, each GnRH neuron has an intrinsic capacity to generate electrical bursting, and it is this intrinsic capacity that is the major focus of our modeling efforts.

4.2   Previous models of GnRH neurons

Much of the previous modeling work on GnRH neurons has been based not on data from GnRH neurons themselves, but on data from analogous cell lines, such as GT1 cells. Although these early models, thus, have only limited direct applicability to GnRH neurons in slice preparations, they still remain the basis for all subsequent modeling work.

The earliest models of electrical spiking in GT1 cells were those of Van Goor *et al.* (2000) and LeBeau *et al.* (2000). These models have the same basic structure as the Hodgkin–Huxley equations. Thus,

$$C\frac{dV}{dt} + I_{\text{ionic}} = 0$$

where C is the membrane capacitance and V is the potential difference across the cell membrane. (For an introductory discussion of the Hodgkin–Huxley model and a brief look at the mathematical theory of that model, see Keener and Sneyd (2008).)

In the LeBeau model, there were nine different ionic conductances:

$$I_{\text{ionic}} = I_{\text{Na}} + I_{\text{CaL}} + I_{\text{CaT}} + I_{\text{KDR}} + I_{\text{M}} + I_{\text{ir}} + I_{\text{SK}} + I_{\text{SOC}} + I_{\text{d}}$$

where I_{Na} is a TTX-sensitive Na$^+$ current, I_{CaL} and I_{CaT} are L-type and T-type Ca^{2+} currents, and I_{KDR}, I_{M}, and I_{ir} are delayed-rectifier, M-type, and inward-rectifier K$^+$ currents. I_{SK} is a Ca^{2+}-activated K$^+$ current, while I_{SOC} is a store-operated Ca^{2+} channel, that is, a Ca^{2+} channel that opens when the endoplasmic reticulum is depleted of Ca^{2+}. Finally, I_{d} is a nonselective inward cation current.

Each of these currents is modeled as the product of a conductance, some gating variables, and a linear current–voltage curve. Thus, for example,

$$I_{\text{CaL}} = g_{\text{CaL}} m_{\text{CaL}}^2 (V - V_{\text{Ca}})$$

where m_{CaL} is a time-dependent gating variable satisfying the equation

$$\tau_m \frac{dm_{\text{CaL}}}{dt} = m_{\text{CaL},\infty} - m_{\text{CaL}}$$

g_{CaL} is the channel conductance, and V_{Ca} is the Nernst potential of Ca^{2+}. Many of the gating variables were set at their steady states, for simplicity.

In the model of Van Goor *et al.* (2000), there was no detailed model of the intracellular Ca^{2+} dynamics, but this was substantially improved in the subsequent version of LeBeau *et al.* (2000). In the LeBeau model, spiking was essentially caused by the Na^+ and K^+ currents, with the frequency modulated by the three pacemaker currents, I_{SK}, I_{SOC}, and I_d, all three currents being coupled to the intracellular Ca^{2+} concentration, and thus to the Ca^{2+} influx through I_{CaL} and I_{CaT}.

One of the most interesting results of the LeBeau model was their prediction of the existence of a nonselective cation current, I_d, activated by cAMP and inhibited by Ca^{2+}. Although they were unable to confirm the existence of this current experimentally, the model still demonstrated the components needed to explain the experimental results.

The Ca^{2+} handling in this model was further improved by Fletcher and Li (2009), who constructed a spatial model of the intracellular Ca^{2+}, as well as simplifying the currents in the model.

In a series of papers, Roberts and Suter and others (Roberts *et al.*, 2006, 2008b; Roberts and Suter, 2008; Roberts *et al.*, 2008a; 2009; Hemond *et al.*, 2012) constructed a GnRH model of a rather different type. Although their model was also based to an extent on the earlier work of LeBeau and van Goor, Roberts and Suter constructed a more complex compartmental model using the software package GENESIS (http://www.genesis-sim.org), and determined some of the parameters (the membrane resistance, the membrane capacitance and the axial resistance) by fitting to experimental data. The other parameters were taken from previous work, mostly from the LeBeau and van Goor models. GENESIS is a tool for constructing compartmental models of spatially distributed neurons, and was used to construct a model that gave excellent agreement with the shape of the individual action potentials in each burst. They also performed an elementary bifurcation analysis on a single-compartment version of the model, although their analysis did not focus on the mechanisms of bursting.

Possibly the most comprehensive model to date of GnRH neurons *in vivo* is that of Csercsik *et al.* (2012). They incorporated the earlier models of van Goor and LeBeau with the later model of Lee *et al.* (2010) to provide a single integrated model that reproduced the shape of the action potentials in detail, as well as incorporating the mechanisms that controlled burst length and interburst interval. Finally, the Csercsik model incorporated a simple form of soma–dendrite interaction, thus including, in a simplified form, the approach of Roberts and Suter.

Overall, these models fall into two main groups. The earlier models of Van Goor *et al.* (2000) and LeBeau *et al.* (2000), as well as the model of Fletcher and Li (2009), are based on data from GT1 cells, while the later models of Roberts and Suter (Roberts *et al.*, 2006, 2008b; Roberts and Suter, 2008), Csercsik *et al.* (2012), and Lee *et al.* (2010) are based on data from hypothalamic slices, and are, thus, presumably, more applicable to GnRH neurons *in vivo*. Nevertheless, the later models still rely to a large extent on the earlier modeling work based on GT1 cells, as there are few detailed measurements of electrophysiological parameters of the ion channels in GnRH neurons in brain slices.

4.3   A model of GnRH neurons in hypothalamic slices

Given the plethora of existing models of GnRH neurons, it is natural to ask why another model is needed. To answer this question, it is important first to make clear exactly which data the model is designed to explain, and what is the purpose of the model. Essentially, we are less concerned with the detailed structure of each individual action potential, but are more interested in the mechanisms that determine the bursting structures such as the interburst interval, or the number of action potentials in each burst.

Our original model (Lee *et al.*, 2010) was also designed to answer these same questions, and was successful (at least partially) in doing so. However, the complexity of our original model is such as to make it difficult to extract and understand the important mechanisms that control the bursting. This motivates the construction of a simpler model which nevertheless incorporates the important control mechanisms. Here, we discuss this simpler version of the model.

Because of this particular focus, our simplified model is not a good quantitative description of a single action potential. In this respect, it can compete neither with the work of Roberts and Suter, nor with the integrated model of Csercsik *et al.* However, the full model has already led to an increased understanding of behaviors on the longer time scale of the bursts, and has led to the discovery of long-lasting Ca^{2+}-sensitive hyperpolarising currents which appear to set the interburst interval. Because of this success, it is a worthwhile exercise to simplify the model, so that its underlying structure and behavior can be better understood.

From the typical experimental results shown in Figure 4.1, we conclude:

- Bursting is a spontaneous feature of GnRH neurons, and does not need to be initiated by synaptic input from outside the cell.
- The apamin-sensitive, $[Ca^{2+}]$-dependent SK channel is responsible for termination of the electrical bursting.
- The $[Ca^{2+}]$ transients consist principally of Ca^{2+} released from internal stores via the IP_3 receptor.

However, a number of questions remain. Most importantly,

- Which comes first, the $[Ca^{2+}]$ transient or the electrical bursting? On the one hand, the TTX result indicates that the AC bursting initiates the

[Ca^{2+}] transient, as blocking the bursting also stops the [Ca^{2+}] transients. On the other hand, the 2-APB (and Xestospongin) result indicates the reverse, that the [Ca^{2+}] transient initiates the bursting, as the blockage of the [Ca^{2+}] transients also prevents bursting.

- Why does a zero external [Ca^{2+}] solution increase burst frequency?
- The response to apamin shows that the SK channel plays an important role in the termination of bursting. However, what stops the activity between bursts, when [Ca^{2+}] is sitting at its baseline? In the presence of 2-APB, why does the bursting stop at all?

Our mathematical model is designed to answer these questions, at least partially. However, as we shall see, the model not only provides plausible answers to these questions, it also predicts that a previously unsuspected Ca^{2+}-gated K$^+$ channel plays a major role in the control of the interburst interval. Experimental investigation subsequently confirmed the existence of this channel in GnRH neurons, and thus the model has also played a useful predictive role.

It is worthwhile considering briefly just how these questions determine, at least partially, the structure of the model that we use to answer them. Firstly, our questions are qualitative, rather than quantitative, and thus we do not aim to build a model that reproduces the exact shape of individual action potentials. We will need to get the statistics of the bursts (histograms of interburst interval, burst length, number of spikes in a burst, etc.) as accurately as possible, but individual spikes are less important for our goals. Secondly, the questions do not address the question of spike propagation, and are thus (possibly) relatively unaffected by spatial considerations. For this initial model, we thus omit any spatial dependencies. (Interestingly, later work by Chen *et al.* (2013) shows that spatial considerations can be important, but that is not our current goal.) Finally, from the extensive earlier modeling work on GT1 cells and GnRH neurons we have a rough *a priori* idea of which ionic currents are likely to play a role, and, thus, our model has only limited freedom in which components it may use.

The model equations and parameters are based, to a greater or lesser extent, on the earlier models of Van Goor *et al.* (2000) and LeBeau *et al.* (2000). Although we have no *a priori* reason to believe that the ionic channels in GnRH neurons *in situ* are the same as those in GT1 cells, neither do we have detailed measurements of these channels in GnRH neurons, and thus our options are limited. Thus, our initial model (Lee *et al.*, 2010; Duan *et al.*, 2011) used, to a large extent, the same channels and parameters as the earlier models. However, in subsequent work, it has become clear that the full array of channels is not necessary in order to study the mechanisms underlying the interburst interval. Instead, a simpler model can be constructed to do the same job, and it is this simpler model that we mostly discuss here.

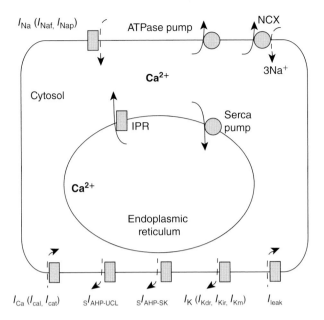

Figure 4.2   Schematic diagram of the model. I_{Na} amalgamates two different Na$^+$ currents, while I_K amalgamates three different K$^+$ currents. The I_K currents combine with the I_{Na} currents to generate oscillatory AC spiking, in the manner of the Hodgkin–Huxley model. sI_{AHP-SK} is a [Ca^{2+}]-sensitive and apamin-sensitive K$^+$ current that is activated when [Ca^{2+}] is raised, while $sI_{AHP-UCL}$ is a [Ca^{2+}]-sensitive and time-dependent K$^+$ current that is activated by raised [Ca^{2+}] and turns off only gradually, in a [Ca^{2+}]-independent manner. An inward leakage current (I_{leak}) is also included. There are five influx or efflux pathways for Ca^{2+}; the Na$^+$-Ca^{2+} exchanger, the plasma membrane ATPase pump, the IP$_3$ receptor, membrane Ca^{2+} channels and the SERCA pump. The dashed lines represent the direction of net ionic fluxes and the Ca^{2+} fluxes are denoted by solid lines.

4.3.1   The full model

Before we can discuss how our simplified model is constructed, it is first necessary to discuss briefly the construction of the full model (see Figure 4.2 for a schematic diagram). Full details can be found in Lee *et al.* (2010) and Duan *et al.* (2011).

The original GnRH neuron model consists of a membrane potential (V) submodel and a Ca^{2+} submodel, which simulate the electrical activity and Ca^{2+} dynamics, respectively. Each submodel can affect the other; the voltage submodel can affect the Ca^{2+} dyamics via the entry of Ca^{2+} through voltage-gated channels, while the Ca^{2+} submodel can affect the voltage via Ca^{2+}-gated K$^+$ channels.

Most of the currents included in the V submodel are defined by gating equations, as in the Hodgkin–Huxley model. With one exception, they are standard currents, of the type found in a variety of electrophysiological models. The exception is $I_{\text{AHP-UCL}}$, which is central to our model construction and results, and shall be discussed in more detail later.

The equation for V is of the standard form

$$C_m \frac{dV}{dt} = -I_{\text{ionic}}(V, t)$$

where $I_{\text{ionic}}(V, t)$ is the sum of all the ionic currents in the model. More precisely, $I_{\text{ionic}}(V, t)$ is the sum of 10 different ionic currents: two types of Na$^+$ current (I_{Naf} and I_{Nap}), three types of K$^+$ current (I_{Kdr}, I_{Kir} and I_{Km}), two types of Ca^{2+} current (I_{CaL} and I_{CaT}), a passive membrane leakage current (I_{leak}), and two pacemaker K$^+$ currents ($I_{\text{AHP-SK}}$ and $I_{\text{AHP-UCL}}$).

Although it looks like that there is only a single equation for V, this is deceptive, as each of the currents making up I_{ionic} is modeled by gating variables, each with their own differential equation. We do not give all these equations here in detail; the interested reader is referred to Lee *et al.* (2010) and Duan *et al.* (2011).

The Ca^{2+} submodel using two spatially homogeneous compartments, the cytosol and the ER, again using standard equations that are found in a variety of Ca^{2+} models (Keener and Sneyd, 2008). Thus, the Ca^{2+} dynamics are modeled in a simple way, but one that is sufficient for our purposes. Five Ca^{2+} fluxes are included in the Ca^{2+} submodel: influx through plasma-membrane channels (J_{in}), efflux through the Ca^{2+}-ATPase (J_{pm}) and NCX (J_{NCX}), and release (J_{release}) and uptake (J_{SERCA}) of Ca^{2+} from the ER.

The most important Ca^{2+} flux is J_{release}, which models release of Ca^{2+} from the ER through the IPR, and thus mediates the Ca^{2+}-induced Ca^{2+} release that is a central feature of the model. We assume that the flux through the IPR is an algebraic function of [Ca^{2+}], and thus all dynamic aspects of IPR modulation by Ca^{2+} are ignored.

In summary, the equations for the Ca^{2+} submodel are

$$\frac{dc}{dt} = \rho \left(J_{\text{in}} - J_{\text{pm}} - J_{\text{NCX}} \right) + J_{\text{release}} - J_{\text{SERCA}},$$

$$\frac{dc_e}{dt} = \gamma \left(J_{\text{SERCA}} - J_{\text{release}} \right)$$

where c is the cytoplasmic [Ca^{2+}], and c_e is the ER [Ca^{2+}]. The constant γ is the ratio of the ER volume to the cytoplasmic volume, and is necessary because c_e has units of moles per unit ER volume, while c has units of moles per unit cytoplasmic volume. The constant ρ is a scaling factor that describes the rate of Ca^{2+} transport across the plasma membrane compared to the rate of Ca^{2+} transport across the membrane of the ER. It is not strictly necessary to include ρ explicitly, but it is often convenient to do so, particularly for any analysis of the model.

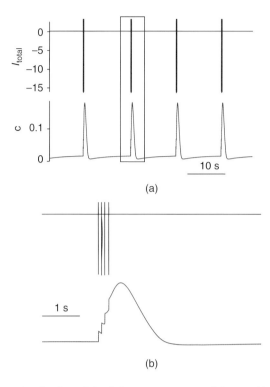

Figure 4.3 **Bursting in the original GnRH neuron model**. (a and b) Regular AC bursting and associated [Ca^{2+}] (c; drawn as blue lines) transients (panel b shows the area boxed in panel a). Four spikes can be seen in each burst, and c increases after the end of the burst.

Before we look at how this model can be simplified, it is useful first to gain a qualitative understanding of how the model behaves. Each of these channels and Ca^{2+} fluxes has a specific role to play. The Na$^+$ and K$^+$ currents generate electrical spiking, and bring in Ca^{2+} through the voltage-gated Ca^{2+} channels. This Ca^{2+} entry causes the release of more Ca^{2+} through the IPR (Ca^{2+}-induced Ca^{2+} release modeled by $J_{release}$), which activates the pacemaker currents, I_{AHP-SK} and $I_{AHP-UCL}$. I_{AHP-SK} acts relatively quickly to increase K$^+$ current, hyperpolarize the cell and stop the spiking, while $I_{AHP-UCL}$ is a slower and longer lasting K$^+$ current that prevents bursting for a longer time. Thus, to a good approximation, I_{AHP-SK} determines the length of the burst, while $I_{AHP-UCL}$ sets the interburst interval.

The most significant thing about our model is that it predicted the existence of a new channel (new for GnRH neurons at least) before it was found experimentally in that cell type. Our initial modeling efforts did not include the $I_{AHP-UCL}$ current, and were unable to reproduce the observed bursting properties. This led us to propose the existence of an additional

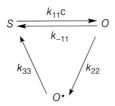

Figure 4.4 Schematic diagram of the $sI_{\text{AHP-UCL}}$ channel model. O and $O^{\star}$ are the two open states and S is the closed state. k_{11}, k_{-11}, k_{22} and k_{33} are the corresponding rate constants. This model is not based on experimental data, but is purely heuristic, being based solely on the need to have a channel that opens when $[Ca^{2+}]$ increases, but then takes a long time to close.

Ca^{2+}-activated K^+ current, that we now call $I_{\text{AHP-UCL}}$, for reasons that shall become clear later.

$I_{\text{AHP-UCL}}$ is central to how the model behaves, and is modeled in a different way from the other channels. The purpose of our $I_{\text{AHP-UCL}}$ model is to construct a channel that opens when $[Ca^{2+}]$ rises, but takes a long time to close, as these properties are necessary for setting a long interburst interval. The model is entirely heuristic, designed solely to behave in a given way. It is not based on biophysical data, or measured properties of any known channel. Thus, the model should not be interpreted as a literal biophysical mechanism, but rather as a way of representing in a Markov model the properties that are required to explain the data. A schematic diagram of the $I_{\text{AHP-UCL}}$ model is shown in Figure 4.4.

The open states are O and $O^{\star}$. The closed state is denoted as S. The transition from closed to open is dependent on $[Ca^{2+}]$, and the rate constant k_{33} is small, so that inactivation is slow.

The current through the $sI_{\text{AHP-UCL}}$ channel is modeled as

$$sI_{\text{AHP-ucl}} = g_{\text{ucl}}(O + O^{\star})(V - V_K)$$

and the kinetic equations for O and $O^{\star}$ are

$$\frac{dO}{dt} = k_{11}cS - k_{-11}O - k_{22}O$$

$$\frac{dO^{\star}}{dt} = k_{22}O - k_{33}O^{\star}$$

where k_{11}, k_{-11}, k_{22}, and k_{33} are the rate constants for the corresponding transitions, and $O + O^{\star} + S = 1$.

This full model behaves in a way that is qualitatively similar to experimental data (Duan *et al.*, 2011). In the absence of any pacemaker currents, the cell spontaneously spikes. This spiking brings in a little Ca^{2+}, which in turn stimulates Ca^{2+}-induced Ca^{2+} release from the IPR, giving a large Ca^{2+}

transient, of a characteristic form. This Ca^{2+} transient turns on the sI_{AHP-SK} channel and stops the spiking, but also turns on a second, much slower K^+ channel, the $sI_{AHP-UCL}$ channel, which remains on for a much longer time, giving a large interburst interval. Figure 4.3a shows a deterministic simulation of the regular AC behavior and the associated Ca^{2+} transients. A detailed plot of one burst is shown in Figure 4.3b. The burst consists of four spikes, and all spikes occur before the Ca^{2+} reaches its peak. More detail can be found in Duan *et al.* (2011).

4.3.2 Simplifying the model

Since the full model appears to work well, the question arises as to why one would wish to simplify it. To answer this question it is necessary to be clear about what purpose the model is supposed to serve. Our model is not designed to reproduce each individual action potential flawlessly. Instead, the focus is on trying to understand the length of the burst, and the interburst interval. Thus, the precise details of the currents that shape the action potentials are of less interest than the currents that shape the burst length and interburst interval. Similarly, our model of Ca^{2+} dynamics is a simple one, designed to give whole-cell Ca^{2+} transients, and paying no attention to spatial heterogeneities in $[Ca^{2+}]$. Again, this is because we are not here interested in detailed Ca^{2+} spatial distributions, but rather in a macroscopic view of how the whole-cell Ca^{2+} transients can shape the bursts. In keeping with this approach, it would seem that a simple model of Ca^{2+} influx through voltage-gated channels is sufficient.

Furthermore, the simpler the model is, the easier it is to analyse and to extract the important dynamical features that are causing the behavior of interest. Since this is the ultimate goal of the model, the simpler we can make the model, the better chance we have of success. Of course, this comes with the caveat that there is no point in simplifying the model past the point of physiological relevance. Simpler is not better if the physiology is lost. However, there is, unfortunately, no magic wand that we can use to simplify the model while ensuring we retain the relevant behaviors. Instead, such simplifications are approached mostly by trial and error. There are certain well-established principles and methods, but they come with no guarantee of success, and so the simplification process must be approached with great care.

As a side issue, any readers who are interested in the reasons for model simplification, and the ways in which it can be done, should study the Hodgkin–Huxley equations and their simplification, the FitzHugh–Nagumo (FHN) equations. A good reference for this is Keener and Sneyd (2008). By extracting the essential behaviors from the Hodgkin–Huxley model and recasting them in a simple two-variable form, FitzHugh constructed a model that still stands today as the pre-eminent example of an excitable system. (Related work by Rinzel (1978) and Rinzel and Keener (1983) is also highly relevant.) The FitzHugh–Nagumo model is one of the most widely studied models in applied mathematics, has played a crucial role in the theory of excitability, and is a testament to how useful a simplification can be, when done cleverly.

Returning to GnRH neurons, we seek ways to extract the principal model features that generate the behaviors of interest, while omitting detail that is unnecessary at this stage. Our simplifications focus mainly on the many different currents in the model; the Ca^{2+} submodel is already about as simple as it can be, without losing essential features.

Firstly, we decrease the number of similar currents, since we believe it will be sufficient to model GnRH neuron bursting by having just one type each of Na^+, K^+ and Ca^{2+} channels. For example, in the original model there are three types of K^+ currents (I_{Kdr}, I_{Kir} and I_{Km}). For the sake of simplicity, we omit I_{Kir} and I_{Km} and increase the conductance of I_{Kdr}. Thus, in the simplified model, I_{Kdr} is actually a combination of all the K^+ currents. Na^+ and Ca^{2+} currents are similarly simplified.

We then simplify the model further by setting fast variables to their quasi-steady states. This is not done by a formal and rigorous non-dimensionalization and time-scale reduction. Instead, the simplified model is constructed by a process of trial and error, ensuring always that the fundamental behaviors are preserved in the simpler model. In addition, physiological reasoning indicates certain variables that should remain, such as voltage, cytosolic Ca^{2+}, and ER Ca^{2+}.

The final major simplification is the observation that two variables in the full model are linearly related to one another. The H- gating variable of I_{Naf} (i.e., H_{Naf}; the analogous variable in the simplified model is H_{Na}. The use of gating variables is discussed in the appendix) and the N gating variable of I_{Kdr} (i.e., N_{Kdr}; the analogous variable in the simplified model is N_K) are related by the linear relation

$$H_{Naf} = -0.42 N_{Kdr} + 0.205$$

This can be seen in Figure 4.5 which shows the graph of H_{Naf} against N_{Kdr} over time, plotted over one burst period. There is no obvious biophysical reason for the linear relationship, it is merely something we can observe and use.

In summary, the V subsystem of the simplified model is given by

$$-C_m \frac{dV}{dt} = I_{Na} + I_K + I_{Ca} + sI_{AHP\text{-}SK} + sI_{AHP\text{-}UCL} + I_{leak}$$

$$\tau_{N_k} \frac{dN_K}{dt} = N_{K\infty} - N_K$$

where C_m is the membrane capacitance and I_{Na}, I_K, and I_{Ca} represent the Na^+, K^+, and Ca^{2+} currents, respectively. The two pacemaker currents, an

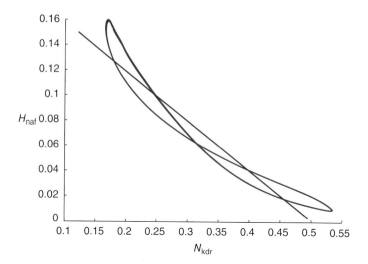

Figure 4.5 The graph of H_{Naf} against N_{Kdr} from the original GnRH neuron model. In our simplified model, these variables are denoted by H_{Na} and N_{K}, as discussed in the appendix. The butterfly shape of the graph indicates the fixed relationship between H_{Naf} and N_{Kdr}. In the simplified model, we have used the simplest form, a linear equation ($H_{\text{Naf}} = -0.42N_{\text{Kdr}} + 0.205$, the red straight line), to model this relationship.

SK-type [Ca^{2+}]-activated K$^+$ current ($sI_{\text{AHP-SK}}$) and a slow [Ca^{2+}]-activated after hyperpolarization current ($sI_{\text{AHP-UCL}}$), remain in the simplified model since they are crucial for controlling the interburst dynamics.

The SK channel model remains unchanged in the simplified model, but the $I_{\text{AHP-UCL}}$ channel model has been simplified to contain only a single dynamic variable. This was done by assuming a fast equilibrium between states S and O. In this case, we have

$$k_{11}cS = k_{-11}O$$

Then, setting $X = S + O$ we have

$$X = O\left(1 + \frac{k_{-11}}{k_{11}c}\right)$$

from which it follows that

$$\frac{dO^*}{dt} = k_{22}O - k_{33}O^*$$

$$= \frac{k_{22}k_{11}cX}{k_{11}c + k_{-11}} - k_{33}O^*$$

$$= \frac{k_{22}k_{11}c}{k_{11}c + k_{-11}}(1 - O^*) - k_{33}O^*$$

Note that $I_{AHP\text{-}UCL}$ is proportional to $O + O^*$. However, $X + O^* = 1$, from which it follows that

$$O = \frac{1 - O^*}{1 + \frac{k_{-11}}{k_{11}c}}$$

Thus, O can be written in terms of O^*, leaving us with a single dynamic variable in the model for $I_{AHP\text{-}UCL}$.

The Ca^{2+} submodel of the simplified model is unchanged from the original model. Detailed equations and all parameter values are listed in the appendix. Simulations were done with the differential equation solver ODE15s in Matlab.

4.4 Model results

As shown by the model simulations of Figure 4.6a, the regular interburst period is about 27–30 s on average, AC spikes are from −6 to 1.8 pA, and $[Ca^{2+}]$ transients vary from 0.01 to 1.1 µM. A detailed graph of one burst is shown in Figure 4.6b; just like the full model, the burst consists of four spikes, and all spikes occur before the $[Ca^{2+}]$ transient reaches its peak.

The simplified model also reproduces the responses to the same pharmacological perturbations that were studied in the full model. These results are all qualitatively similar to the experimental observations shown in Figure 4.1. TTX blocks all spiking (Figure 4.6c), while the removal of extracellular Ca^{2+} leads to continuous spiking and no Ca^{2+} transients (Figure 4.6d). This is because, if Ca^{2+} cannot enter during an action potential, there is no trigger to stimulate further Ca^{2+} release from the ER, and thus no Ca^{2+} transient to activate the K^+ channels and terminate the spiking. Apamin, which inhibits $I_{AHP\text{-}SK}$, gives longer bursts without changing the interburst interval (Figure 4.6e and f).

Blocking the SERCA pumps with CPA decreases the interburst interval, increases the number of spikes in each burst, and decreases the amplitude of the Ca^{2+} transient (Figure 4.7a). This is because the addition of CPA leads to the depletion of the ER, smaller Ca^{2+} transients, and thus less activation of the pacemaker K^+ currents. Blocking the IPR by 2-APB is slightly more complicated, as 2-APB exerts multiple effects, including blocking the IPR as well as decreasing the activity of the Ca^{2+} ATPases (Figure 4.7b). Blockage of the IPR alone has little effect. Rather it is the inhibition of the Ca^{2+} ATPases that is more important, as intracellular $[Ca^{2+}]$ rises, the pacemaker currents are activated, and the bursting stops.

The most interesting prediction to come from this model (or, more precisely, from the full model) is that, in order to get the correct interburst intervals, there has to be a Ca^{2+}-activated K^+ current that activates in a

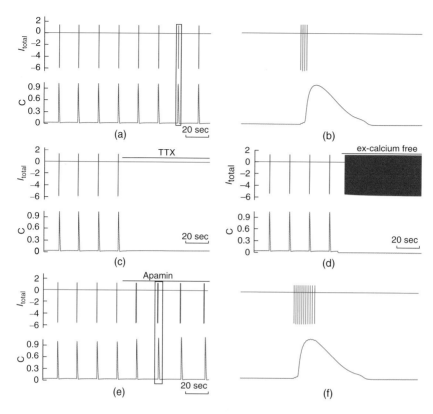

Figure 4.6 Model simulations. I_{total} denotes the total membrane current, and c denotes $[Ca^{2+}]$. (a and b) Regular AC bursting and associated $[Ca^{2+}]$ transients with the indicated detail shown in panel B. Four spikes can be seen in the burst and $[Ca^{2+}]$ increases after the end of the burst. (c) TTX simulation result, obtained by setting $g_{Na} = 0$ nS. (d) The solution in the presence of low extracellular $[Ca^{2+}]$, obtained by setting $g_{Ca} = 0$ nS. (e and f) Apamin simulation result, obtained by setting $g_{sk} = 0$. One burst after the addition of apamin is shown in panel f.

few seconds, and inactivates over a longer period. It turns out that such a current can be found experimentally (Lee *et al.*, 2010). A compound called UCL2077 is known to selectively block an after-hyperpolarization (AHP) current in hippocampal cells, and this motivated the use of UCL2077 in GnRH neurons. Application of apamin and UCL2077 to GnRH cells shows that the AHP current in GnRH neurons has two components: one mediated by the apamin-sensitive SK channel (I_{AHP-SK}) and the other current being blocked by UCL2077, but not by apamin. It is this latter channel that we call $I_{AHP-UCL}$. As predicted by the model, $I_{AHP-UCL}$ has slower kinetics than I_{AHP-SK}, and thus causes a long interburst interval. When $I_{AHP-UCL}$ is blocked, the interburst interval decreases in both the model (Figure 4.7c and d) and experiment (Lee *et al.*, 2010).

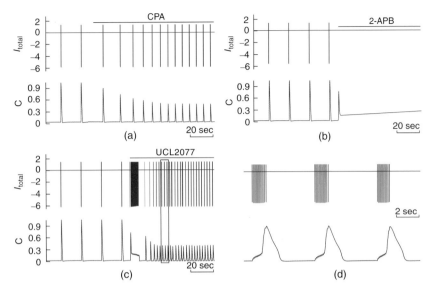

Figure 4.7 **More model simulations**. As before, I_{total} denotes the total membrane current, and c denotes $[Ca^{2+}]$. (a) The addition of the SERCA pump blocker, CPA, is simulated by setting $P_{rate} = 0$ μM pL ms^{-1}. (b) Response to the addition of 2-APB, which blocks IPR, SERCA pumps and membrane Ca-ATPase pumps. This is simulated by setting $[IP_3] = 0$, and setting the rates of the SERCA pump and the membrane Ca-ATPase pumps to 0 and 0.0005 μM pL ms^{-1}, respectively. (c) The result of blocking $sI_{AHP\text{-}UCL}$ partially. After changing the conductance of $sI_{AHP\text{-}UCL}$ (g_{ucl}) from 1050 to 750 nS, the bursting frequency gets much higher and the $[Ca^{2+}]$ amplitudes decrease. Three bursts are shown in detail in panel d.

We have, thus, now answered all the questions that we previously posed.
- It is now clear that the electrical bursting is the trigger event that initiates the Ca^{2+} transients. Although the 2-APB experiment seemed initially to be in contradiction to this result, it turns out not to be so. The model predicts that the major effect of 2-APB is through its effect on the Ca^{2+} ATPases, not through its blockage of the IPR. Thus, if it were possible to block the IPR, but without changing the activity of the Ca^{2+} ATPases, the model predicts that bursting would not disappear, but would become continuous. As yet we have not been able to test this prediction, as it is not an easy matter to block only the IPR without affecting other cellular components.
- Zero external $[Ca^{2+}]$ increases the burst frequency through the effect on voltage-gated Ca^{2+} entry. If Ca^{2+} cannot enter through the voltage-gated Ca^{2+} channels then no rise in intracellular Ca^{2+} is possible. The pacemaker currents remain unactivated, and the spiking continues indefinitely.

- Between the burst, the electrical spiking is stopped by the slower pacemaker current, $I_{\text{AHP-UCL}}$. The existence of this current was predicted by the model, which also predicted that it would have slower kinetics than the SK current. Experimental data confirmed this prediction, and showed that it is indeed a long-lasting Ca^{2+}-activated K^+ current that sets the interburst interval. In the presence of 2-APB, intracellular $[Ca^{2+}]$ increases, the two pacemaker currents are activated, and spiking is eliminated.

Our simple model contains only five differential equations, for V, N_k, O^*, c, and c_e. V and N_k form a two-dimensional fast subsystem that generates electrical spiking, while c and c_e form a two-dimensional slow subsystem that modulates the spiking over a longer time scale. O^* is a variable that connects the fast subsystem to the slow subsystem. Each of the subsystems can oscillate independently of the other, and it is the connection between these oscillatory subsystems that generates the bursting behavior.

The bifurcation structure of the simplified model turns out to be very similar to that of the original model (which is one of the reasons we believe that the simplified model contains all the important dynamic behavior of the full model).

It is possible to replace both fast and slow subsystem with generic oscillatory models, such as FHN models (Keener and Sneyd, 2008), and connect the FHN models with a variable analogous to O^* to obtain qualitatively similar bursting behavior (computations not shown). Thus, it appears that our simple model is a biophysical realization of a generic bursting mechanism based on two coupled oscillators, similar to that seen by Kopell and Ermentrout (1986) and Rinzel and Lee (1987). However, more work is needed on the exact bifurcation structure of our model before we will fully understand how the structure of our model relates to the structure of previous bursting models based on coupled oscillators.

4.5   Conclusions and future work

So far, the model has been a useful tool for helping us to understand the mechanisms that control electrical bursting in GnRH neurons. Interestingly, many of the complications of the original model turn out to be unnecessary. For example, to answer these questions, it is not necessary to include multiple types of Na^+, K^+, and Ca^{2+} channels; amalgated models of these channels suffice. Although by constructing a simplified model, we have sacrificed the ability to reproduce the exact shape of each action potential (which, to be fair, the original model does not do well either), we have gained a simpler model that can be analyzed more effectively and easily.

Many questions remain.

- Our model of $I_{\text{AHP-UCL}}$ was not based on biophysical data, and it is unlikely that it provides an accurate description of the channel's actual behavior. The description we used here is useful, but a more accurate understanding of this crucial pacemaker channel will be important for a more quantitative understanding of bursting.

- In the same vein, neither our original full model, nor the simplified model presented here, provide an accurate quantitative description of the action potentials. For a model that does a better job in this respect, the reader is referred to the work of Roberts and Suter (2008) or Csercsik *et al.* (2012). Although such quantitative accuracy is not necessary for the questions we pose here, the differences between our model and the data may well yet prove to be important, and should not be forgotten.

- Even though the experimental results clearly have a significant stochastic component, here we have used a fully deterministic model. This is mostly for convenience. A stochastic version of the same model exhibits the same qualitative behavior (Duan *et al.*, 2011) but the deterministic version provides an easier platform for the study of the model's underlying dynamic behavior.

- Although we know that GABA/glutamate inputs are not important for bursting, the possible effect of other afferent inputs is not clear. Thus the assumption that bursting in the GnRH neuron is entirely self-generated will need to be continually re-examined. However, we still have only limited understanding of the relationship between intrinsic bursting mechanisms and synaptic input. Such understanding awaits both more experimental work and a more sophisticated model.

- Real GnRH neurons are spatially distributed, and we now know that the electrical spiking is initiated at a place some 100 μm away from the soma (Iremonger and Herbison, 2012). Although preliminary computations have shown that this spatial organization of the GnRH neuron appears to be of only minor importance (Chen *et al.*, 2013), a full spatially realized model of the neuron, including the synapses, has the potential to increase our understanding of how the neuron behaves on a larger spatial scale.

4.6 Appendix: the model equations and parameters

4.6.1 The *V* submodel

In the model, the equation for the membrane potential (V) is given by

$$-C_{\text{m}}\frac{dV}{dt} = I_{\text{Na}} + I_{\text{K}} + I_{\text{Ca}} + sI_{\text{AHP-SK}} + sI_{\text{AHP-UCL}} + I_{\text{leak}} \quad (4.1)$$

where C_m is the membrane capacitance, and I_{Na}, I_K, and I_{Ca} represent the Na^+, K^+, and Ca^{2+} currents, respectively. The two pacemaker currents are an SK-type $[Ca^{2+}]$-activated K^+ current ($sI_{AHP\text{-}SK}$) and a slow $[Ca^{2+}]$-activated after hyperpolarization current ($sI_{AHP\text{-}UCL}$), which are both defined in the same way as the original GnRH neuron model (Lee *et al.*, 2010; Duan *et al.*, 2011). I_{leak} is the passive membrane leakage current.

A conventional Hodgkin–Huxley-type model for I_K is used. Thus,

$$I_K = g_K N_K^4 (V - V_K) \tag{4.2}$$

where g_K is the conductance, N_K is the activation gating variable, and V_K is the reversal potential for K^+. Similar equations govern the other voltage-dependent currents:

$$I_{Na} = g_{Na} M_{Na\infty}^3 H_{Na} (V - V_{Na})$$

$$I_{Ca} = g_{Ca} M_{Ca\infty}^2 H_{Ca\infty} (V - V_{Ca})$$

Note that H_{Na} is modeled as a linear function of N_K,

$$H_{Na} = -0.42 N_K + 0.205$$

The equation for the N_K gating variable is

$$\tau_{N_k} \frac{dN_K}{dt} = N_{K\infty} - N_K \tag{4.3}$$

where the time constant, τ_{NK} (in units of ms) is

$$\tau_{NK} = 21 (\exp((V + 30)/15) + \exp(-(V + 30)/15))^{-1} + 1.4 \tag{4.4}$$

The gating variables M_{Na}, M_{Ca}, and H_{Ca} are set to their steady-state values:

$$M_{Na\infty} = (1 + \exp(-(V + 40)/4.3))^{-1}$$

$$M_{Ca\infty} = (1 + \exp(-(V + 56.1)/10))^{-1}$$

$$H_{Ca\infty} = (1 + \exp((V + 86.4)/4.7))^{-1}$$

The equation for $sI_{AHP\text{-}SK}$ is

$$sI_{AHP\text{-}SK} = g_{sk} \left(\frac{c^{n_{sk}}}{c^{n_{sk}} + K_{sk}^{n_{sk}}} \right) (V - V_K) \tag{4.5}$$

The $sI_{AHP\text{-}UCL}$ is modeled by the same reaction scheme as in the original GnRH neuron model (Lee *et al.*, 2010; Duan *et al.*, 2011). It has two open states (O and $O^\star$), and one closed state (S), but states O and S are amalgamated using a fast equilibrium approximation (as described in detail in the text). The current through the $sI_{\text{AHP-UCL}}$ channel is modeled as

$$sI_{\text{AHP-ucl}} = g_{\text{ucl}}(O + O^{\star})\left(V - V_{\text{K}}\right)$$

where

$$\frac{dO^*}{dt} = \frac{k_{22}k_{11}c}{k_{11}c + k_{-11}}(1 - O^*) - k_{33}O^*$$

and where

$$O = \frac{1 - O^*}{1 + \frac{k_{-11}}{k_{11}c}}$$

4.6.2 The Ca^{2+} submodel

The Ca^{2+} submodel of the simplified physiological model is described in the same way as the original GnRH neuron model,

$$\frac{dc}{dt} = \rho(J_{\text{in}} - J_{\text{pm}} - J_{\text{NCX}}) + J_{\text{release}} - J_{\text{serca}}$$

$$\frac{dc_e}{dt} = \gamma(J_{\text{serca}} - J_{\text{release}})$$

where ρ is the scaling factor between plasma fluxes and ER fluxes, and γ is the ratio of the ER volume to the cytoplasmic volume. The individual Ca^{2+} flux terms are: influx via plasma membrane channels (J_{in}), efflux via the plasma membrane Ca-ATPase (J_{pm}), efflux via the Na–Ca exchanger (J_{NCX}), release and uptake of $[Ca^{2+}]$ from the ER (J_{release}, J_{serca}, respectively). These terms are exactly the same as the original GnRH neuron model (Lee *et al.*, 2010; Duan *et al.*, 2011), so we omit the details here.

The open probability of the IPR model is taken from Gin *et al.* (2009). This simplification approach has been used in the bifurcation analysis in Duan *et al.* (2011).

All the parameter values are identical to those in Duan *et al.* (2011) and Lee *et al.* (2010), so we do not give them in detail here.

References

Bertram R, Satin LS, Pedersen MG, Luciani DS and Sherman A (2007a). Interaction of glycolysis and mitochondrial respiration in metabolic oscillations of pancreatic islets. *Biophys J.* **92**(5): 1544–1555.

Bertram R, Satin L, Zhang M, Smolen P and Sherman A (2004). Calcium and glycolysis mediate multiple bursting modes in pancreatic islets. *Biophys J.* **87**(5): 3074–3087.

Bertram R, Sherman A and Satin LS (2007b). Metabolic and electrical oscillations: partners in controlling pulsatile insulin secretion. *Am J Physiol Endocrinol Metab.* **293**(4): E890–E900.

Chay TR and Keizer J (1983). Minimal model for membrane oscillations in the pancreatic β-cell. *Biophys J.* **42**: 181–190.

Chen X, Iremonger K, Herbison A, Kirk V and Sneyd J (2013). Regulation of electrical bursting in a spatiotemporal model of a GnRH neuron. *Bull Math Biol.* **75**(10): 1941–1960.

Csercsik D, Farkas I, Hrabovszky E and Liposits Z (2012). A simple integrative electrophysiological model of bursting GnRH neurons. *J Comput Neurosci.* **32**(1): 119–136.

Duan W, Lee K, Herbison AE and Sneyd J (2011). A mathematical model of adult GnRH neurons in mouse brain and its bifurcation analysis. *J Theor Biol.* **276**(1): 22–34.

Fletcher PA and Li YX (2009). An integrated model of electrical spiking, bursting, and calcium oscillations in GnRH neurons. *Biophys J.* **96**(11): 4514–4524.

Gin E, Falcke M, Wagner LE, Yule DI and Sneyd J (2009). Markov chain Monte Carlo fitting of single-channel data from inositol trisphosphate receptors. *J Theor Biol.* **257**(3): 460–474.

Hemond PJ, O'Boyle MP, Roberts CB, Delgado-Reyes A, Hemond Z and Suter KJ (2012). Simulated GABA synaptic input and L-type calcium channels form functional microdomains in hypothalamic gonadotropin-releasing hormone neurons. *J Neurosci.* **32**(26): 8756–8766.

Hodgkin A and Huxley A (1952). A quantitative description of membrane current and its application to conduction and excitation in nerve. *J Physiol.* **117**: 500–544.

Iremonger KJ and Herbison AE (2012). Initiation and propagation of action potentials in gonadotropin-releasing hormone neuron dendrites. *J Neurosci.* **32**(1): 151–158.

Keener J and Sneyd J (2008). *Mathematical Physiology* second edn. Springer-Verlag, New York.

Kopell N and Ermentrout GB (1986). Subcellular oscillations and bursting. *Math Biosci.* **78**: 265–291.

LeBeau AP, Van Goor F, Stojilkovic SS and Sherman A (2000). Modeling of membrane excitability in gonadotropin-releasing hormone-secreting hypothalamic neurons regulated by Ca^{2+}-mobilizing and adenylyl cyclase-coupled receptors. *J Neurosci.* **20**(24): 9290–9297.

Lee K, Duan W, Sneyd J and Herbison AE (2010). Two slow calcium-activated afterhyperpolarization currents control burst firing dynamics in gonadotropin-releasing hormone neurons. *J Neurosci.* **30**(18): 6214–6224.

Lee K, Liu X and Herbison AE (2012). Burst firing in gonadotrophin-releasing hormone neurones does not require ionotrophic GABA or glutamate receptor activation. *J Neuroendocrinol.* **24**(12): 1476–1483.

Rinzel J (1978). On repetitive activity in nerve. *Federation Proc.* **37**: 2793–2802.

Rinzel J and Keener J (1983). Hopf bifurcation to repetitive activity in nerve. *SIAM J Appl Math.* **43**: 907–922.

Rinzel J and Lee YS (1987). Dissection of a model for neuronal parabolic bursting. *J Math Biol.* **25**(6): 653–675.

Roberts CB, Best JA and Suter KJ (2006). Dendritic processing of excitatory synaptic input in hypothalamic gonadotropin releasing-hormone neurons. *Endocrinology.* **147**(3): 1545–1555.

Roberts CB, Campbell RE, Herbison AE and Suter KJ (2008a). Dendritic action potential initiation in hypothalamic gonadotropin-releasing hormone neurons. *Endocrinology.* **149**(7): 3355–3360.

Roberts CB, Hemond P and Suter KJ (2008b). Synaptic integration in hypothalamic gonadotropin releasing hormone (GnRH) neurons. *Neuroscience.* **154**(4): 1337–1351.

Roberts CB, O'Boyle MP and Suter KJ (2009). Dendrites determine the contribution of after depolarization potentials (ADPs) to generation of repetitive action potentials in hypothalamic gonadotropin releasing-hormone (GnRH) neurons. *J Comput Neurosci.* **26**(1): 39–53.

Roberts CB and Suter KJ (2008). Emerging methodologies for the study of hypothalamic gonadotropin-releasing-hormone (GnRH) neurons. *Integr Comp Biol.* **48**(5): 548–559.

Van Goor F, Krsmanovic LZ, Catt KJ and Stojilkovic SS (2000). Autocrine regulation of calcium influx and gonadotropin-releasing hormone secretion in hypothalamic neurons. *Biochem Cell Biol.* **78**(3): 359–370.

CHAPTER 5

Modeling Spiking and Secretion in the Magnocellular Vasopressin Neuron

Duncan J. MacGregor and Gareth Leng
Centre for Integrative Physiology, University of Edinburgh, Edinburgh, UK

5.1 Background

5.1.1 Neurons, physiology, and modeling

Magnocellular vasopressin neurons, together with their oxytocin-secreting neighbors, have been important "model systems" in neuroscience because of circumstances that make them exceptionally open to experimental study. The supraoptic nucleus contains only oxytocin and vasopressin neurons, and this greatly facilitates identifying these neurons to make recordings of their electrical activity. Most importantly, however, these neurons all project to the pituitary gland, so their primary output can be measured directly, in their respective plasma oxytocin and vasopressin concentrations. Thus, these systems are a "window on the brain", they allow us to look directly at the relationship between spiking activity and physiological function.

The first recordings of vasopressin cells announced an enigma that has provoked speculation ever since. In the rat, vasopressin cells display a distinctive phasic firing pattern that is not seen in oxytocin neurons (Figure 5.1). Many types of neurons fire in bursts, but the slow, intrinsic, phasic bursting of vasopressin cells was different from that of other neuronal populations, which mostly exhibit much faster, or network-dependent, bursting. Understanding *how* vasopressin cells burst, thus, became an important modeling target. Moreover, because of the transparency of their physiological function, combined with diverse opportunities for prediction and testing, it should also be possible, aided by models, to answer *why* these cells burst.

There have thus been many attempts to model these neurons, and both the successes and failures have formed useful steps in learning how to

Computational Neuroendocrinology, First Edition. Edited by Duncan J. MacGregor and Gareth Leng.
© 2016 John Wiley & Sons, Ltd. Published 2016 by John Wiley & Sons, Ltd.
Companion Website: www.wiley.com/go/Leng/Computational

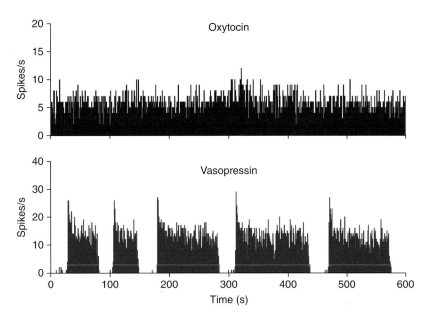

Figure 5.1   Spiking in oxytocin and vasopressin neurons. These traces show 10 min of spiking recorded from typical oxytocin and vasopressin neurons. The activity in the oxytocin neuron is mostly random. The vasopressin neuron shows a "phasic" pattern of long bursts and silences, with a distinctive peak at the start of each burst.

apply modeling to spike and pattern generation. We have developed a computational model which can reproduce the detailed firing behavior of vasopressin cells (MacGregor and Leng, 2012).

5.1.2   History matters

Most modeling papers present the finished product. This is fine if you want to know what it contributes to the physiology, or to use it as a tool, but to learn how to model, or to assess how good a model is, it helps to understand exactly how the model ended up in its final form. The final model would have been preceded by many earlier versions, even whole previous models which never made it to publication. These hidden parts can be useful to other modelers, and can also help give more confidence in the final model to the physiologists. Here, we present this story for the vasopressin neuron.

5.1.3   Detection and recording

The rat hypothalamus contains about 9000 magnocellular vasopressin neurons, mostly within the supraoptic and the paraventricular nuclei. The supraoptic nucleus contains *only* magnocellular neurons, about 70% of which make vasopressin and 30% oxytocin. Because all magnocellular neurons project to the posterior pituitary gland, and because *only* magnocellular neurons project there, it is possible to identify these neurons *antidromically*: if a stimulating electrode is placed on the neural stalk through which all axons en route to the pituitary pass, then stimuli will trigger spikes in those axons; these spikes are propagated antidromically to invade the cell bodies, with a latency that reflects the axonal length and the propagation speed.

Oxytocin cells and vasopressin cells can be distinguished from each other not only by their responses to various stimuli, but also by their spontaneous firing patterns (Figure 5.1). Most importantly, many supraoptic neurons fire in a phasic pattern, and these are almost always vasopressin cells. Phasic bursts typically begin with a rapid acceleration to a peak firing rate as high as 30 spikes/s; this peak only lasts a few seconds, subsiding to a plateau firing rate of at least 4 spikes/s and up to 10 spikes/s. The bursts usually last for 10–60 s, end abruptly, and are followed by (typically) 10–30 s of silence, punctuated by just the occasional spike. In any one cell, the pattern tends to be quite consistent, though with more variability in burst duration than in silence duration.

During lactation, oxytocin neurons also fire in bursts, but these are very unlike the bursts of vasopressin cells. In response to suckling, at intervals of several minutes, oxytocin cells synchronize to produce a short (1–3 s) and intense (50–100 spikes/s) burst of spikes that leads to a large pulse of oxytocin secretion, driving milk ejection. In contrast, the phasic firing in vasopressin neurons is *asynchronous*; even adjacent cells show no correlation in their spiking activity. Therefore, the population output is not phasic, and so if there is any *purpose* to phasic firing, it is not for generating patterning in the final output.

5.1.4   *In vivo* versus *in vitro*

Our focus is on modeling the activity of vasopressin neurons *in vivo* (in anaesthetized rats), but our model must be reconciled with data obtained both *in vivo* and *in vitro*. However, there are differences between the behavior of vasopressin cells *in vivo* and *in vitro* (and differences between *in vitro* hypothalamic slice preparations, hypothalamic explants, isolated cell preparations, and organotypic cultures). Many of these differences relate to the sparseness of synaptic input *in vitro*. The few intracellular recordings that have been made *in vivo* confirm that supraoptic neurons *in vivo* receive intense synaptic input, whereas vasopressin neurons *in vitro* typically receive very little. In slice preparations, magnocellular neurons have truncated dendrites, few of their sources of input remain within the slice, those that are may not still be connected to the vasopressin neurons, and those that do remain are themselves deafferented. The neurons still generate spikes in response to direct depolarization, but show little spontaneous spiking unless the bathing medium is adjusted by, for instance, an increase in K^+ concentration or by the addition of glutamate.

This is a general issue with *in vitro* recordings; an intact neuron in the brain may receive 10000 synaptic inputs, and if most come from active neurons, then they receive a massive barrage of excitatory and inhibitory synaptic potentials (EPSPs and IPSPs). Because most classical neurotransmitters open ligand-gated ion channels, the overall conductance state of the neuron at rest is different *in vivo* and *in vitro*; a high rate of input results in extensive opening of ion channels, reducing the cell's input resistance, with consequences for many membrane properties. The *effect* of the voltage-gated opening of ion channels depends on the cell's input resistance; if this is high, then a given change in conductance will produce a larger change in membrane voltage. Accordingly, activity-dependent mechanisms are exaggerated in *in vitro* preparations; these preparations give good access to the components of the spiking mechanism, but properties such as the magnitude and time course of voltage-dependent conductances may be altered.

Over and above this, the membrane noise that synaptic input provides can change how neurons process information. We often assume that noise is undesirable, but in complex nonlinear systems "stochastic resonance" can occur. Stochastic resonance is when an increase in levels of unpredictable fluctuations *improves* the quality of signal transmission or detection performance, rather than degrading it, raising the possibility that the brain has evolved to utilize random noise as part of the "neural code." Stochastic resonance is an essential part of osmoresponsiveness in vasopressin neurons. Vasopressin neurons possess stretch-sensitive ion channels that support depolarization in response to the cell shrinkage that accompanies a rise in extracellular osmolarity. In the physiological range of osmotic stimuli, this depolarization is too small to result in spike activity in vasopressin cells that are isolated from a synaptic input. However, the presence of fluctuations in membrane potential changes this – even a small depolarization will increase the probability that fluctuations will exceed spike threshold, allowing small sustained depolarizations to translate into increased spiking activity.

Thus, synaptic "noise" is not merely something that adds imprecision to the behavior of a neuron; it can alter how the neuron processes information. To model vasopressin cells as they operate physiologically, we must include a realistic simulation of synaptic noise. We can incorporate intrinsic mechanisms as established by *in vitro* experiments, but must be aware that the magnitude and dynamics of conductance changes will be different *in vivo* from those observed *in vitro*.

5.1.5   Outputs

Vasopressin cells project to the posterior pituitary gland, where spike activity triggers exocytosis of hormone-containing vesicles. The peptide secreted from the nerve terminals of the 9000 vasopressin cells forms a relatively smooth summed signal, which passes into the bloodstream and on to targets across the body. This is the important output, the population signal, and to understand the function of the phasic firing pattern, we must recognize that the pattern of secretion from any single cell is lost in the output of a large and asynchronous population.

In many neuronal network models, it is assumed that the output of neurons is synonymous with their spike activity. But the biologically relevant output of any neuron is *not* its spike activity, but the chemicals that it secretes. This secretion is regulated by spike activity, but the relationship is not linear, is state dependent, and often is subject to retrograde modulation by factors secreted from the post-synaptic target. Thus, the presumption that spike activity is an adequate representation of the information transmitted from a neuron is *always* unsafe. However, for vasopressin cells, we know the properties of stimulus–secretion coupling, and so we can relate our understanding of spiking behavior to the real output of these neurons.

5.1.6   Asynchronous bistability

Vasopressin cells *in vivo* are not spontaneously active; without synaptic input, they remain silent. With low rates of synaptic input, they exhibit very slow (<1 Hz) or irregular spiking. However, given enough synaptic input, they fire phasically. This is *not* because the input comes in a phasic pattern. Phasic firing involves a combination of *activity-dependent excitation* and a delayed *activity-dependent inhibition*. *Activity-dependent excitation* of bursts can be demonstrated by perturbing a vasopressin cell during its silent period with a stimulus strong enough to trigger just a few spikes. Such stimuli will trigger the onset of a burst depending (a) on the intensity and (b) on the time that has elapsed since the end of the previous burst: it becomes progressively easier to trigger a burst with increasing time. *Activity-dependent inhibition* can be observed similarly, by delivering stimuli during a burst. Stimuli will stop a burst depending (a) on the intensity and (b) on the time that has elapsed since the beginning of the burst: it becomes progressively easier to stop a burst with increasing time. Thus, *the same stimulus can stop or start bursts depending on exactly when in the burst cycle it is delivered*. This identifies the vasopressin cell as a *bistable oscillator* – it has two relatively stable states, activity and silence, and even small perturbations can "flip" the cell from either state into the other.

Knowing that vasopressin cells fire asynchronously, we can see that a brief stimulus may activate some cells, inhibit others, and have no effect on many – and which cells it activates and which it inhibits depend purely on the state of the different cells at the time of application. Phasic activity in vasopressin cells, therefore, does not depend critically on the *patterning* of their inputs and must be generated by an intrinsic mechanism. However, excitatory inputs are essential for *any* spiking in vasopressin cells *in vivo*, and these inputs can be modulated by several retrograde signals that are released from the dendrites of vasopressin cells. So in some circumstances, the input to vasopressin cells is correlated with the phasic activity, but it is the phasic activity that determines the input pattern, not the input pattern that determines the phasic pattern.

5.2 Modeling

5.2.1 Inputs, and a good place to start a model

The inputs to vasopressin cells are diverse, reflecting the multiple functions of vasopressin. Some inputs come from osmoresponsive neurons of the forebrain, including from two "circumventricular organs" – the subfornical organ (SFO) and the organum vasculosum of the lamina terminalis (OVLT). These inputs involve both excitatory inputs mediated by the neurotransmitter glutamate and inhibitory inputs mediated by gamma-aminobutyric acid (GABA).

Synaptic input consists of many small events. We expect a typical neuron to receive inputs from many different neurons, via as many as perhaps 10000 synapses. Assuming that these inputs are independent on a short timescale (tens of milliseconds), the timing of each synaptic event is essentially random. This gives us a simple way to simulate the spontaneous inputs for a model neuron, by using a random number generator to generate inputs, using a defined mean rate. Each input event generates a postsynaptic potential (PSP) which rises rapidly over 1–2 ms, to a magnitude of ~1–5 mV and then decays more slowly, over 10–20 ms. These PSPs can be either excitatory (depolarizing) EPSPs or inhibitory (hyperpolarizing) IPSPs. Because the rise is rapid, we can simplify the PSP to an instantaneous step and model the decline using a single exponential decay. PSP magnitude varies between synapses and events, and also depends on the difference between the membrane potential and the reversal potential for the ion that carries the PSP (usually mainly Na^+ for EPSPs and Cl^- for IPSPs). Just after a spike, IPSPs are smaller because the vasopressin cell is hyperpolarized, but because of this hyperpolarization, the vasopressin cell is not spiking then, so the difference in IPSP size has no consequences for spike activity. Otherwise, changes in PSP magnitude are small, and if we simplify by using a fixed magnitude for PSPs, we do not affect anything noticeably. It is always worth checking conclusions using a detailed model with variable PSP magnitudes and half-lives, and with realistic reversal potentials, but in our models of vasopressin cells, qualitative behavior is robust to such changes. Hence, in our working model, synaptic input is defined by just three parameters for EPSPs and three for IPSPs: event rate, magnitude, and decay rate. If we make these the same for EPSPs and IPSPs, we can study the neuron under conditions where the input is, on average, an exact balance between inhibition and excitation – the state at which we expect neurons generally to be, in resting conditions *in vivo*, given that we know that inhibitory synapses and excitatory synapses are approximately equally abundant on magnocellular neurons.

Box 5.1 The basic model - inputs, summation, and threshold

To simulate synaptic input, we use twin Poisson random processes to generate counts of EPSP and IPSP events (e_n and i_n) at each time step (usually 1 ms), using the mean rates I_{re} and $I_{ri} = I_{re}I_{ratio}$ (usually $I_{ratio} = 1$):

$$I = e_h e_n + i_h i_n \qquad (5.1)$$

where e_h and i_h are the PSP magnitudes, usually both 2 mV:

$$\frac{dV_{syn}}{dt} = -\frac{V_{syn}}{\tau_{syn}} + I \qquad (5.2)$$

Time constants (τ) are calculated from half-life parameters (λ) using

$$\tau_x = \frac{\lambda_x}{\ln 2} \qquad (5.3)$$

The new input I is added to the summed synaptic variable V_{syn} which decays exponentially with a half-life of usually 7.5 ms, translated into time constant τ_{syn}. This is then summed with the resting potential V_{rest} to generate the membrane potential V:

$$V = V_{rest} + V_{syn} \qquad (5.4)$$

If at time t, $V > V_{thresh}$, then spike at time t. Typically, $V_{rest} = -56$ mV and $V_{thresh} = -50$ mV.

5.2.2 Membrane potential

Hodgkin–Huxley-type models model a cell's membrane potential in detail, using representations of the dynamics driving individual ionic conductances. In contrast, in the *integrate-and-fire* (or *spike-response*) model, we only model influences on the neuron's ability to fire a spike (its "excitability"). The first of these "influences" are the PSPs. Each of these perturbs the membrane potential, which starts at a fixed resting value (the resting potential). If the membrane potential reaches a spike threshold, we record a spike. We do not model the spike's rapid changes in the membrane potential, only record its time of occurrence, but we do model the slower changes in the membrane potential which follow.

5.2.3 Post-spike potentials

The other "influences" consist of potentials generated by the cell after a spike. Vasopressin neurons express several types of voltage-gated Ca^{2+} channels, and every spike is accompanied by Ca^{2+} entry. Accordingly, repetitive spiking results in a large increase in intracellular (cytosolic) Ca^{2+} concentration ($[Ca^{2+}]_i$). This is cleared quite slowly, and it functions as a short-term memory of spike activation, influencing membrane properties via Ca^{2+}-sensitive channels. There are several types of Ca^{2+}-sensitive channels, and their time course and magnitude of activation differ, depending on channel properties, spatial distribution, proximity to the Ca^{2+} entry channels, and variable Ca^{2+} dynamics within the cell.

In vasopressin neurons, we can recognize three phases of post-spike-altered excitability that we can relate to these channels (Figure 5.2). Immediately after, and for about 30–40 ms, is a period of relative inexcitability, which reflects a *hyperpolarizing afterpotential* (HAP), mediated by a voltage- and Ca^{2+}-dependent K^+ current. This is succeeded by relative hyperexcitability, which is the result of a voltage- and Ca^{2+}-dependent *depolarizing afterpotential* (DAP), which has both a fast and a slow components. Finally, trains of spikes activate a long-lasting reduction in excitability, identified with a Ca^{2+}-dependent *afterhyperpolarization* (AHP)

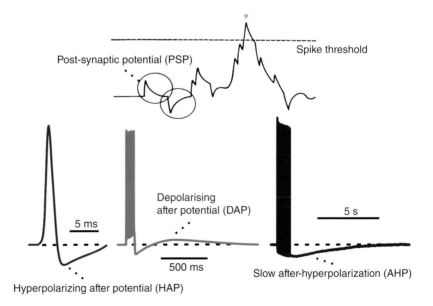

Figure 5.2 Integrate-and-fire and afterpotentials. Model simulated excitatory and inhibitory PSPs summate and trigger a spike when the sum (the membrane potential) crosses the spike threshold. Following the spike, the HAP, DAP, and AHP are simulated by decaying exponentials with varied magnitude and half-life.

that has both an apamin-sensitive, medium duration component and a slower, apamin-insensitive component.

We can either model these post-spike potentials as conductances in a Hodgkin–Huxley-type model, or model the changes in excitability as a function of spike activity in a spike-response model. Which approach we choose depends on exactly what data we are using to fit the model and what behaviors we are trying to explain. Here, we are interested in understanding the genesis of spike-activity patterns and their role in information processing, and our data come from extracellular recordings of spike activity *in vivo*. Accordingly, we are not primarily interested in the shape of spikes and are less interested in how the HAP, DAP, and AHP are formed than in their influence on spike patterning. We want a model that is inspired by the biophysical understanding from mechanistic *in vitro* studies, but quantitative data derived from *in vitro* studies cannot easily be used in a model of *in vivo* behavior because of the caveats referred to above.

A spike-response model uses deterministic functions that describe the *effects* of spike activity, rather than the underlying mechanisms, and hence can be computationally concise. Such a model aims only to match spike-timing data. For vasopressin neurons, the HAP, DAP, and AHP are the result of a superposition of spike-triggered conductance changes that have different dynamics. In a spike-response model, we model these as exponentially decaying changes in the membrane potential, and, for any given vasopressin cell, we can choose parameters for these that generate a model that is effectively indistinguishable from the recorded cell by statistical measures of spike activity.

Box 5.2 The basic model - post-spike potentials

We can model the HAP, DAP, and AHP using exponentially decaying variables, each defined by a step parameter k, defining the increase after each spike, and a time course parameter τ, defining their decay rate:

$$\frac{dHAP}{dt} = -\frac{HAP}{\tau_{HAP}} + k_{HAP}s \qquad (5.5)$$

$$\frac{dDAP}{dt} = -\frac{DAP}{\tau_{DAP}} + k_{DAP}s \qquad (5.6)$$

$$\frac{dAHP}{dt} = -\frac{AHP}{\tau_{AHP}} + k_{AHP}s \qquad (5.7)$$

where $s = 1$ if a spike is fired at time t, and $s = 0$ otherwise.

5.2.4   Spike analysis

We fit the model by applying the same analysis techniques that we use to examine the experimental data. Our analysis of experimental data begins with the series of spike times from cells recorded *in vivo*. It is possible to record spike activity from a single vasopressin cell for several hours, and, because extracellular recording does not involve damaging the cells membrane integrity, activity patterns are very stable. For a cell firing at a mean rate of 5 spikes/s (about average for vasopressin cells recorded *in vivo*), 1 h of recording yields a time series of about 18000 spike events.

From the spike times, we calculate the interspike intervals (ISIs) and generate an ISI histogram, showing the ISI distribution (Figure 5.3). If a cell has an equal chance of firing a spike at any time, that is, if spikes occur purely randomly, then the ISIs will follow a *Poisson distribution* – the number of ISIs of a given length declines exponentially with increasing length. However, this cannot be exactly true for any neuron: every neuron has an absolute refractory period when it cannot fire again after a spike, and there can be no ISIs less than about 2 ms. After the absolute refractory period, neurons have a relative refractory period, but the duration of this varies considerably between neuron types. A refractory period manifests as an obvious gap at the front of the ISI distribution (Figure 5.4), but other effects on the ISIs tend to be lost in the curved Poisson tail of the distribution, and are better detected using the *hazard function*. The hazard function is generated by transforming the ISI distribution into a plot of the probability of a spike occurring as a function of the time elapsed since the last spike

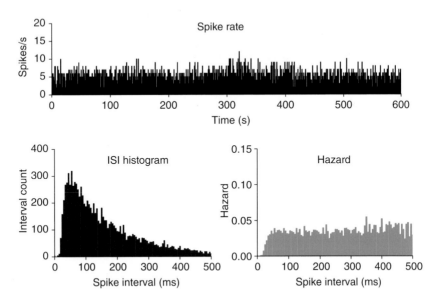

Figure 5.3 Inter-spike interval (ISI) histogram and hazard oxytocin cell example. These show short-term patterning in the spike activity. The hazard becomes less reliable at longer intervals, but a good hazard function can usually be generated for up to ~500 ms, subject to the firing rate and number of spikes in a recording.

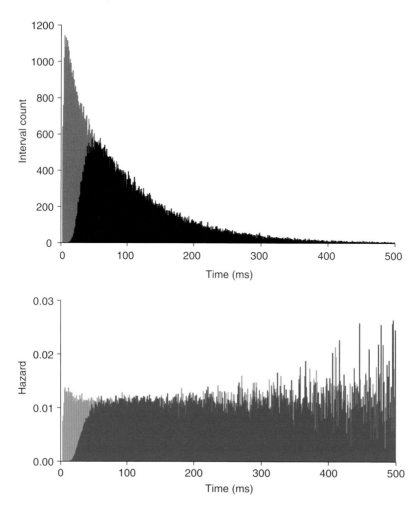

Figure 5.4   Model fitted to oxytocin cell. The dark shaded histogram and hazard show the basic model with an HAP fitted to the oxytocin cell of Figure 5.3. The light shade shows the effect of removing the HAP (hyper-polarizing afterpotential). Spiking is then only limited by the absolute refractory period (2 ms). The small peak early in the hazard shows a small increase in post-spike excitability due to the persistence of EPSPs (excitatory post-synaptic potentials).

(Sabatier *et al.*, 2004). The curved Poisson tail becomes a flat plateau, and any deviation from a constant hazard value indicates an effect of the spike on neuronal excitability (Figure 5.4).

5.2.5   A simple model

The HAP, in both oxytocin and vasopressin cells, is a spike-triggered hyperpolarization which decays over about 30–40 ms (Figure 5.2). The

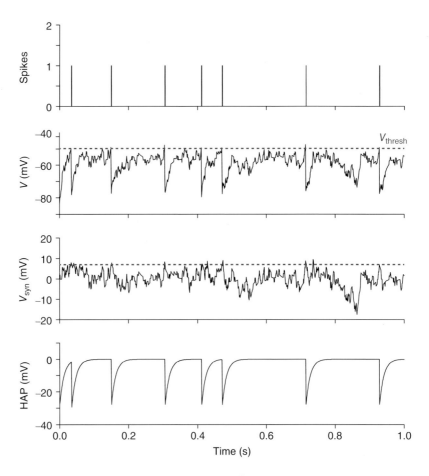

Figure 5.5   Traces of the simple oxytocin cell model. V_{syn} shows the summed random EPSPs and IPSPs. These are summed with the fixed V_{rest} to generate the membrane potential V. When this crosses V_{thresh} the model records a spike and increments the HAP, which is also summed with V, generating a post-spike refractory period.

first published spiking model studying these cells (Leng *et al.*, 2001) focussed initially on the simpler spike patterning in oxytocin neurons, represented synaptic input as randomly generated PSPs and the HAP as a fixed, step change, that occurs instantaneously with a spike, which subsequently decays exponentially (Figure 5.5), and defined by just two parameters, step magnitude and half-life (k_{HAP} and λ_{HAP}). This simple model matched the ISI distributions and hazard functions of oxytocin cells indistinguishably, showing that a simple HAP is sufficient to explain the observed refractoriness in oxytocin cells.

Box 5.3 The oxytocin cell model

Taking our basic model elements from above, we can assemble the simple oxytocin cell model:

$$V = V_{rest} + V_{syn} - \text{HAP} \tag{5.8}$$

with example parameters fitted to a recorded cell in Table 5.1. This model can be improved by adding an AHP:

$$V = V_{rest} + V_{syn} - \text{HAP} - \text{AHP} \tag{5.9}$$

fitted to the same cell using parameters in Table 5.2.

Table 5.1 Simple oxytocin model parameters.

Name	Description	Value	Units
I_{re}	Excitatory input rate	210	Hz
I_{ratio}	Inhibitory input ratio	1	–
e_h	EPSP amplitude	2	mV
i_h	IPSP amplitude	−2	mV
λ_{syn}	PSP half-life	7.5	ms
k_{HAP}	HAP amplitude per spike	30	mV
λ_{HAP}	HAP half-life	7.5	ms
v_{rest}	Resting potential	−56	mV
v_{thresh}	Spike threshold potential	−50	mV

Table 5.2 Simple oxytocin model with AHP.

Name	Description	Value	Units
I_{re}	Excitatory input rate	315	Hz
k_{AHP}	AHP amplitude per spike	0.5	mV
λ_{AHP}	AHP half-life	350	ms

5.2.6 Slower effects: the AHP

Slower effects that last beyond a single ISI and summate over a train of spikes may not be apparent in the ISI distribution, and are still difficult to distinguish in the hazard. The AHP is much smaller than the HAP, but has a much longer half-life (>500 ms), and its effects can be identified by plotting ISI duration against the mean preceding ISI duration (MacGregor *et al.*, 2009). If ISIs are independent of previous activity, then this will show no correlation (Figure 5.6); but in oxytocin cells, there is a weak inverse correlation, indicating that short ISIs are more likely to be followed by longer ISIs and vice versa. This effect accumulates, so a train of short ISIs is increasingly

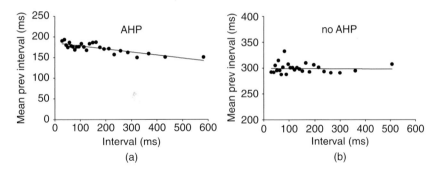

Figure 5.6 Detecting the AHP's influence using spike train analysis. Adding an AHP to the simple model and applying spike train analysis to the spike times shows a negative correlation (a), matching the same analysis applied to a recorded cell. With no AHP the model can still match the ISI histogram and hazard, but not the negative correlation (b).

likely to be followed by a long ISI. The HAP, in comparison, is usually much shorter than a single ISI, and so cannot summate during a train of spikes. Thus, although both the HAP and AHP are hyperpolarizing influences, their different magnitudes and time courses give them different roles.

The role of the AHP in this "spike ordering" effect was tested with the model (MacGregor *et al.*, 2009), using the same decaying exponential form as the HAP. The model fitted to cell data with just an HAP matches the ISI histogram and hazard, but does not show the spike-ordering effect. Adding an AHP to the model had a greater negative effect on the spike rate than expected, requiring a higher rate of synaptic input to refit the cell data, but otherwise had little effect on the fit to the ISI histogram and hazard function. It did, however, reproduce the spike-ordering effect observed in the oxytocin cell data, suggesting that it is indeed the AHP which is responsible. Functionally, the AHP in oxytocin cells acts to stabilize a cell's firing rate in that randomly occurring flurries of spikes are immediately compensated for by a counterbalancing depression of activity.

5.3 Bursting in a spiking model

5.3.1 Detecting bursting

The same type of model can also be fitted to the spike rate, ISI histogram and hazard of vasopressin neurons. However, it only matches the short timescale patterning, not the bursting. Approaching this problem first of all requires quantitative detection. Analysis techniques such as the hazard function and spike train analysis can be used to detect short timescale spike patterning which cannot be visually observed. Longer timescale patterning,

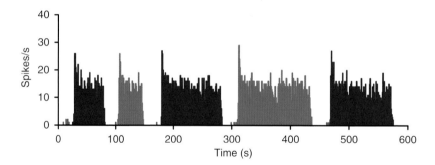

Figure 5.7 Using coloring to visualize burst detection. If you are developing your own software then simple coloring is a very useful tool for visualizing bursts and adjusting the detection parameters. The alternating green and blue make it easier to see where detected bursts begin and end.

such as phasic firing, can be crudely detected visually, by counting the number of spikes per second and plotting spike rate against time (Figure 5.1). However, for quantitative detection and analysis of phasic bursts, we use an algorithm which scans through the whole sequence of spike intervals, defining a burst by two criteria:

- a burst contains at least X spikes
- no ISI within the burst is greater than Y ms.

For vasopressin cells, we use $X = 25$ and $Y = 1500$, but by varying X and Y, this method can be adapted to detect bursting on multiple timescales, even when bursting exists at multiple scales within a single recording, such as in mitral olfactory neurons. A useful visual analysis technique is to use the time points of the detected bursts to color the spike rate plot, so that the algorithm can be checked against visual identification (Figure 5.7).

5.3.2 How does bursting work?

The key mechanism underlying phasic bursting is the DAP, which is slow enough to summate across ISIs, and by causing faster spiking, acts as a positive feedback. The presence of a DAP in vasopressin cells (but not generally in oxytocin cells) can be recognized from the hazard function, where the DAP is reflected by a peak following the HAP. The hazard function shows the sequence of post-spike effects: first the HAP, then the DAP, eventually followed by the AHP, which if large enough can be observed in the hazard as a slow, positive gradient (Figure 5.8).

The earliest hypothesis for the burst mechanism was that the DAP generates a "plateau potential" which maintains the burst. The positive-feedback effect would initially generate a rapid increase in the spike rate, which would then reach a limit at a level sufficient to allow enough spiking to maintain the "plateau." However, to explain bursting, there must also

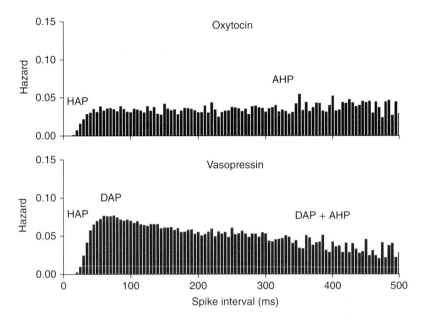

Figure 5.8   **Oxytocin versus vasopressin hazard – post-spike influence of the DAP**. The DAP generates a peak in the hazard, observed in vasopressin, but not oxytocin neurons. The peak indicates a period of increased post-spike excitability following the decay of the HAP. At longer intervals the influence of the DAP in the vasopressin hazard competes with the AHP. In the oxytocin hazard, the AHP manifests as a very gradual positive slope following the HAP.

be a mechanism for terminating the burst, and the key to this is a novel mechanism that may be particular to vasopressin cells – activity-dependent dendritic release of an autocrine inhibitory substance.

Vasopressin is not only secreted at the posterior gland but it is also released from dendrites within the hypothalamus, in an activity-dependent manner, and the endogenous opioid peptide dynorphin is co-packaged and co-secreted with vasopressin. Vasopressin cells have receptors for both vasopressin (V1a and V1b receptors) and dynorphin (which acts at kappa opioid receptors), so these peptides act as local feedback signals. Vasopressin acts mainly as a paracrine "population" signal, providing negative feedback proportional to the overall level of activity in the population. Dynorphin is released in much lower amounts (it is present at about 0.3% of the vasopressin content), but has an important role as an autocrine signal, acting on its cell of origin (Brown *et al.*, 1998). Specifically, dynorphin inhibits the effect of the DAP. Because dynorphin has modest but persistent effects, a burst can go on for tens of seconds before enough dynorphin accumulates to terminate it (Brown and Leng, 2000).

The DAP and the inhibitory action of dynorphin provide the classic pairing for generating bursts: a positive feedback, and a slower negative feedback. Positive feedback triggers and sustains the burst; eventually, it gets suppressed; the drop in activity kills the suppressor, and then the cycle repeats. Testing whether this would explain phasic firing provides a strong target for modeling.

5.3.3   Measuring, testing, and failing

In vivo (unlike *in vitro*), spiking in vasopressin cells is never fully regenerative. The DAP never brings the membrane potential of a vasopressin cell above spike threshold, but merely facilitates the depolarizing effects of membrane fluctuations. We can add a DAP to our spike-response model using the same form of decaying exponential as that for the HAP (but with opposite sign), and the parameters for magnitude and decay can be fitted to match the peak in the hazard function. This match predicts a DAP with a half-life of ~150 ms. However, models with this DAP show no bursting: the half-life is too short. *In vivo*, the ISI histogram shows that ISIs of >300 ms are common in vasopressin cells – and a modestly sized DAP (that does not lead to regenerative spiking) decays considerably in this time. We can simulate the effects of dynorphin by adding another, slower variable to suppress the DAP, but this is of no use if the DAP cannot sustain a burst in the first place. Accordingly, it seems that this type of DAP cannot explain the burst mechanism, at least not within a spike-response model.

5.3.4   Explicit bistability

Bursting and silence are two distinct activity states, both of which can be maintained for tens of seconds. When the neuron shifts between these states, the change is rapid, occurring over just a few seconds. Such bistability can be represented most simply by a differential equation for the membrane potential (v), $dv/dt = v(v - a)(v - b)$, where $1 < a < b$ (as used in Brown *et al.* (1994) to model LHRH neurons). This defines a system with two stable states ($v = 0$ and $v = b$) separated by an unstable equilibrium ($v = a$), and gives a simple way of producing phasic bursting. This was used in a bursting model, with the DAP still included to match the short-term patterning detected in the hazard, but not part of the bursting mechanism. However, while this could produce bursting, it was too simple a model to reproduce the detailed features of bursts observed *in vivo*. The next attempt (Clayton *et al.*, 2010) retained this explicit bistability, but made it more dependent on spiking activity, using a more sophisticated form informed by dynamic systems theory. This created a model with 14 parameters, and fitting the parameters by hand was replaced with fitting using a genetic algorithm along with fit measures designed to detect the match to the histogram, hazard, and measures of the bursting, including shape, mean burst duration and mean silence duration. This model produced extremely close qualitative and quantitative fits to the *in vivo* data, matching the spiking to the point of being difficult to distinguish between the model and the cell.

It could also fit a range of cells with highly varied spike rates and forms to their bursting.

5.3.5   When is a model good enough?

The focus thus far had been on producing a model that could match the form of bursts *in vivo*. The assumption was that if you could match this in detail, then the important dynamics of how the model cell responds to input would follow. Vasopressin cells only fire phasically under intense osmotic challenge when they receive a high rate of synaptic input. At low input rates, they show slow firing, and as input increases, they progress to an irregular pattern, before transitioning into full phasic firing. As input continues to increase, the bursts intensify and may lengthen, until the cells eventually shift to continuous firing. These transitions are functionally important, because phasic firing is much more effective at triggering hormone secretion than continuous spiking. The secretion mechanism is very nonlinear, and in particular, subject to fatigue: it can only maintain a high secretion rate in response to sustained spiking for about 20 s before dropping to a low rate of response, and it requires a period of silence to recover. This makes the phasic pattern optimal at triggering secretion. The Clayton *et al.* (2010) model was good at reproducing the shift from slow firing through irregular spiking into a phasic pattern and came close to matching the shift into continuous spiking but would still tend to drop into silent or slow firing periods. This could be fixed, but only by adjusting the sensitivity of the bistable mechanism. This was problematical; the model would reproduce the response of a vasopressin cell to increasing input only if we assumed that parameters of the bistable mechanism were themselves activity dependent.

5.3.6   Emergence

The problem with the Clayton model is the explicit bistability. Instead of using representations of the cell's mechanisms to reproduce bursting behavior, it abstracts directly at the required behavioral level: the resulting model thus reproduces the outward appearance of bursting, but not the underlying mechanism, and matches the *in vivo* spiking response only within a limited input range. Developing a model which reproduces the *emergent* bistability of the neuronal mechanisms, rather than using an explicit mechanism, is more challenging. The original DAP-based bursting model had attempted this and failed.

5.3.7   Two DAPs

The initial hypothesis that a DAP could explain how a burst was maintained failed because in a spike-response model, a single DAP that fits the hazard function decays too quickly to sustain bursting at the intraburst firing rate of 4–10 spikes/s, given the variability of ISI durations observed *in vivo*. Sustaining such a burst needs a slower DAP (with a half-life of ~2 s), and to avoid runaway positive feedback, there must be a "cap" on its amplitude. Adding a slow (half-life >5 s) activity-dependent decaying exponential to represent the inhibitory effect of dynorphin on the DAP can then produce bursting (Figure 5.9). The model then still needs another "fast" DAP to match the hazard function, predicting that the vasopressin cell has two DAPs: a fast DAP that dominates the effect observed in the

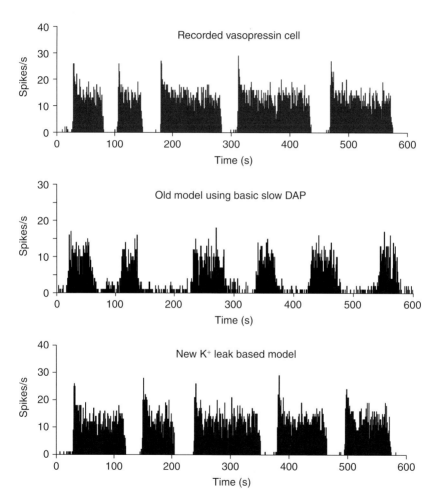

Figure 5.9   The phasic cell and the old and new model. The top panel shows the target phasic pattern, as in Figure 5.1. The old model extends the oxytocin cell model by adding a fast DAP, and a simple dynorphin opposed slow DAP. It produces bursts, but without proper silent periods, or the sharp transitions observed *in vivo* (parameters in Table 5.3). The new model uses an improved form, replacing the slow DAP with a K^+ leak current based mechanism, combining the action opposing action of dynorphin and Ca^{2+} (parameters in Table 5.4).

hazard function, and a slow DAP that is responsible for the plateau state. Recent *in vitro* recordings indicate that there are indeed two DAPs in vasopressin cells, with the fast DAP matching our predicted time course (Armstrong *et al.*, 2010).

However, bursts with this model still do not show the sharp transitions of phasic activity observed *in vivo*, and the silent period is not particularly silent; this can be improved by using a very hyperpolarized resting potential, but this affects the patterning of intraburst spiking. In a model that is subject to sustained synaptic input and that generates depolarization, it is actually more difficult to explain the silent periods than to explain the burst activity.

Box 5.4 The basic two DAP + dynorphin model

Based on the model of Box 5.3, we can match the vasopressin cell hazard by adding a DAP:

$$V = V_{rest} + V_{syn} - HAP - AHP + DAP \tag{5.10}$$

This model is sufficient to match the ISI histogram hazard, but produces no bursting. Bursting requires adding dynorphin (*D*) and a second slow DAP (DAP$_{slow}$):

$$\frac{dD}{dt} = -\frac{D}{\tau_D} + k_D s \tag{5.11}$$

Table 5.3 Basic two DAP phasic model parameters.

Name	Description	Value	Units
I_{re}	Excitatory input rate	210	Hz
I_{ratio}	Inhibitory input ratio	1	–
e_h	EPSP amplitude	2	mV
i_h	IPSP amplitude	−2	mV
λ_{syn}	PSP half-life	7.5	ms
k_{HAP}	HAP amplitude per spike	30	mV
λ_{HAP}	HAP half-life	7	ms
k_{AHP}	AHP amplitude per spike	0.25	mV
λ_{AHP}	AHP half-life	350	ms
k_{DAP}	DAP amplitude per spike	0.5	mV
λ_{DAP}	DAP half-life	150	ms
$k_{DAP_{slow}}$	Slow DAP amplitude per spike	0.75	mV
$\lambda_{DAP_{slow}}$	Slow DAP half-life	2000	ms
DAP_{cap}	Maximum for slow DAP	7	mV
k_D	Dynorphin activation per spike	0.002	a.u.
λ_D	Dynorphin half-life	25000	ms
v_{rest}	Resting potential	−62.5	mV
v_{thresh}	Spike threshold potential	−50	mV

D acts against the accumulation of DAP$_\text{slow}$:

$$\frac{\text{dDAP}_\text{slow}}{dt} = -\frac{\text{DAP}_\text{slow}}{\tau_{\text{DAP}_\text{slow}}} + (k_{\text{DAP}_\text{slow}} - D)sc \qquad (5.12)$$

where $c = 1$ if DAP$_\text{slow}$ < DAP$_\text{cap}$ and $c = 0$ otherwise.

These are assembled to give the two DAP phasic model:

$$V = V_\text{rest} + V_\text{syn} - \text{HAP} - \text{AHP} + \text{DAP} + \text{DAP}_\text{slow} \qquad (5.13)$$

Parameters for the example in Figure 5.9 are given in Table 5.3.

5.3.8 Hodgkin–Huxley

Contemporary to the spike-response model, Hodgkin–Huxley-type models (Roper *et al.*, 2004, 2003) were developed that could reproduce the *in vitro* cell activity. Although vasopressin cells *in vitro* have little synaptic input, they still fire phasically when bathed in a depolarizing medium. The conductance-based model of Roper *et al.* (2004) using a combined DAP and a dynorphin-based mechanism was able to produce bursting, although with bursts of a shorter and more regular duration than experimentally observed: in their model, the bursts are regenerative and do not depend on synaptic input. The bursting is (in some respects) unlike that seen *in vivo* – spiking is regenerative because of a large DAP, and intraburst firing is very regular (as observed *in vitro*). However, even if the quantitative behavior of vasopressin cells is different *in vitro*, the underlying mechanisms must be similar. The DAP had been thought of as an active depolarization, lifting the membrane potential to a plateau; but the Roper model (and the experimental work of Li and Hatton (1997), on which its mechanism is based) suggests the opposite: the plateau potential is the passive state, and the silent state is the one that is actively created. In other words, the DAP is not an active depolarization, but the turning off of a hyperpolarization. Could this idea, and the Roper model's formulation of the mechanisms, be used to build a better spike-response model?

5.3.9 Translation

Spike-response- and conductance-based models both model the membrane potential, but they use very different representations of the underlying mechanisms, and it is not obvious how to map them. However, in vasopressin cell models, there is a close correspondence between the spike-response model's post-spike influences, such as the HAP and DAP, and the Ca^{2+}-dependent conductances in the Hodgkin–Huxley model. In particular, the decay rates of the post-spike influences, and the conductance model's distinct Ca^{2+} compartments, use a similar set of time constants. This suggested that other elements of the more detailed model could be translated to the spike-response model.

It has not been established what channel-type underlies the slow, burst generating DAP: two suggestions are a Ca^{2+}-activated cation current and a Ca^{2+} suppressed K^+ leak current. The Roper conductance-based model uses the K^+ leak current, generating a slow DAP by suppressing a hyperpolarization instead of an active depolarization. Translated to the spike-response model, this might be able to generate both bursts and silences using a single mechanism. Its equation form (Box 5.5 in the following section) also neatly combines the effects of Ca^{2+} and dynorphin.

5.3.10 The spiking model

Adding a representation of the K^+ leak current to the spike-response model (Figure 5.10) produces the sharp transitions, and the required silent periods (Figure 5.9). It also reproduces the variation in burst duration seen *in vivo*, and most importantly, as an advance on the explicitly bistable model, matches the shift to continuous spiking at high rates of synaptic input (Figure 5.11). The model is simple enough to fit by hand: first by matching an *in vivo* cell's hazard to fit the HAP and fast DAP, and then by adjusting the AHP, Ca^{2+}, and dynorphin parameters to match the cell's mean burst form (Figure 5.12). Thus, we have our current model that provides a close quantitative match to all of the *in vivo* data that are available with us. With an apparently good enough model that can

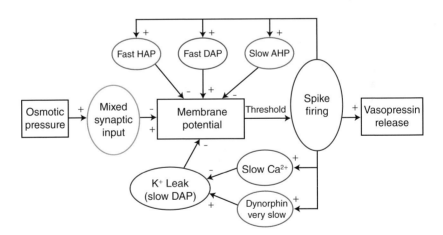

Figure 5.10 **The vasopressin spike firing model**. Input is a Poisson random timed mix of excitatory and inhibitory pulses, simulating PSPs. These are summed to generate a membrane potential which is also modulated by a set of spike triggered Ca^{2+}-based potentials. The HAP, fast DAP, and AHP are based on simple decaying exponentials, similar to a previous oxytocin cell model. The K^+ leak-current-based slow DAP which generates bursting is based on the mechanism of the Hodgkin–Huxley-type model of Roper *et al*. Spikes are generated when the membrane potential crosses a threshold value. Reproduced from MacGregor and Leng (2012) under Creative Commons Attribution (CC BY) license.

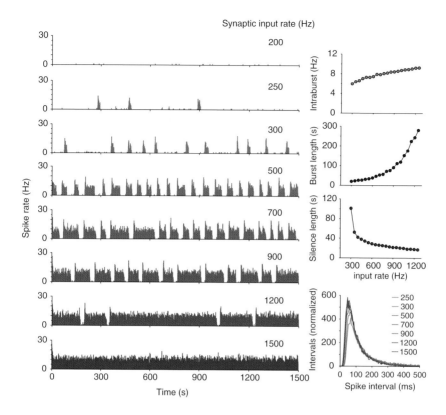

Figure 5.11   Model cell behavior with increasing synaptic input. When osmotic pressure is increased *in vivo*, we see a shift to phasic firing followed by increases in intraburst firing rate and burst duration, eventually shifting to continuous firing. Here, we reproduce this in the model by increasing synaptic input. Intraburst firing rate increases fairly linearly, whereas the increase in burst duration is much more nonlinear. Silence duration shows a fairly linear decline after phasic firing is established. Reproduced from MacGregor and Leng (2012) under Creative Commons Attribution (CC BY) license.

simulate normal activity, work since has focused on using it to further understand the mechanism and function of bursting, including how the spike activity translates into hormone secretion.

Box 5.5 The K+ leak based model

Starting from the basic two DAP model, the slow DAP variable is replaced by $[Ca^{2+}]_i$ (C):

$$\frac{dC}{dt} = -\frac{C - C_{rest}}{\tau_C} + k_C S \qquad (5.14)$$

where C_{rest} is used to scale C to physiological concentrations. This is combined with the inhibitory dynorphin variable D to generate the K+ leak-current-based on the form from the Roper model:

$$L_{act} = \tanh\left(\frac{C - C_{rest} - D}{k_L}\right) \qquad (5.15)$$

where tanh is used to produce a sigmoidal activation curve scaled by the parameter k_L.

$$V_L = g_L(1 - L_{act}) \qquad (5.16)$$

gives the final K^+ contribution to V, scaled by the conductance parameter g_L. The AHP is adapted to make it dependent on C:

$$\frac{dAHP}{dt} = -\frac{AHP}{\tau_{AHP}} + k_{AHP}s(C - C_{AHP}) \quad (0 \text{ if } C < C_{AHP}) \qquad (5.17)$$

where the parameter C_{AHP} gives a minimum $[Ca^{2+}]_i$ for AHP activation. The new V equation is then

$$V = V_{rest} + V_{syn} - HAP - AHP + DAP + V_L \qquad (5.18)$$

Parameters in Table 5.4

5.3.11 Balance and collapse

The model is based on the knowledge of the underlying mechanisms and can reproduce the observed spiking behavior under a wide range of conditions. Studying the model's $[Ca^{2+}]_i$ and dynorphin variables, Figure 5.13 shows how these evolve during the burst cycle, and how they interact with the AHP to produce the typical burst profile. At the start of the burst, both $[Ca^{2+}]_i$ and dynorphin concentration are low. The first spikes increase $[Ca^{2+}]_i$ sufficiently to trigger a positive feedback cascade that rapidly shifts the cell into fast spiking activity, which produces a rapid increase in $[Ca^{2+}]_i$. The positive feedback is limited to a plateau by the maximum conductance of the K^+ leak current. The AHP also accumulates at the start of the burst but more slowly than the activity-dependent depolarization, so after the early peak in spiking activity, there is a decline to a relatively stable intraburst plateau, as the hyperpolarizing and depolarizing influences come into balance. Dynorphin release also increases, but much more slowly, until eventually it accumulates to a level where it begins to weaken the ability of $[Ca^{2+}]_i$ to maintain the burst, and the burst becomes more vulnerable to random variation in the spiking rate. Either a distinct drop, or an increase, in depolarizing input may be sufficient to terminate the burst. A drop will further reduce $[Ca^{2+}]_i$, while an increase may temporarily strengthen the burst by increasing $[Ca^{2+}]_i$, but will also increase dynorphin release, leading to a burst termination after a few seconds of delay.

5.3.12 Antidromic challenge

These observations in the model can be used to explain the ability of stimulation *in vivo* to start and stop bursts. We can reproduce these experiments

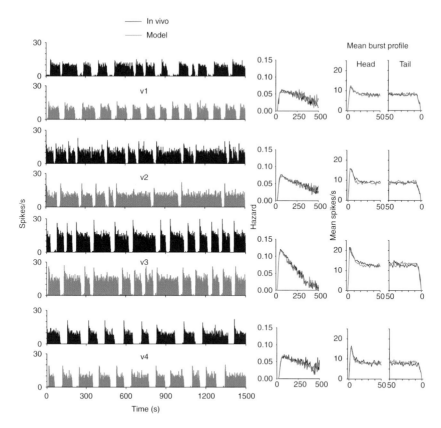

Figure 5.12   The model fitted to four typical phasic cells recorded *in vivo*. On the left, we show pairs of matched *in vivo* and model generated spike rate data, and on the right, the fitted hazard and burst profiles. The model closely matches burst profile, mean burst length, mean silence length, intraburst firing rate, and the intraburst hazard, showing post-spike excitability and patterning. A subset of eight of the model's 21 parameters were varied to match the cells. The fit parameters vary synaptic input rate, HAP half-life, AHP magnitude, fast DAP magnitude, dynorphin magnitude, Ca^{2+} magnitude, and K^+ leak conductance. The parameter values are given in MacGregor and Leng (2012), Tables 1 and 2. Adapted from MacGregor and Leng (2012) under Creative Commons Attribution (CC BY) license.

by simulating antidromic stimulation, adding extra spikes to the model's output (Figure 5.14). With the model, we have the advantage of being able to repeat an experiment with an identical pattern of synaptic input. From the model, it was predicted that stimulation should be able to stop a burst, but that this would occur with a delay – something that had not been reported previously. This prediction was accordingly tested *in vivo* and was confirmed by new experiments, providing further evidence that the model is a good representation of the real cells. The ability to start bursts by stimulating during a silent period can also be explained by the model. Following

Table 5.4 K^+ leak-based phasic model parameters.

Name	Description	Value	Units
I_{re}	Excitatory input rate	920	Hz
I_{ratio}	Inhibitory input ratio	1	–
e_h	EPSP amplitude	2	mV
i_h	IPSP amplitude	−2	mV
λ_{syn}	PSP half-life	7.5	ms
k_{HAP}	HAP amplitude per spike	60	mV
λ_{HAP}	HAP half-life	9.5	ms
k_{DAP}	DAP amplitude per spike	1.2	mV
λ_{DAP}	DAP half-life	150	ms
k_{AHP}	AHP activation factor	0.00005	mV/nM
λ_{AHP}	AHP half-life	10000	ms
C_{AHP}	Minimum $[Ca^{2+}]_i$ to activate AHP	200	nM
C_{rest}	rest $[Ca^{2+}]_i$	113	nM
k_C	$[Ca^{2+}]_i$ increase per spike	12	nM
λ_C	$[Ca^{2+}]_i$ half-life	2500	ms
k_D	Dynorphin activation per spike	3.10	–
λ_D	Dynorphin half-life	7500	ms
k_L	K^+ leak calcium sensitivity	36	nM
g_L	K^+ leak maximum voltage	8	mV
v_{rest}	Resting potential	−56	mV
v_{thresh}	Spike-threshold potential	−50	mV

burst termination, $[Ca^{2+}]_i$ falls rapidly, but dynorphin takes longer to clear, making it more difficult to trigger a burst, by requiring a larger increase in $[Ca^{2+}]_i$ to act against dynorphin. When dynorphin levels have fallen enough, triggering a burst again depends on random increases in the input depolarization.

5.3.13   Yes, but what does it do?

The importance of the antidromic results (Figure 5.14) is that they demonstrate the neurons' (and the model's) bistability. The *same* stimulus can either trigger an increase or a decrease in spike activity, depending on the current activity state, and this has a strong effect on shaping the signal response. We tested this by plotting the spiking model's mean output spike rate against increasing rates of synaptic input. Individual spikes are all-or-nothing events, and typical neurons such as the oxytocin cell (Leng *et al.*, 2001) increase their firing rate nonlinearly in response to increasing input. At first, the firing rate increases slowly, as random synaptic inputs only occasionally push the cell beyond the firing threshold, then it increases more quickly as input becomes sufficient to hold the cell close to the firing threshold. This relationship is complicated by post-spike influences, such as the AHP, which eventually slows the increase in response, generating

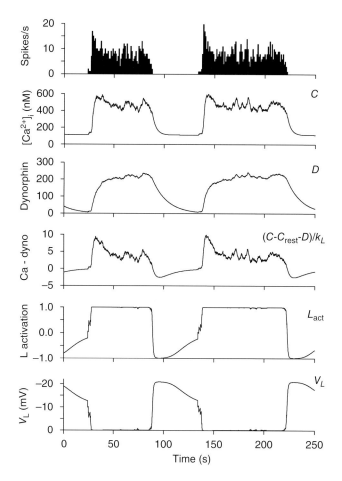

Figure 5.13   The model's burst firing mechanism. The data here show two typical bursts from the model fitted to cell v4. The burst mechanism is driven by the spike-triggered accumulation of $[Ca^{2+}]_i$ and dynorphin. The $[Ca^{2+}]_i$ signal inhibits the hyperpolarizing K^+ leak current, increasing firing and creating a positive feedback that sustains a burst. The more slowly accumulating dynorphin signal opposes the effect of $[Ca^{2+}]_i$, eventually causing burst termination and driving a silent period of sustained hyperpolarization. The positive feedback combined with the two opposing effects acting on different timescales creates an emergent bistability, shown in the rapid shifts of the K^+ leak activation (L_{act}) and the resulting effect on membrane potential (V_L). Reproduced from MacGregor and Leng (2012) under Creative Commons Attribution (CC BY) license.

a sigmoidal response curve. This is what we see in nonphasic model cells (Figure 5.15) (made so by switching off the K^+ leak current). However, the full phasic model produces a remarkably linear response over a large part of its physiological output range.

Conventionally, the "purpose" of phasic firing in vasopressin cells is to optimize their secretion response (see in the following section), but this

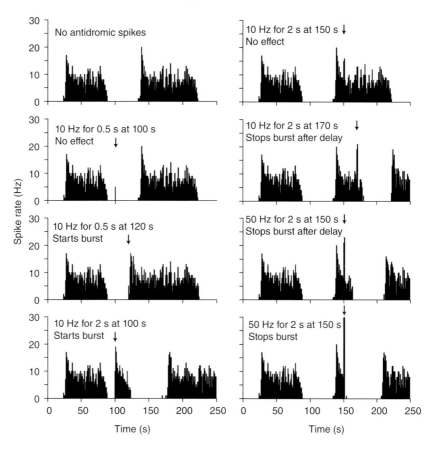

Figure 5.14   Using simulated antidromic spikes to trigger and terminate bursts. The data here use the model fitted to cell v4, repeated using the same random synaptic input. Antidromic stimulation is simulated by adding spikes to the model, at a specified frequency and time. In the left column, spikes are added during the silent period, attempting to trigger a burst. In the right column, spikes are added during the second burst, attempting to terminate the burst. Burst triggering occurs more likely when it is stimulated later into the silent period, or using a more intense stimulation. Generally, burst termination requires a more intense stimulation than burst triggering. Successful termination is more likely later into the burst, when there is more dynorphin accumulation, or with a more intense stimulation. The competing effects of spike-triggered increases in $[Ca^{2+}]_i$ and dynorphin cause a delay before termination occurs, unless the stimulation is sufficiently intense to trigger a large AHP, which immediately terminates spike firing. Reproduced from MacGregor and Leng (2012) under Creative Commons Attribution (CC BY) license.

linear response suggests that there may be another important advantage of phasic firing; for signal processing. However, as previously stated, the important output of the neurons is hormone secretion, and studying this requires another component for the model, to turn spike output into secretion.

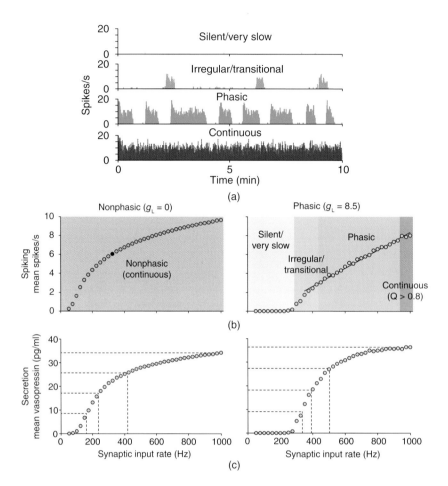

Figure 5.15 Single-cell spike rate and secretion response to increasing synaptic stimulation. The spiking model (parameters in Table 5.1) is coupled to the fitted secretion model (Table 5.2). Nonphasic spiking is generated by setting $g_L = 0$. (a) Examples of the four different modes of spike patterning generated by the same phasic spiking model with varied input rates. (b) The nonphasic model (left) shows a nonlinear increase in spike rate with increased input. The phasic spiking model (right), after very little response at low input rates, shows a more linear increase in spike rates. The rate of increase is initially steep as the patterning transitions from irregular firing to full phasic spiking, but this is followed by a wide range of very linear increase as bursts lengthen and intraburst firing rate increases. (c) The nonphasic model (left) shows a similarly nonlinear secretion response to increasing spike rate, showing a slow increase in secretion at low frequencies, followed by a facilitation driven rapid increase, which then slows along with the reduced spike rate response. The phasic secretion profile (right) shows an initial steep increase which slows as the intraburst spike rate reaches the optimal response frequency, and longer bursts allow less recovery from fatigue. Reproduced from MacGregor and Leng (2013) under Creative Commons Attribution (CC BY) license.

5.4 Modeling spike-triggered secretion

5.4.1 Secretion

Vasopressin is synthesized in the cell body and packaged into large, dense core vesicles which are transported down the axon to the secretory terminals, of which each cell has about 2000. A few vesicles at each terminal are docked close to the membrane in a releasable pool, the rest are part of a reserve pool (store). Spike activity conducted down the axon produces Ca^{2+} entry as the spike invades the terminal, and this triggers vesicle exocytosis. A simple model might make secretion proportional to the mean spiking rate over some time window, or just a fixed amount of secretion per spike, but the relationship between spiking activity and secretion is much more complex. Spikes do not always successfully invade the terminal, and terminal spike duration varies, changing the amount of Ca^{2+} entry, and the rate of secretion in response to Ca^{2+} entry depends on the size of the releasable pool. All of these influences are activity dependent, and thus stimulus–secretion coupling is highly nonlinear, subject to both *frequency facilitation*, increasing secretion per spike, and *fatigue* – a vasopressin cell can only maintain a high secretion rate in response to sustained spiking for about 20 s before dropping to a low rate of response, and it requires a period of silence to recover.

In MacGregor and Leng (2013), we modeled secretion from a single vasopressin cell as though it came from one compartment, rather than from the thousands of individual terminals and swellings, and fitted it to experimental data in which secretion from the isolated pituitary was evoked by electrical stimulation, using either a regular pattern or patterns recorded from neurons *in vivo*.

In the model, as in the biological system, secretion is triggered by spike-generated Ca^{2+} entry, and as spike frequency increases, the spikes at the terminal broaden (due to the voltage sensitive suppression of a K^+ conductance), increasing Ca^{2+} entry. At higher spike rates, this facilitation effect is opposed by a Ca^{2+}-dependent Ca^{2+} channel inactivation, acting as a fast negative feedback. Thus, as the frequency of stimulation increases, there is an initial increase in vasopressin secretion per spike, which peaks at about 15 Hz before slowly declining. However, when the axon terminals are subject to sustained stimulation, another slower negative feedback generates the fatigue effect. At 13 Hz stimulation (the most common experimental protocol), the amount of vasopressin secreted declines progressively after about 10 s, but if stimulation is interrupted for 10 s or longer, the secretory response recovers. We modeled this slow suppression of secretion as due to a long-lasting Ca^{2+}-activated K^+ conductance, which hyperpolarizes the terminals, leading to an increase in the failure of spike invasion.

5.4.2 The secretion model

The secretion model (Figure 5.16) comprises a set of differential equations which take as input the spikes generated by the spiking model. Exocytosis occurs at sites that are close to clusters of voltage-gated Ca^{2+} channels that experience high Ca^{2+} concentrations in response to spike activity, so secretion is modeled as proportional to a "fast" variable e that represents the submembrane Ca^{2+} concentration. Spike broadening (b) affects secretion by producing a larger rise in e, limited by the Ca^{2+}-dependent inactivation of Ca^{2+} channels: b is incremented by k_b, and decays exponentially with half-life λ_b (converted to time constant τ_b). The fatigue effect acts through a "slow" variable c, representing intracellular (cytosolic) Ca^{2+} accumulation, acting on the slowly activating Ca^{2+}-activated K^+ conductance. These effects, which reflect both increased spike propagation failure and the inactivation of Ca^{2+} channels, are represented in a simplified form as a reduction in the Ca^{2+} entry per spike. The model also has a finite vesicle store with two pools: a large reserve (r) and a smaller releasable pool (p).

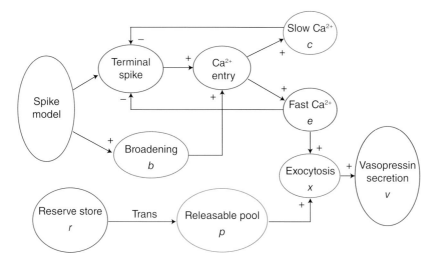

Figure 5.16 The vasopressin secretion model. Schematic illustrating the structure of the differential-equation-based single-neuron secretion model. The model takes as input either a regular spike protocol or the output from the integrate-and-fire-based spiking model. For a single vasopressin cell, secretion occurs from about 2000 terminals and swellings; in the model, secretion is represented as coming from a single compartment; thus secretion is treated as a single continuous variable rather than many discrete stochastic variables. In the model, Ca^{2+} entry is modulated by both fast (e) and slow (c) Ca^{2+} variables through their modulation of axonal terminal excitability, and is also a function of spike broadening (b). The secretion rate (vesicle exocytosis) is the product of the releasable pool (p) and the fast Ca^{2+} variable (e). When depleted, pool p is refilled from a reserve store (r) at a rate dependent on the store content. Reproduced from MacGregor and Leng (2013) under Creative Commons Attribution (CC BY) license.

The spiking model interacts with the secretion model through variables b, c, and e, which are incremented with every spike. Thus,

$$\frac{db}{dt} = -\frac{b}{\tau_b} + k_b s \tag{5.19}$$

where $s = 1$ if a spike is fired at time t, and $s = 0$ otherwise. c and e are incremented at a rate governed by Ca^{2+} entry (Ca_{ent}), with the similar exponential decay

$$\frac{dc}{dt} = -\frac{c}{\tau_c} + k_c Ca_{ent} s \tag{5.20}$$

$$\frac{de}{dt} = -\frac{e}{\tau_e} + k_e Ca_{ent} s \tag{5.21}$$

Ca^{2+} entry depends on b and is subject to Ca^{2+}-dependent inactivation (e_{inhib}) and spike failure (c_{inhib}):

$$Ca_{ent} = e_{inhib} c_{inhib} (b + b_{base}) \tag{5.22}$$

where b_{base} gives a basal level for b. Entry is inhibited by c and e using two inverted Hill equations with the threshold and coefficient parameters, c_θ, e_θ, c_n, and e_n:

$$c_{inhib} = 1 - \frac{c^{c_n}}{c^{c_n} + c_\theta^{c_n}} \tag{5.23}$$

$$e_{inhib} = 1 - \frac{e^{e_n}}{e^{e_n} + e_\theta^{e_n}} \tag{5.24}$$

The releasable pool (p) is depleted with secretion, x, and refilled at a rate proportional to r, unless it is full ($p = p_{max}$). The refill rate is scaled by β:

$$\frac{dp}{dt} = -x + \beta \frac{r}{r_{max}} \tag{5.25}$$

where $p < p_{max}$, $-x$ otherwise. The reserve (r) is depleted as it refills p, with its maximum (and initial) value defined by r_{max}:

$$\frac{dr}{dt} = -\beta \frac{r}{r_{max}} \tag{5.26}$$

where $p < p_{max}$, 0 otherwise. The rate of secretion (x) is the product of the cube of e (Ca^{2+} activation of exocytosis is thought to be cooperative) and the releasable pool (p):

$$x = e^3 \alpha p \tag{5.27}$$

Parameter α scales secretion to units that match experimental data. The final output, vasopressin plasma concentration (v), increases with secretion (x) and decays with half-life λ_v, the value of which is fixed as the experimentally determined half-life of vasopressin in plasma:

$$\frac{dv}{dt} = -\frac{v}{\tau_v} + x \tag{5.28}$$

Table 5.5 Secretion model parameters

Name	Description	Value (units)
k_b	Broadening per spike	0.05
λ_b	Broadening half-life	2000 (ms)
b_{base}	Basal spike broadening	0.5
k_c	Max cytosolic Ca^{2+} per spike	0.0003
λ_c	Cytosolic Ca^{2+} half-life	20000 (ms)
k_e	Max submembrane Ca^{2+} per spike	1.5
λ_e	Submembrane Ca^{2+} half-life	100 (ms)
c_θ	Threshold, terminal inhibition by c	0.07
c_n	Gradient, terminal inhibition by c	5
e_θ	Threshold, terminal inhibition by e	2.8
e_n	Gradient, terminal inhibition by e	5
β	Pool refill rate scaling factor	50 (units/s)
r_{max}	Reserve store maximum	1000000 (pg)
p_{max}	Releasable pool maximum	5000 (pg)
α	Secretion rate scaling factor	0.0005 (pg/unit/s)
λ_v	Plasma vasopressin half-life	120 (s)

The parameter values are given in Table 5.5. The model variables are initialized to 0, except $c = 0.03$, $p = p_{max}$, and $r = r_{max}$.

5.4.3 Signal response and the single cell

The model was fitted against *in vitro* experiments which measure the facilitation and fatigue effects (Figure 5.17), and the resulting dependence of the secretion rate on both spike frequency *and* patterning (Figure 5.18). A fit of the model parameters was chosen which makes a close quantitative match to spike frequency response, and the time course and magnitude of fatigue and recovery. Combined with the spiking model, this gives a complete single-cell model, taking us from synaptic input to secretion, and we can now begin to examine how the properties of the cells relate to their function.

In both rats and humans, vasopressin secretion increases linearly with osmotic pressure above a set point. Although this appears to be a simple relationship, the nonlinear properties of the neuronal spiking and secretion mechanisms make this difficult to achieve. Phasic firing helps to linearize the spiking response, but this is still subject to the nonlinearities (facilitation and fatigue) of the secretion mechanism. As a result, although the single-cell model's spike response to increasing osmotic input is linear, the secretion response is not (Figure 5.15). To solve this, we need to look beyond the single cell.

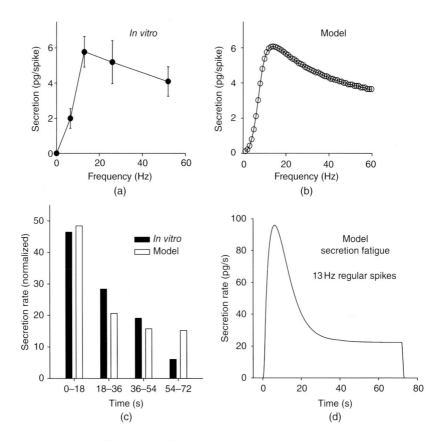

Figure 5.17   Facilitation and fatigue: the secretion model fitted to experimental data. (a) Data (redrawn from Bicknell (1988)) show vasopressin secretion per spike from an isolated rat posterior pituitary stimulated with a fixed number of stimulus pulses (156) at varied frequencies, producing a frequency response profile showing an initial climb to a peak at 13 Hz followed by a slower decline. (b) The same experiment reproduced in the model with frequency ranging from 1 to 60 Hz in 1 Hz steps. The model combines frequency facilitation and competing fast negative feedback modulating Ca^{2+} entry to match the *in vitro* data. (c) Experimental data (redrawn from Bicknell *et al.* (1984)) show secretion rate measured in four consecutive 18 s periods during regular stimulation at 13 Hz, showing a progressive fatigue of the secretion response. The model tested with the same protocol shows a similar decline, though fails to match the last point. The experimental data come from a series of experiments in which glands were stimulated repeatedly for different durations with different orders of presentation. (d) The same model run as C, plotted to show a detailed temporal profile. This shows the initial facilitation of secretion, followed by a slow fatigue. Reproduced from MacGregor and Leng (2013) under Creative Commons Attribution (CC BY) license.

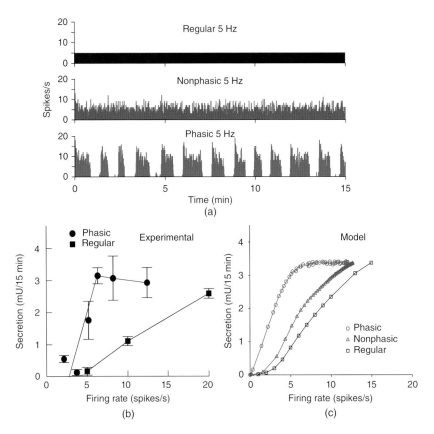

Figure 5.18 Secretion response comparing regular and phasic stimulation with increasing frequency. (a) Examples of regular, nonphasic, and phasic model-generated spiking used to stimulate the secretion model, all with the same 5 Hz mean rate. (b) Data (redrawn from Dutton and Dyball (1979)) show total secretion over 15-min stimulation, using regular stimulation, and stimulation triggered by recorded activity from phasic vasopressin cells. Phasic stimulation evokes much more secretion than regular stimulation at the same frequency; this is a consequence of greater facilitation of secretion at the higher intraburst firing rates, while the effects of fatigue are minimized by recovery during the silent intervals between bursts. (c) The model tested with a similar protocol matches the more optimal response to phasic patterned spiking, here also comparing randomly patterned nonphasic spiking. The nonphasic stimulus with periods of faster spiking at the same mean rate takes more advantage of facilitation than the regular patterned stimulus. Reproduced from MacGregor and Leng (2013) under Creative Commons Attribution (CC BY) license.

5.5 Population modeling

5.5.1 Strength among numbers

To properly understand the regulation of secretion, we need to look not at individual cells, but at the whole population – vasopressin neurons vary considerably in their intrinsic properties, and accordingly their spontaneous firing rates and patterns vary substantially. To do this, we generated populations of 100 independent model cells to look at the relationship between the mean level of synaptic input to the population (assumed to be representative of osmotic pressure) and the total secretion. The problem of how to generate a linear output response gives an objective for such a population model.

5.5.2   The heterogeneous population

Testing a *homogeneous* population (of 100 identical model cells, differing only in that they receive independent random inputs) has the expected smoothing effect of an averaged population signal, but otherwise reproduces the features of the single-cell response. To simulate a *heterogeneous* population like that observed *in vivo*, we have to choose *how* to vary the model cells.

A simple way of producing a heterogeneous population is to ensure that different cells in the population receive different levels of synaptic input. To achieve this, matching the spike rate variation observed *in vivo*, we randomly varied the rates of synaptic input received by each model cell, using a log-normal distribution. Testing how this heterogeneous population responds to increasing synaptic input shows a marked linearization of the population response (compared to the response of the homogeneous population), along with a large increase in the dynamic range (Figure 5.19), producing a profile much closer to the linear secretion response observed *in vivo* (Figure 5.20). Interestingly, this linearization effect only works using the phasic cell model: nonphasic cells showing very little difference between homogeneous and heterogeneous populations.

5.5.3   State of the art

At this point, we have a heterogeneous population of input-spiking-secretion neuronal models that can explain the robust linear vasopressin secretion response observed *in vivo*. The next challenge is to incorporate the consequences of depletion of the cells' vasopressin stores. Heterogeneity of spiking and secretion rates means that cells will deplete their stores at varying rates. This is a system that must continue to robustly respond to challenges that may last for days. The path for future work to tackle this problem will be to move from a disconnected population, sharing only a common input and output, to a full network model with dendritic release-based communication between the cells, somehow acting to balance activity and maintain response (MacGregor *et al.*, 2013).

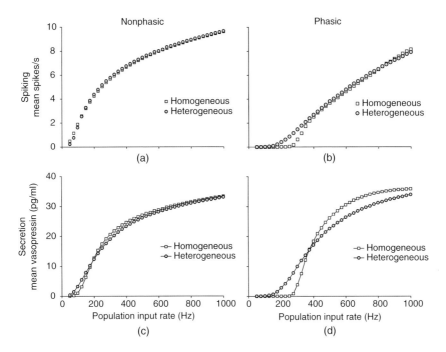

Figure 5.19   Homogeneous and heterogeneous 100 neuron population spike rate and secretion response to increasing synaptic stimulation. (a) Introducing heterogeneity to the population of nonphasic cells makes little difference to the mean spike rate response. (b) In contrast, introducing equivalent heterogeneity to the phasic cell population results in an increased linearity of the mean response to stimulation. (c) Introducing heterogeneity to the population of nonphasic cells produces a modest increase in the linearity of the secretory response to stimulation. (d) In contrast, introducing heterogeneity to the population of nonphasic cells markedly enhances the linearity of secretion. Reproduced from MacGregor and Leng (2013) under Creative Commons Attribution (CC BY) license.

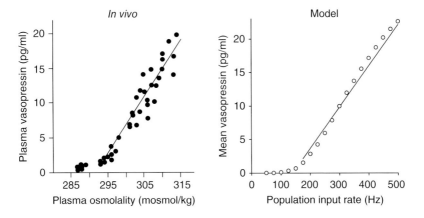

Figure 5.20   Heterogeneous phasic model cell population matched to *in vivo* secretion response. The summed population secretion data of Figure 5.19d plotted on a reduced range (0–4 Hz mean spike rate) show a close match to the experimentally observed relationship between plasma osmotic pressure and vasopressin secretion in rats (Dunn *et al.*, 1973). Reproduced from MacGregor and Leng (2013) under Creative Commons Attribution (CC BY) license.

5.6 Conclusion

We have presented here the story of a modeling project looking at a particular cell. However, many of the properties we have attempted to simulate
and explain exist in many other neurons. The spike-response model does
not replicate as much of the detailed knowledge on the underlying mechanisms that generate spike activity as other more complex models, but its
simplicity can make it a more agile tool for studying the spike patterning
and signal-processing properties that result from these mechanisms, especially when dealing with the more limited data available *in vivo*.

Ultimately, any model of cell activity must consider secretion, since in
most neurons this forms the functioning output. We are studying an accessible example with large hormone releasing terminals, but any neuron
which signals by synaptic transmission is dependent on Ca^{2+}-based exocytotic secretion. The complexity of these mechanisms means that there is
not necessarily a straightforward relationship between spike activity and
secretion. Hopefully, we have given some insight into the path from the
thinking of a physiologist to a modeler, which should be useful to those
going in either direction.

References

Armstrong WE, Wang L, Li C, Teruyama R (2010). Performance, properties and plasticity of identified oxytocin and vasopressin neurones *in vitro*. *J Neuroendocrinol.* **22**(5):
330–342.

Bicknell RJ (1988). Optimizing release from peptide hormone secretory nerve terminals.
J Exp Biol. **139**: 51–65.

Bicknell RJ, Brown D, Chapman C, Hancock PD, Leng G (1984). Reversible fatigue of
stimulus–secretion coupling in the rat neurohypophysis. *J Physiol.* **348**: 601–613.

Brown D, Herbison AE, Robinson JE, Marrs RW, Leng G (1994). Modelling the luteinizing
hormone-releasing hormone pulse generator. *Neuroscience* **63**(3): 869–879.

Brown CH, Leng G (2000). *In vivo* modulation of post-spike excitability in vasopressin
cells by κ-opioid receptor activation. *J. Neuroendocrinol.* **12**(8): 711–714.

Brown CH, Ludwig M, Leng G (1998). Kappa-opioid regulation of neuronal activity in
the rat supraoptic nucleus *in vivo*. *J. Neurosci.* **18**(22): 9480–9488.

Clayton TF, Murray AF, Leng G (2010). Modelling the *in vivo* spike activity of
phasically-firing vasopressin cells. *J Neuroendocrinol.* **22**(12): 1290–1300.

Dunn FL, Brennan TJ, Nelson AE, Robertson GL (1973). The role of blood osmolality and
volume in regulating vasopressin secretion in the rat. *J Clin Invest.* **52**(12): 3212–3219.

Dutton A, Dyball RE (1979). Phasic firing enhances vasopressin release from the rat neurohypophysis. *J Physiol.* **290**(2): 433–440.

Leng G, Brown CH, Bull PM, Brown D, Scullion S, Currie J, Blackburn-Munro RE, Feng J,
Onaka T, Verbalis JG, Russell JA, Ludwig M (2001). Responses of magnocellular neurons to osmotic stimulation involves coactivation of excitatory and inhibitory input:
an experimental and theoretical analysis. *J Neurosci.* **21**(17): 6967–6977.

Li Z, Hatton GI (1997). Reduced outward K$^+$ conductances generate depolarizing after-potentials in rat supraoptic nucleus neurones. *J Physiol.* **505**(Pt 1): 95–106.

MacGregor DJ, Clayton TF, Leng G (2013). Information coding in vasopressin neurons: the role of asynchronous bistable burst firing. *Bio Syst.* **112**(2), 85–93.

MacGregor DJ, Leng G (2012). Phasic firing in vasopressin cells: understanding its functional significance through computational models. *PLoS Comput Biol.* **8**(10): e1002740.

MacGregor DJ, Leng G (2013). Spike triggered hormone secretion in vasopressin cells; a model investigation of mechanism and heterogeneous population function. *PLoS Comput Biol.* **9**(8): e1003187.

MacGregor DJ, Williams CKI, Leng G (2009). A new method of spike modelling and interval analysis. *J Neurosci Methods* **176**(1): 45–56.

Roper P, Callaway J, Armstrong W (2004). Burst initiation and termination in phasic vasopressin cells of the rat supraoptic nucleus: a combined mathematical, electrical, and calcium fluorescence study. *J Neurosci.* **24**(20): 4818–4831.

Roper P, Callaway J, Shevchenko T, Teruyama R, Armstrong W (2003). AHP's, HAP's and DAP's: how potassium currents regulate the excitability of rat supraoptic neurones. *J Comput Neurosci.* **15**(3): 367–389.

Sabatier N, Brown CH, Ludwig M, Leng G (2004). Phasic spike patterning in rat supraoptic neurones *in vivo* and *in vitro*. *J Physiol.* **558**(Pt 1): 161–180.

Further Reading

Biophysical properties of vasopressin cells: reviews

Armstrong WE, Stern JE (1998). Phenotypic and state-dependent expression of the electrical and morphological properties of oxytocin and vasopressin neurones. *Prog Brain Res.* **119**: 101–113.

Bourque CW (2008). Central mechanisms of osmosensation and systemic osmoregulation. *Nat Rev Neurosci.* **9**: 519–523.

Brown CH *et al.* (2008). Multi-factorial somato-dendritic regulation of phasic spike discharge in vasopressin neurons. *Prog Brain Res.* **170**: 219–28.

Brown CH, Ruan M, Scott V, Tobin VA, Ludwig M (2004). Rhythmogenesis in vasopressin cells. *J Neuroendocrinol.* **16**: 727–733.

Cunningham JT, Bruno SB, Grindstaff RR, Grindstaff RJ, Higg KH, Mazella D, Sullivan MJ (2002). Cardiovascular regulation of supraoptic vasopressin neurons. *Prog Brain Res.* **139**: 257–273.

Leng G, Brown C, Sabatier N, Scott V (2008). Population dynamics in vasopressin cells. *Neuroendocrinology.* **88**: 160–72.

Leng G, Ludwig M (2008). Neurotransmitters and peptides: whispered secrets and public announcements. *J Physiol.* **586**: 5625–5632.

Richard P, Moos F, Dayanithi G, Gouzènes L, Sabatier N (1997). Rhythmic activities of hypothalamic magnocellular neurons: autocontrol mechanisms. *Biol Cell* **89**: 555–560.

Models of vasopressin cells

Armstrong WE, Gallagher MJ, Sladek CD (1986). Noradrenergic stimulation of supraoptic neuronal activity and vasopressin release *in vitro*: mediation by an alpha 1-receptor. *Brain Res.* **365**: 192–197.

Komendantov AO, Trayanova NA, Tasker JG (2007). Somato-dendritic mechanisms underlying the electrophysiological properties of hypothalamic magnocellular neuroendocrine cells: a multicompartmental model study. *J Comput Neurosci.* **23**: 143–168.

Leng G, Macgregor DJ (2008). Mathematical modelling in neuroendocrinology. *J Neuroendocrinol.* **20**: 713–718.

Nadeau L, Arbour D, Mouginot D (2010). Computational simulation of vasopressin secretion using a rat model of the water and electrolyte homeostasis. *BMC Physiol.* **10**: 17.

Nadeau L, Mouginot D (2012). Quantitative prediction of vasopressin secretion using a computational population model of rat magnocellular neurons. *J Comput Neurosci.* **33**: 533–545.

Phasic firing

Ghamari-Langroudi M, Bourque CW (2004). Muscarinic receptor modulation of slow afterhyperpolarization and phasic firing in rat supraoptic nucleus neurons. *J Neurosci.* **24**: 7718–726.

Sabatier N, Leng G (2007). Bistability with hysteresis in the activity of vasopressin cells. *J Neuroendocrinol* **19**: 95–101.

Scott V, Brown CH (2010). State-dependent plasticity in vasopressin neurones: dehydration-induced changes in activity patterning. *J Neuroendocrinol.* **22**: 343–354.

Wakerley JB *et al.* (1975). Activity of phasic neurosecretory cells during haemorrhage. *Nature* **258**: 82–84.

The DAP and dynorphin

Bourque CW (1991). Activity-dependent modulation of nerve terminal excitation in a mammalian peptidergic system. *Trends Neurosci.* **14**: 28–30.

Brown CH, Bourque CW (2004). Autocrine feedback inhibition of plateau potentials terminates phasic bursts in magnocellular neurosecretory cells of the rat supraoptic nucleus. *J Physiol.* **15**: 557: 949–960.

Brown CH, Leng G, Ludwig M, Bourque CW (2006). Endogenous activation of supraoptic nucleus kappa-opioid receptors terminates spontaneous phasic bursts in rat magnocellular neurosecretory cells. *J Neurophysiol.* **95**: 3235–3244.

Ghamari-Langroudi M, Bourque CW (2002). Flufenamic acid blocks depolarizing afterpotentials and phasic firing in rat supraoptic neurones. *J Physiol.* **545**: 537–542.

Li C, Tripathi PK, Armstrong WE (2007). Differences in spike train variability in rat vasopressin and oxytocin neurons and their relationship to synaptic activity. *J Physiol.* **581**: 221–240.

Teruyama R, Armstrong WE (2007). Calcium-dependent fast depolarizing afterpotentials in vasopressin neurons in the rat supraoptic nucleus. *J Neurophysiol.* **98**: 2612–221.

Neural signal processing

McDonnell MD, Abbott D (2009). What is stochastic resonance? Definitions, misconceptions, debates, and its relevance to biology. *PLoS Comput Biol.* **5**(5): e1000348.

CHAPTER 6

Modeling Endocrine Cell Network Topology

David J. Hodson[1,2,3,4], Francois Molino[1,2,3,5], and Patrice Mollard[1,2,3]

[1] CNRS, UMR-5203, Institut de Génomique Fonctionnelle, F-34000 Montpellier, France
[2] INSERM, U661, F-34000 Montpellier, France
[3] Universités de Montpellier 1 & 2, UMR-5203, F-34000 Montpellier, France
[4] Department of Medicine, Section of Cell Biology and Functional Genomics, Imperial College London, Imperial Centre for Translational and Experimental Medicine, Hammersmith Hospital, Du Cane Road, London W12 0NN, UK
[5] Centre National de la Recherche Scientifique, Unité Mixte de Recherche 5221, Laboratoire Charles Coulomb, University Montpellier 2, F-34095 Montpellier, France

6.1 Introduction

6.1.1 Overview of pituitary networks

A long-standing conundrum in endocrinology has been the observation that two-dimensional culture of cells results in impaired hormone secretion compared with measures taken from the intact pituitary gland. From this, an important role of tissue context for endocrine cell function has been inferred. However, until recently, the *in situ* assessment of endocrine cell function has been restricted to immunohistochemistry alongside functional assays that rely on the crude identification of cells using nonspecific secretagogues. To circumvent these problems, a range of transgenic animals with cell-specific tags have been created, opening up the possibility of mapping and recording the structure and function of cells within their native environment using two-photon and allied imaging approaches. By applying these methods to intact tissue, we have so far provided evidence for network organization of four endocrine (*gonadotrope, corticotrope, lactotrope, and somatotrope*) (Bonnefont *et al.*, 2005; Budry *et al.*, 2011; Hodson *et al.*, 2012b) and two nonendocrine (*folliculostellate, sex determining region Y-box 2 (SRY2 or SOX2)*) (Fauquier *et al.*, 2001; Mollard *et al.*, 2012) pituitary cell populations, with consequences for hormone release (Figure 6.1). In this chapter, we will concentrate on the experimental techniques and the data analysis tools available to investigate functional network organization in endocrine tissues.

Computational Neuroendocrinology, First Edition. Edited by Duncan J. MacGregor and Gareth Leng.
© 2016 John Wiley & Sons, Ltd. Published 2016 by John Wiley & Sons, Ltd.
Companion Website: www.wiley.com/go/Leng/Computational

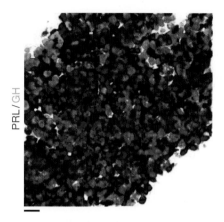

PRL/GH

Figure 6.1   High-resolution snapshot of two intermingled pituitary networks (PRL, prolactin; GH, growth hormone) (scale bar = 20 μm).

6.1.2   Free cytosolic calcium as a determinant of endocrine network dynamics

To determine a functional network, a population measure of cell activity is required. In large organs, such as the brain, *functional magnetic resonance imaging* (*fMRI*) signals tend to be used to map interactions between distant areas (Bullmore and Sporns, 2009), whereas *calcium* (Ca^{2+})-imaging is used to monitor the contribution of individual neurons to the function of discrete neural circuits (e.g., hippocampus) (Peterlin *et al.*, 2000). As the pituitary is a small organ – the size of a pea in humans – large swathes can easily be mapped using the latter approach. Moreover, basal- and secretagogue-stimulated hormone release from most neuroendocrine cells depends on action potential-driven extracellular Ca^{2+}-entry through voltage-gated ion channels (a notable exception being mammalian gonadotropes) (Mollard and Schlegel, 1996; Schlegel *et al.*, 1987; Stojilkovic *et al.*, 2005). Thus, simultaneous assessment of cytosolic free Ca^{2+} from hundreds of individual endocrine cells allows the activity dynamics underlying hormone secretion to be reasonably estimated. This technique has been widely used in assessing network organization in discrete brain regions.

6.1.3   Problem: defining contributions of endocrine cell networks to hormone release

Decoding the complex network dynamics underlying hormone release is challenging because of our limited knowledge about the nature, strength, extent, and rapidity of cell–cell communication. For example, paracrine couplings mediated by readily diffusible molecules will be subject to different temporal/spatial limitations compared to those that rely on next-neighbor gap junction linkages. Indeed, both exist inside the pituitary, but their exact details remain largely obscure (reviewed in (Hodson *et al.*, 2012a)). Are the coupling mechanisms of short- or long range? Do they necessitate precise orchestration of cell activity? Are cell–cell communications predominantly homo- or hetero-typic? Consequently, the investigation of structural and functional endocrine cell connectivity is necessarily statistical and descriptive.

The following sections will describe how the mathematical language of graph theory can be used to analyze correlations in position and activity, providing information about the physiologically relevant cell–cell interactions which may contribute to hormone secretion from the pituitary. These tools will then be used in a worked example to analyze spontaneous activity of a pituitary endocrine cell population *in situ*.

6.2 Networks

6.2.1 Network science

A branch of statistical physics has emerged in recent years to probe the characteristics of complex systems. Relying principally on *graph theory*, algorithms have been developed to identify the various components of networks, and derive a better understanding of the interactions that occur across multiple scales (μm; seconds to years) to generate complex behavior. Such analyses have deepened our understanding of how network topology permeates seemingly complex scenarios ranging from scientific publishing (e.g., a few influential authors are responsible for the majority of citations) (Price, 1965) to the world wide web (e.g., just a few websites are referred to in the majority of hyperlinks) (Barabási and Albert, 1999) to biology (e.g., protein–protein networks where some key targets such as p53 have wide-ranging effects by virtue of their multiple interactions) (Barabási and Oltvai, 2004). A critical aspect of understanding networks is borne from the observation that, although the constituents can be different (people versus cells) the resultant behaviors/topologies are highly conserved (e.g., random, scale-free and small world).

6.2.2 Network criteria

For a system to behave as a *complex biological system*, a set of criteria, as adapted from Alon (Alon, 2003), must be fulfilled (see Text Box 6.1).

Box 6.1 Classification criteria for complex biological networks

Robustness: The resilience of a network to operational failure is a consequence of its underlying topology.

Plasticity: Refers to the predisposition of a system to display both reversible and irreversible changes to structure and/or function in response to demand. This can be either physiological (e.g., GH network plasticity during puberty) or pathological (e.g., formation of a pituitary tumour).

Modularity: The presence of biological- or algorithm-identified building blocks (e.g., hubs, GH cell clusters, lactotrope honeycomb motifs) that typify the network and which adapt in response to changing demand.

Connectivity: Mechanisms must exist to allow cells to communicate over both short and long distances. Within endocrine cell networks these are usually chemical (e.g., paracrine) and electrical linkages (e.g., gap junctions).

Coordination: A network gain of function must exist in the form of either coordinated cell behavior to support hormone release (Hodson *et al.*, 2010), or more complex activity patterns which underlie transcriptional processes (Harper *et al.*, 2010).

Box 6.2 Features of endocrine cell networks identified to date

The growth hormone and lactotrope lineages are the most studied networks to date, and using a variety of structural and functional mapping techniques, they have been shown to possess features consistent with their behavior as complex systems (see Le Tissier *et al.* (2012) for further information). Whilst gonadotropes are organized three-dimensionally, functional characterization of the gonadotrope network has predominantly relied on observations of connectivity/coordination in cell populations identified using gonadotropin-releasing hormone (GnRH), and measures of robustness are lacking. *In situ* functional challenge of corticotropes has yet to be achieved.

Network	Robustness	Plasticity	Modularity	Connectivity	Coordination
Growth Hormone	X	X	X	X	X
Lactotrope	X	X	X	X	X
Gonadotrope		X	X	X	X
Corticotrope			X	X	

6.2.3 Network jargon

Nodes and edges: A network is constructed of nodes connected by edges. In biology, the nature of nodes can vary from individual cells to distinct tissue regions responsible for a particular function.

Node degree (k): The number of edges emanating from each node. The population degree distribution probability largely determines network topology.

Node association: A measure of similarity between nodes which determines node degree. This is normally based upon statistical observations of nonrandom behavior such as cell–cell correlation measures.

Adjacency matrix: Usually a binary table (i.e., "0" or "1") specifying whether cell 1 is statistically connected/associated to cell 2,....,x. It contains all possible pairwise permutations and allows the calculation of the node degree.

Network topology: A characteristic description of the network structure drawn from the degree distribution in combination with various other network measures (see network jargon heading).

Undirected network: No inference is made about the line origins, that is, both nodes are considered to potentially give rise to the interaction.

Directed network: Lines originate from a specified node. Requires statistical measures of association which can take into account directionality, for example, *Granger causality*.

6.2.4   Network metrics

Quantitative analysis of network topology is critical for a better understanding of how functional connectivity influences network performance. For example, do just a few endocrine cells possess most of the edges, thus acting as hubs, or do all cells contribute equally to network architecture? What are the consequences of this for cell–cell communications, robustness in the face of insults, and downstream outputs, such as hormone secretion and transcription? To aid this, some common metrics are listed in the following with explanations of what their values mean. The necessary input data are derived from the correlation matrix and Euclidean distances (see later for how to derive this information).

Degree distribution (*P(k)*): The proportion of nodes in the network which possess degree (k). It is otherwise known as the probability distribution of degrees across the population *P(k)*. The value can be derived from summing the columns of the correlation matrix. Cells with the maximum k-value are considered to possess 100% of the connections. The degree distribution is an important indicator of network topology and geometry. For example, if the distribution obeys a power law, then the network is scalefree, i.e., a hub and spoke architecture. Conversely, if *P(k)* follows a Poisson or Gaussian distribution, then the network is random, that is, all nodes have identical degrees (or edge number).

Average path length (*L*): The shortest path between two nodes, averaged for all pairwise combinations, is determined by the following formula:

$$L = 1/N(N-1) \sum d_{ij}$$

where N is the total number of nodes, and d_{ij} is the shortest distance between nodes i and j (summed over all possible node pairs).

In general, the shorter the average path length, the more efficient the information transfer through the network.

Clustering coefficient (*C*): The number of neighboring edges hosted by a node i as a function of total possible edges (ranging from 0 to 1) and can be calculated using:

$$C = 2k/(j(j-1))$$

where j is the number of neighboring nodes and k is the number of edges with all neighbors (i.e., degree). The network clustering coefficient is simply the average for all nodes in the population.

High values indicate increased local connectedness with neighbors, streamlining communications due to a tendency toward decreased path length.

Degree centrality (*D*): A measure of how connected a node's neighbors are. Degree D centrality of a given node i can be summarized by the following:

$$D_i = \sum i,j$$

where $i,j = 1$ if an edge exists between node i and j.

Nodes with high centrality have neighbors with low degree and, thus, act as relays for information flow, minimizing average path length.

Closeness centrality (*CC*): The sum of the inverses of the distances between a node and all other nodes:

$$CC_i = \sum j[d_{i,j}]^{-1}$$

where i is the node under examination and $d_{i,j}$ is the shortest distance between nodes i and j. Information transfer is most efficient if routed through a central node that is close to all other nodes.

6.2.5 Network topologies

Random: For a total of n nodes, the probability P that an edge (i,j) exists for all i, j is equal and is denoted by the random graph process $G(n,P)$. That is, all nodes have the same chance of being connected, and the resulting degree distribution is binomial/Poisson (Figure 6.2a).

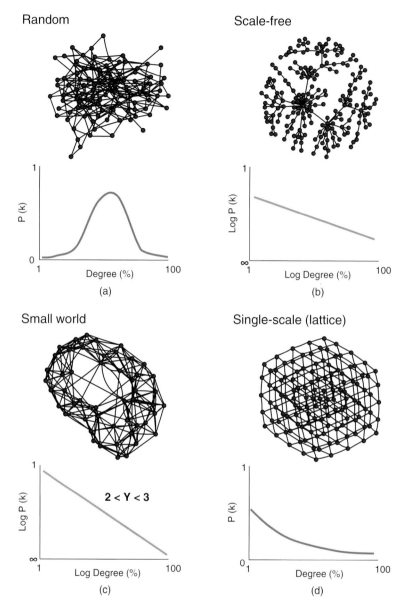

Figure 6.2 Common network topologies based upon degree (or edge number) distribution. (a) A random network (above) has a Gaussian degree distribution (i.e., the proportion of nodes in a network which possess degree k) (below) meaning nodes, on average, possess a similar degree. (b) Degree distribution of a scale-free network (above) follows a power law (below) giving rise to a topology typified by a hub and spoke arrangement. (c) A small-world network (top) has a similar degree distribution probability to a scale-free network, but an exponent value $2 < \gamma < 3$ (below) and high clustering coefficient which results in a shorter average path length. (d) A single-scale network (above) has a lattice like structure determined by its scaling factor k_0 (below).

Pros:

- Short average path length between any two nodes ensures efficient parallel communication.
- Can maintain function in the face of a targeted insult, since information will be re-routed via other equally connected nodes.

Cons:

- Large wiring costs.
- Random and targeted attack will equally disrupt network function, since all nodes contribute to communications.

Scale-free: The k degree distribution follows a power law and $P(k) = k^{-\gamma}$. Scale-free networks are characterized by a "hub and spoke" arrangement whereby a few nodes possess disproportionately many connections. They are ubiquitous throughout science and engineering (e.g., scientific citations, social networks and neural networks possess scale-free topology) (Figure 6.2B).

Pros:

- Low wiring costs.
- Distant nodes can be connected via hubs with high centrality/closeness, maintaining a reasonable path length.
- Most nodes have a low degree, rendering the network more resistant to disruption by a random attack.

Cons:

- Vulnerable to disintegration following targeted attacks against hubs (i.e., nodes with a high degree).
- Average path length is still longer than in a random network.

Small world: These are scale-free networks, with $2 \leq \gamma \leq 3$ and high clustering and *assortativity* indices. Since the distance d between two edges increases logarithmically with node number ($d \propto \log(i,j)$), subnetworks or cliques tend to be formed and most nodes are linked via common neighbours. Small worldness is best epitomized by the six degrees of separation concept (i.e., any two people can always be linked via six contacts) (Figure 6.2C).

Pros:

- A high clustering coefficient result in a lattice-like structure but with random graph-like path lengths.
- Increased robustness to network perturbation.

Cons:

- As for scale-free networks.

Single-scale: The degree distribution (k) follows $P(k) = e^{k/k_0}$, where k_0 is the scaling factor. Single-scale networks are lattice-like and possess *pros* and *cons* somewhere between random and scale-free networks. They are observed in the nervous system of lower mammals such as *Caenorhabditis elegans* (Figure 6.2D).

6.3 Step-by-step experimental and analytical protocol

6.3.1 Identification of specific cell populations

The use of transgenic animals allows the identification of signals arising from specific pituitary cell populations/lineages. A variety of strains exist which contain fluorophores driven by specific promoters (e.g., prolactin-Discosoma red fluorescent protein (DsRed), luteinizing hormone-Cerulean, growth hormone-enhanced green fluorescent protein (eGFP)). It is important to consider any excitation/emission overlap between the fluorescent tag and Ca^{2+} indicator when designing imaging protocols.

6.3.2 Pituitary slice preparation

- Prepare bicarbonate buffer (see Table 6.1) and bubble for 10 min with 95% O_2/5% CO_2 (*! critical: ensure that appropriate local and national ethical approval for animal experimentation is obtained*).
- Remove pituitary and embed in 4–5% low melting point agarose diluted in bicarbonate buffer and allow them to solidify on ice.
- Using a scalpel, carefully remove a 1.5×1.5 cm^2 block of agarose containing the pituitary, secure to the vibratome chuck with superglue and mount in the vibratome bath containing bicarbonate buffer at 4°C (bubbled with 95% O_2/5% CO_2). Use a fresh blade for each experiment and slice 150–200 μm sections at 60 Hz using the slowest speed setting (*! critical: maintain bath at 4°C for optimal slices otherwise agarose can become unstable*).
- Use a paintbrush or 5 ml plastic pipette (tip widened with scissors) to retrieve the section. Place on a poly-L-lysine coated (1 mg/ml) coverslip (de-greased with acetone followed by ethanol rinse; size will depend on microscope chamber characteristics) and carefully aspirate excess solution until the section is adherent. Remove excess agarose if still present using two 23G needles (*! critical: for best adherence, place*

Table 6.1 Bicarbonate buffer constituents

NaCl (mM)	KCl (mM)	NaH$_2$PO$_4$ (mM)	NaHCO$_3$ (mM)	Glucose (mM)	CaCl$_2$ (mM)	MgCl$_2$ (mM)
125	2.5	1.25	26	12	2	1

50 μl 1 mg/ml poly-L-lysine in centre of a coverslip and allow to dry at 37°C overnight before attaching pituitary sections).

- Allow sections to recover for 1 h at 37°C, 95% O_2/5% CO_2 in bicarbonate buffer.

6.3.3   Load with a Ca^{2+} indicator

- Mix 50 μg *fura-2AM* with 5 μl DMSO + 10 μl 20% pluronic acid (w/v in DMSO) and sonicate for 3 min. Add 500 μl bicarbonate buffer and sonicate for a further 3 min to disperse micelles. Make up to 2 ml and incubate slice in fura-2-containing solution for 1–2 h at 37°C/5% CO_2. Rinse sections twice with bicarbonate buffer and reincubate for 30 min without fura-2 to allow cleavage and activation of fura-2 intracellular esterases *(! critical: do not over-incubate slice to avoid buffering of cytosolic free calcium by fura-2).*
- Mount slices on/in microscope chamber and perfuse with bicarbonate buffer at 34–36°C *(! critical: ion channel kinetics are temperature-dependent).*
- Use a 10–40× water immersion objective depending on desired size of imaged field. Capture a snapshot of the fluo-tagged cell population under investigation. A 20× NA 0.95 water immersion objective allows pituitary slices to be imaged with single-cell resolution whilst retaining a large field of view.
- Proceed to functional multicellular imaging (fMCI).

6.3.4   Functional multicellular calcium imaging (fMCI)

- Perform excitation at 780–800 nm and record emission at 525/50 nm for nonratiometric *two-photon* imaging of fura-2. Multiphoton microscopy has many advantages over single photon modalities including better depth penetration, less photoxicity and improved axial resolution (see Glossary) *(! critical: due to fura-2 excitation above the isosbestic point, increased $[Ca^{2+}]_i$ will present as decreased signal intensity).*
- Acquire a three-dimensional reconstruction of the cell population under investigation. This will allow functional connectivity (based on association measures) to be directly correlated with structural connectivity (based on physical linkages) (see later).
- Image fura-2 in the second cell layer. This avoids artifacts due to recording at the cut surface and ensures optimal overlap with the cell fluo-tag. Generally, Ca^{2+} indicators will penetrate three to four cell layers deep.
- According to the *Nyquist sampling theorem*, the frame rate should be twice the highest frequency which needs to be resolved for analysis purposes. For example, 1 Hz will be required to detect events at 0.5 Hz. For long-term time lapses (>15 min), reduce laser power, and frame rate at the expense of spatial resolution/image quality *(! critical: phototoxicity introduces artefacts into signal analysis).*

- Use binning to average intensity for 2×2 pixels if using the an EM-CCD-based system.

Note: Fura-2 is ideal for both one- and two-photon imaging modalities as it possesses nonoverlapping excitation/emissions spectra with commonly used eGFP cell-tags, loads pituitary cells better than equivalent Ca^{2+} indicators, and possesses a dissociation constant ($K_d \sim 145\,nM$) compatible with resolution of both spontaneous and secretagogue-driven Ca^{2+} events in pituitary cells. Since fura-2 can exit cells via chloride channels, "leak resistant" forms are recommended for long time-lapse experiments.

6.3.5 Data extraction

- Export time-lapse sequences as .tif files and open in ImageJ or Fiji (both NIH, USA) (Supplemental Movie 1).
- Obtain an average image of the movie using the Stacks->Z project (mean) function.
- Manually delineate fluo-tagged, fura-2-loaded cells using a region of interest (ROI) accessible from the ROI Manager (Ctrl + T) (Supplemental Figure 6.1 and Supplemental File 1).
- Ensure the correct parameter to be measured is selected in the Set Measurement menu (Analyze->Set Measurement->Mean Gray Value). On the ROI Manager, toggle Show All and then Multi Measure to extract intensity over time traces for ROI 1....x. Save ROI and intensity-over-time data as .xls/.csv and .zip files, respectively.

6.3.6 Signal processing

Hilbert–Huang empirical mode decomposition (EMD)

This method relies on decomposing nonlinear nonstationary signals into static intrinsic mode functions (IMF) of varying frequencies, which together are responsible for the observed Ca^{2+} trace. Briefly, the IMFs are extracted using a sifting process of m means determined by a cubic-spline interpolation of the local minima and maxima. The instantaneous frequency of the function $f(x)$ can then be calculated using a Hilbert transform:

$$F(t) = \frac{1}{\pi} \int_{-\infty}^{\infty} \frac{f(x)}{t-x} dx$$

Since the lowest and highest frequency IMFs are likely to be introduced by processes such as photobleaching and sudden movement, respectively, they can be filtered to reduce artifacts which may confound further analysis (Figure 6.3). This form of detrending has advantages over regression-based techniques which tend to discard signals whose characteristics (frequency and amplitude) are dynamic. Further details can be located here: http://perso.ens-lyon.fr/patrick.flandrin/emd.html.

Raw trace

High-frequency IMF removed (denoise)

Low-frequency IMF

Low-frequency IMF removed (detrend)

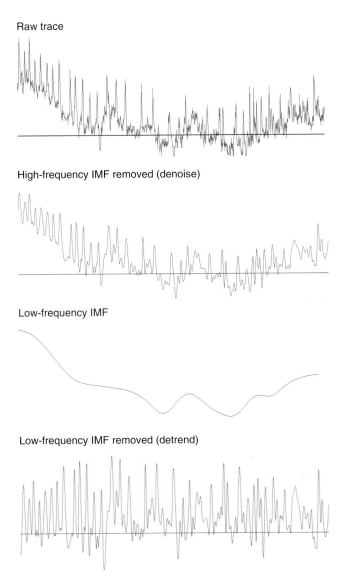

Figure 6.3   Empirical mode decomposition (EMD) of cell signals. In this example, the raw Ca^{2+} trace has artifacts introduced by photobleaching and an axial drift. To denoise and detrend the signal, EM is performed to retrieve the intrinsic mode functions (IMF) or more simply, the static frequenices comprising the wave. The highest and lowest frequency IMFs can then be removed to result in a corrected signal which contains the identical information of interest to the source trace.

Least-squares linear regression

Depending on signal characteristics, detrending can also be performed by removing the mean value or linear trend from x using a least-squares fit of a straight line:

$$y - \bar{y} = b(x - \bar{x})$$

where

$$b = \frac{Sxy}{Sxx} = \frac{\sum (x_i - \bar{x})(y_i - \bar{y})}{\sum (x_i - \bar{x})^2} = \frac{\frac{\sum x_i y_i}{n} - \bar{x}\bar{y}}{\frac{\sum x_i^2}{n} - \bar{x}^2}$$

Whilst such methods are simple to perform using common analysis packages, and will suffice in most cases, they will not remove low-frequency nonlinear components and rapid/high-frequency artifacts. This is particularly important for binarization-type analyses (see later), which depend on adequate filtering to avoid inadvertently detecting active phases due to nonintrinsic mechanisms.

6.3.7   Normalize signals

Cell loading with Ca^{2+}-indicators is heterogeneous due to differences in uptake, acetoxymethyl (AM)-cleavage by esterases, and cell size. As a consequence, when using nonratiometric probes (as is usually the case with two-photon microscopy), baseline intensity (F_{min}) varies from cell to cell. To facilitate data handling, each trace can be normalized (F_{norm}) using:

$$F_{norm} = F/F_{min}$$

where F is signal intensity at any given point and F_{min} is the minimum recordedintensity.

Alternatively, the change in signal intensity ($F_{max} - F_{min} = \Delta F$) can be calculated as follows:

$$\Delta F = (F_{n+1} - F_n)/F_n$$

where F_{n+1} is the intensity during a time window after F_n (an extravagant method to calculate ΔF can be found here:

http://www.nature.com/nprot/journal/v6/n1/full/nprot.2010.169 .html).

6.3.8   Exclude artifacts introduced by Ca^{2+} indicators

Because most indicators buffer cytosolic Ca^{2+} in a K_d-dependent manner, it is advisable to carry out control experiments for each state under investigation to ensure that the observed traces are not associated with differential cell loading. In most cases, buffering effects can be reasonably well excluded by plotting dye intensity as a function of Ca^{2+}-spiking frequency; no correlation should be observed. Moreover, heterogeneous dye loading may reflect differing Ca^{2+} baselines. This can be assessed using zero Ca^{2+}

(5 mM EGTA with ionic balance maintained by the equimolar addition of Mg^{2+}). If $[Ca^{2+}]_i$ is comparable between cells, the distribution of steady-state intensity values should remains unchanged from that observed in the presence of 2 mM Ca^{2+}.

6.3.9 Define the node

The individual pituitary endocrine cell constitutes a node. We will herein refer to both entities interchangeably.

6.3.10 Measure and map node associations

To build a topological network from intensity over time plots, a measure of statistical association between all node pairs is required. Since coordinated endocrine cell behavior is generally accepted to underlie hormone release, as inferred from studies of pituitary somatotropes, correlation indices can be used to assess the strength of node association. It should be noted that stochastic processes may also contribute to hormone release, as has been shown for gene expression (Featherstone *et al.*, 2011; Harper *et al.*, 2010), but their influence on endocrine cell output has yet to be tested empirically.

Unlike neurones which predominantly fire single Ca^{2+} events, pituitary endocrine cells display Ca^{2+}-spikes with varying frequencies, amplitudes, and inter-event intervals. This renders algorithms based upon spike detection unreliable. To circumvent these problems, signals should be binarized using arbitrarily set thresholds for each cell (20–30% ΔF is usually sufficient) to account for the signal-to-noise ratio (SNR).

The resulting data set can then be subjected to correlation analyses based upon observations of cell synchrony i.e. the period of time cells are coactive:

$$C_{ij} = \frac{T_{ij}}{\sqrt{T_i T_j}}$$

where C is a correlation coefficient between -1 and $+1$, T_{ij} is the total time spent in the coactive state between node i and j, and T_i and T_j represent the time spent in the active phase for each individual node. To statistically analyze the probability of correlated events occurring due to chance, a *Monte Carlo-based* simulation is used to determine the probability distribution following iterative and random shuffling of inter-event intervals (i.e., permutation testing) (Ikegaya *et al.*, 2004), and a P-value cut-off (usually between $P < 0.01 - 0.05$) imposed to identify nonrandomly correlated cell pairs. A correlation matrix can then be constructed which marks correlated and noncorrelated cell pairs with a "1" and "0," respectively. Although such analyses do not consider spike magnitude, events downstream of Ca^{2+}-signaling are thought to depend more on the frequency of oscillations than on their amplitude.

6.3.11 Plotting network topology

Network plots based upon measures of node association are termed "functional connectivity" maps, since they detail the location and pattern of node–node interactions, but do not invoke any role for the underlying structure. Whilst this may not necessarily present a problem for social networks, it may be an issue for biological networks, as questions about the morphological basis for the observed topology can be raised. For example, what is the substrate linking a group of functionally connected pituitary cells? How do endocrine cells communicate over long distances in lieu of large axonal projections? What are the mechanisms dictating the balance between cell-specific versus cell autonomous responses? Although beyond the scope of the current chapter, these questions can be circumvented by taking a snapshot of the network structure before fMCI, allowing structural features to be correlated with functional topology

Nonetheless, functional connectivity maps provide an easy way to visualize, understand, and manipulate network topology based upon associative measures. To plot the map, the Euclidean (x–y) coordinates of the nodes will first be required (distances will depend on factors such as objective used, the size of the EM-CCD chip, pixel binning). These can easily be obtained from the ROI list previously saved in ImageJ (Analyse->Set Measurements->select Centroid->open the ROI .zip file in ROI Manager->More->Multi Measure). In combination with the correlation matrix, a weighted graph can then be constructed which displays the distribution of edges between nodes (Figure 6.4).

Note: an *undirected network* means that the nodes from which correlated behavior originates cannot be determined. To identify directionality, Granger causality or similar analyses should be performed. A further refinement of this involves determining effective connectivity which requires perturbation of a node to establish the functional impact on its neighbors.

6.4 Worked example

6.4.1 Question

Pituitary lactotropes form a three-dimensionally organized endocrine network tasked with releasing prolactin (PRL), a hormone which supports lactation primarily through enhanced mammary gland development/function (Freeman *et al.*, 2000). Two distinct activity states exist: (1) *basal* in virgin animals and (2) *stimulated* in lactating animals. Is upregulated prolactin secretion during lactation associated with altered network topology/function?

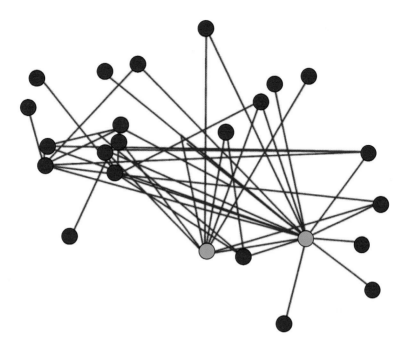

Figure 6.4   Plotting network topology to form a functional connectivity map.
The Euclidean coordinates of the nodes are retrieved and a weighted map depicting the
distribution of edges between nodes constructed on the basis of association measure (in
this case, correlated cell activity). Highly connected cells are displayed in green.

6.4.2 Solution

The following is from two-photon fMCI of pituitary slices obtained from
virgin and lactating animals expressing PRL-DsRed.

1 Delineate fura-2-loaded pituitary lactotropes (DsRed) (Figure 6.5A).
2 Extract intensity over time changes for each cell along with Euclidean
   coordinates (Figure 6.5B).
3 Manually filter cells for artifacts (Supplemental Files 2–5 are filtered
   datasets; please see the legend for more details on how to use these files).
4 Subject to Hilbert–Huang transformation.
5 Binarize traces and subject to correlation analyses to generate the association matrix (Figure 6.5C and D) (Supplemental Files 6 and 7).
6 Construct functional connectivity map (Figure 6.6A).
7 Plot degree distribution (Figure 6.6B).

6.4.3 Conclusions

Lactotropes in virgin animals form a scale-free network in which highly
connected "hub" cells predominate. During lactation, there is an increase
in node association, as measured by indices of correlated activity. Rather

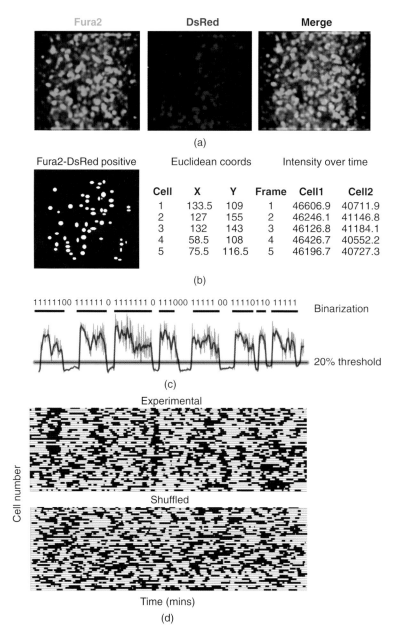

Figure 6.5 Determining network toplogy/function using the lactotrope cell population as an example. (a) Pituitary slices derived from Discosoma red fluorescent protein (DsRed) transgenic animals are loaded with fura-2 and functional multicellular Ca^{2+} imaging (fMCI) performed (DsRed expression is driven by the PRL promoter). Fura-2-DsRed positive cells (merge) are then delineated with a region of interest (ROI). (b) The Euclidean coordinates and intensity over time measure can be extracted from the time series. (c) The resulting traces are subjected to binarization using an arbitariliy determined threshold (dependent on various factors including cell type, experiment duration, and Ca^{2+}-spiking pattern). (d) Correlation analyses are used to determine node association. Here, we have used a measure of coactivity with probability determined using a Monte Carlo statistic. However, other association measures, including Granger causality and principal component analysis, would be equally applicable.

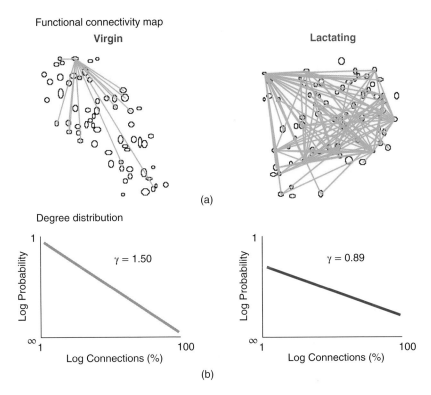

Figure 6.6 **Lactotrope network topology in virgin and lactating females**.
(a) Representative functional connectivity maps demonstrate the presence of a hub and spoke structure in both virgin and lactating animals. (b) Degree distribution probability obeys a power law in both states, but the exponent value is lower during lactation indicating that more cells occupy the medium–high connectivity ranges: i.e., more hubs.

than being added to pre-existing hubs by preferential attachment (the "rich get richer" hypothesis), the resultant extra edges are laid down in the form of new hubs as indicated by the reduced power-law exponent value (i.e., a higher proportion of cells now occupy the high-connectivity range).

6.5 Perspectives

Over the last few decades, network science has facilitated the understanding of complex systems by highlighting the network interactions which underlie emergent, stochastic, or synchronous behavioral states. A striking feature of complex systems is that their topologies are highly conserved throughout nature, irrespective of the processes involved.

Using modeling approaches, it has become evident that various pituitary lineages not only form structural networks, but also functional networks which demonstrate robustness, plasticity, coordination, connectivity, and modularity – all prerequisites of a complex system. Thus, endocrine organs, such as the mammalian pituitary gland, should not be considered as the sum of their parts, but instead a collection of cells which, by virtue of their higher level tissue organization, respond synergistically to a range of inputs. Importantly, these traits result in a network gain of function in terms of hormone release and other related processes.

Specific challenges for the future include: determining how structure influences network function, the interplay between structurally, functionally and developmentally inter-related cell lineages (e.g., GH and PRL cells), whether endocrine cell networks function *in vivo* to generate hormone pulses, how topology can be manipulated in a cell-specific manner to test the contribution to function, and whether similar network phenomena exist in other endocrine tissues, such as the pancreas. With the constant evolution of network science coupled with advances in the imaging arena, these questions should be answered in the not too distant future.

Further reading

Alim Z, Hartshorn C, Mai O, Stitt I, Clay C, Tobet S and Boehm U (2012). Gonadotrope plasticity at cellular and population levels. *Endocrinology* **153**(10): 4729–4739.

Alon U (2007). Network motifs: theory and experimental approaches. *Nat Rev Genet.* **8**(6): 450–461.

Barabasi AL (2009). Scale-free networks: a decade and beyond. *Science* **325**(5939): 412–413.

Berridge MJ, Bootman MD and Lipp P (1998). Calcium – a life and death signal. *Nature* **395**(6703): 645–648.

Berridge MJ, Lipp P and Bootman MD (2000a). Signal transduction. the calcium entry pas de deux. *Science* **287**(5458): 1604–1605.

Berridge MJ, Lipp P and Bootman MD (2000b). The versatility and universality of calcium signalling. *Nat Rev Mol Cell Biol.* **1**(1): 11–21.

Bonifazi P, Goldin M, Picardo MA, Jorquera I, Cattani A, Bianconi G, Represa A, Ben-Ari Y and Cossart R (2009). GABAergic hub neurons orchestrate synchrony in developing hippocampal networks. *Science* **326**(5958): 1419–1424.

Feldt S, Bonifazi P and Cossart R (2011). Dissecting functional connectivity of neuronal microcircuits: experimental and theoretical insights. *Trends Neurosci.* **34**(5): 225–236.

Helmchen F and Konnerth A (2011). *Imaging in Neuroscience: A Laboratory Manual.* Cold Spring Harbor, Cold Spring Harbor, NY.

Koch C and Laurent G (1999). Complexity and the nervous system. *Science* **284**(5411): 96–98.

Lyles D, Tien JH, McCobb DP and Zeeman ML (2010). Pituitary network connectivity as a mechanism for the luteinizing hormone surge. *J Neuroendocrinol.* **22**(12): 1267–1278.

Sanchez-Cardenas C, Fontanaud P, He Z, Lafont C, Meunier AC, Schaeffer M, Carmignac D, Molino F, Coutry N, Bonnefont X, Gouty-Colomer LA, Gavois E, Hodson DJ, Le Tissier P, Robinson ICAF and Mollard P (2010). Pituitary growth hormone network responses are sexually dimorphic and regulated by gonadal steroids in adulthood. *Proc Natl Acad Sci U.S.A.* **107**(50): 21878–21883.

Stojilkovic SS (2012). Molecular mechanisms of pituitary endocrine cell calcium handling. *Cell Calcium* **51**(3-4): 212–221.

Stojilkovic SS, Tabak J and Bertram R (2010). Ion channels and signaling in the pituitary gland. *Endocr Rev.* **31**(6): 845–915.

References

Alon U (2003). Biological networks: the tinkerer as an engineer. *Science* **301**(5641): 1866–1867.

Barabási A and Albert R (1999). Emergence of scaling in random networks. *Science* **286**(5439): 509–512.

Barabási AL and Oltvai ZN (2004). Network biology: understanding the cell's functional organization. *Nat Rev Genet.* **5**(2): 101–113.

Bonnefont X, Lacampagne A, Sanchez-Hormigo A, Fino E, Creff A, Mathieu MN, Smallwood S, Carmignac D, Fontanaud P, Travo P, Alonso G, Courtois-Coutry N, Pincus SM, Robinson ICAF and Mollard P (2005). Revealing the large-scale network organization of growth hormone-secreting cells. *Proc Natl Acad Sci U.S.A.* **102**(46): 16880–16885.

Budry L, Lafont C, El Yandouzi T, Chauvet N, Conéjero G, Drouin J and Mollard P (2011). Related pituitary cell lineages develop into interdigitated 3d cell networks. *Proc Natl Acad Sci U.S.A.* **108**(30): 12515–12520.

Bullmore E and Sporns O (2009). Complex brain networks: graph theoretical analysis of structural and functional systems. *Nat Rev Neurosci.* **10**(3): 186–198.

Fauquier T, Guérineau NC, McKinney RA, Bauer K and Mollard P (2001). Folliculostellate cell network: a route for long-distance communication in the anterior pituitary. *Proc Natl Acad Sci U.S.A.* **98**(15): 8891–8896.

Featherstone K, Harper CV, McNamara A, Semprini S, Spiller DG, McNeilly J, McNeilly AS, Mullins JJ, White MRH and Davis JRE (2011). Pulsatile patterns of pituitary hormone gene expression change during development. *J Cell Sci.* **124**(Pt 20): 3484–3491.

Freeman ME, Kanyicska B, Lerant A and Nagy G (2000). Prolactin: structure, function, and regulation of secretion. *Physiol Rev.* **80**(4): 1523–1631.

Harper CV, Featherstone K, Semprini S, Friedrichsen S, McNeilly J, Paszek P, Spiller DG, McNeilly AS, Mullins JJ, Davis JRE and White MRH (2010). Dynamic organisation of prolactin gene expression in living pituitary tissue. *J Cell Sci.* **123**(Pt 3): 424–430.

Hodson DJ, Molino F, Fontanaud P, Bonnefont X and Mollard P (2010). Investigating and modeling pituitary endocrine network function. *J Neuroendocrinol.* **22**(12): 1217–1225.

Hodson DJ, Romanò N, Schaeffer M, Fontanaud P, Lafont C, Fiordelisio T and Mollard P (2012a). Coordination of calcium signals by pituitary endocrine cells in situ. *Cell Calcium* **51**(3–4): 222–230.

Hodson DJ, Schaeffer M, Romanò N, Fontanaud P, Lafont C, Birkenstock J, Molino F, Christian H, Lockey J, Carmignac D, Fernandez-Fuente M, Le Tissier P and Mollard P (2012b). Existence of long-lasting experience-dependent plasticity in endocrine cell networks. *Nat Commun.* **3**, 605.

Ikegaya Y, Aaron G, Cossart R, Aronov D, Lampl I, Ferster D and Yuste R (2004). Synfire chains and cortical songs: temporal modules of cortical activity. *Science* **304**(5670): 559–564.

Le Tissier PR, Hodson DJ, Lafont C, Fontanaud P, Schaeffer M and Mollard P (2012). Anterior pituitary cell networks. *Front Neuroendocrinol.* **33**(3): 252–266.

Mollard P, Hodson DJ, Lafont C, Rizzoti K and Drouin J (2012). A tridimensional view of pituitary development and function. *Trends Endocrinol Metab.* **23**(6): 261–269.

Mollard P and Schlegel W (1996). Why are endocrine pituitary cells excitable?. *Trends Endocrinol Metab.* **7**(10): 361–365.

Peterlin ZA, Kozloski J, Mao BQ, Tsiola A and Yuste R (2000). Optical probing of neuronal circuits with calcium indicators. *Proc Natl Acad Sci U.S.A.* **97**(7): 3619–3624.

Price DJ (1965). Networks of scientific papers. *Science* **149**(3683): 510–515.

Schlegel W, Winiger BP, Mollard P, Vacher P, Wuarin F, Zahnd GR, Wollheim CB and Dufy B (1987). Oscillations of cytosolic Ca^{2+} in pituitary cells due to action potentials. *Nature* **329**(6141): 719–721.

Stojilkovic SS, Zemkova H and Van Goor F (2005). Biophysical basis of pituitary cell type-specific Ca^{2+} signaling–secretion coupling. *Trends Endocrinol Metab.* **16**(4): 152–159.

CHAPTER 7

Modeling the Milk-Ejection Reflex

Gareth Leng[1] and Jianfeng Feng[2]
[1]Centre for Integrative Physiology, University of Edinburgh, Edinburgh, UK
[2]Department of Computer Science, University of Warwick, UK

When babies suckle at their mother's breast, they are rewarded with a let-down of milk that results from the secretion of the hormone oxytocin (video 1). Oxytocin is synthesized by magnocellular neurons in the hypothalamus. Each of these cells has one axon that projects into the neurohypophysis where it gives rise to about 2 000 nerve endings. Oxytocin is secreted from these in response to action potentials (spikes) generated in the cell bodies and propagated down the axons. Normally, spikes are infrequent and asynchronous, but during suckling, every few minutes, each cell fires a burst of spikes that results in the secretion of a large pulse of oxytocin into the bloodstream. This milk-ejection reflex involves a mechanism that affects the activity of the oxytocin cells, and that a negative feedback that "spaces" the bursts. These involve the dendrites of oxytocin cells. Dendrites are not only sites where neurons receive most of their afferent inputs, but are also the sites of release of factors that influence neuronal excitability. Dendritic oxytocin release has both autocrine effects (on the cell of origin) and paracrine effects (on adjacent cells); it can occur not only in response to spike activity, but can also be triggered independently of spike activity, by stimuli that mobilize intracellular Ca^{2+} stores. Here, we show how synchronized bursting can arise in a neuronal network model that incorporates these features.

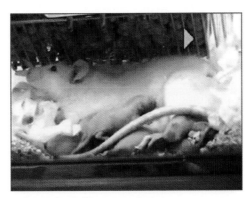

Video 1 The milk-ejection reflex in conscious rats.

7.1 The milk-ejection reflex

In all mammals, oxytocin is made in a few thousand magnocellular neurons whose cell bodies mostly lie within the *supraoptic nuclei* and the paraventricular nuclei of the hypothalamus. Each of these cells has just one axon; this axon extends into the neurohypophysis, giving rise to about 2000 swellings and nerve endings, each of which is packed with *neurosecretory vesicles* that contain oxytocin. Spikes that are generated in the cell bodies of the oxytocin cells and that are propagated down the axons cause some vesicles to fuse with the plasma membrane (*Ca^{2+}-dependent exocytosis*) and release their contents, which then enter the blood. Normally, oxytocin cells fire 1–3 spikes/s, but during suckling, every 5 min or so they all discharge a burst of 50–150 spikes in 1–3 s. These bursts result in the secretion of a pulse of oxytocin that reaches the mammary gland a few seconds later, where it causes milk to release (let down) into a collecting duct from which it can be extracted by suckling.

The background spike activity of oxytocin cells in lactating rats is very similar to that in nonlactating rats; the cells fire slowly, asynchronously, and nearly randomly. At first, suckling produces little change in this activity, except that slowly firing cells tend to speed up slightly, while faster firing cells slow down. However, after a few minutes of suckling, the first bursts occur. The first bursts are small and involve only some cells, but progressively more and more cells are recruited, until all show intense bursts. Bursts are elicited *specifically* by the suckling stimulus; many other stimuli cause oxytocin secretion, but they produce a graded increase in electrical activity that is identical in lactating and nonlactating rats, and which does not entail bursting. The bursts (Figure 7.1) differ in amplitude from cell to cell and according to how many pups are suckling, but they are quite consistent in their shape, especially from one burst to the next in a given cell.

7.1.1 The supraoptic nucleus
The hypothalamus contains two supraoptic nuclei: one at the base of the brain and another adjacent to the optic chiasm on either side. Each nucleus contains about 2000 oxytocin cells (Figure 7.2); in addition to its axon, each cell has 2–5 dendrites, and each dendrite contains more than 10000 vesicles. The cells intercommunicate within "bundles" of 3–8 dendrites; in lactating rats, bundles are separated from each other by glial cell processes (thin, sheet-like processes that "wrap round" the bundles), but within each bundle dendrites are directly apposed to one another. In basal conditions, dendritic oxytocin release is not much influenced by spike activity, but it can be evoked by stimuli that mobilize intracellular Ca^{2+} stores. When oxytocin is released from dendrites, it depolarizes oxytocin cells and also mobilizes intracellular Ca^{2+}, promoting further oxytocin release.

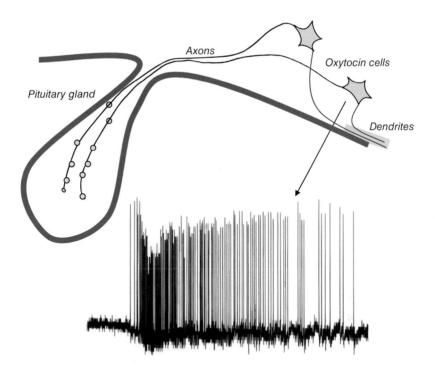

Figure 7.1   Milk-ejection bursts. Magnocellular oxytocin neurons each have one axon that projects into the neurohypophysis from where oxytocin is secreted into the general circulation. During suckling, they display intermittent high-frequency bursts of spikes every few minutes. An example of one bursts is shown – the trace is a 3-s extract from an extracellular recording.

7.1.2   Priming

Mobalization of intracellular Ca^{2+} can "prime" the dendritic stores of oxytocin, making them available for subsequent activity-dependent release (by relocating them to sites adjacent to the plasma membrane where they can be influenced by voltage-gated Ca^{2+} entry to fuse with the plasma membrane; Figure 7.3). During suckling, dendritic oxytocin release has been detected *before* any increase in the spike activity of oxytocin cells, and before any increase in secretion into the blood, so it seems that the suckling input initiates dendritic oxytocin release independently of effects on spike activity. Oxytocin itself is able to prime dendritic stores of oxytocin, so it seems that the suckling stimulus primes the dendritic stores, either purely as a result of evoking oxytocin release or possibly also independently.

7.1.3   Endocannabinoids

Oxytocin cells modulate their afferent inputs by producing *endocannabinoids* (and other substances), which inhibit excitatory inputs presynaptically, and oxytocin itself suppresses inhibitory inputs by attenuating the effects of

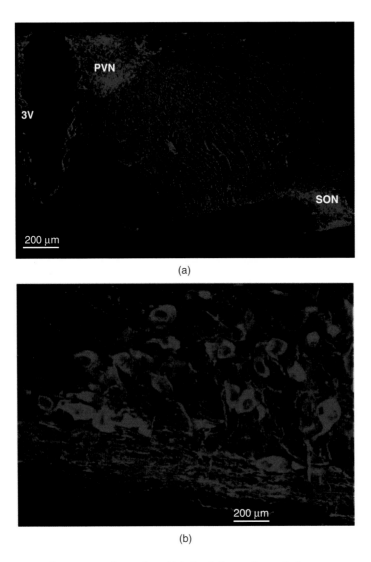

(a)

(b)

Figure 7.2   The supraoptic nucleus (SON) of the rat hypothalamus.
(a) Oxytocin cells in the SON and paraventricular nucleus (PVN) are stained red by
immunohistochemistry, in a coronal section of the rat brain. 3V=third ventricle.
(b) Higher power view of the SON – the mat of fibers at the base of the nucleus are
dendrites. Figure courtesy of Vicky Tobin.

GABA. Endocannabinoid production is activity dependent, and is linked
to increases in intracellular Ca^{2+} concentration. Endocannabinoids act via
specific cannabinoid receptors that are located on afferent endings; oxytocin acts via specific oxytocin receptors which are expressed by oxytocin
cells themselves.

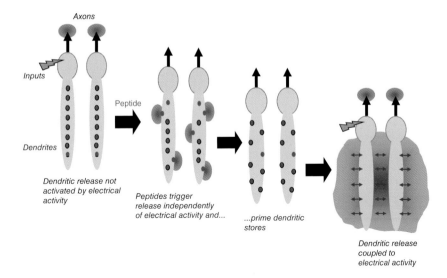

Figure 7.3 **Priming in oxytocin cells**. The dendrites of oxytocin cells contain many vesicles (shown as red organelles). These vesicles are normally located away from the plasma membrane, so stimuli that increase spike activity (indicated as a green stimulus) trigger release of oxytocin from axon terminals (where many vesicles are located adjacent to the plasama membrane) but not from dendrites. Some peptides can cause release from the dendrites without increasing spike activity, by triggering a mobilisation of intracellular calcium release. In addition, some peptides can prime the dendritic stores – moving vesicles close to the plasma membrane. After priming, these vesicles are available for release in response to increases in spike activity.

7.2   The Model

Mathematical modeling involves:
- translating biological statements into differential equations or computational algorithms;
- simulating a biological system by running these equations on a computer to generate "data" that can be compared with observational data;
- "fitting" the model to observations by varying its parameters to ensure that the model data matche *in vivo* data;
- "testing" the model by using it to generate new predictions or insights.

In our model of the milk-ejection reflex, each model cell is a *modified leaky integrate-and-fire model* (Figure 7.4), sometimes called a *spike-response model*. Such models describe a system that translates synaptic input (transient perturbations of voltage) into spikes by a threshold function. They *integrate* synaptic inputs over time, calculating the cumulative balance of excitation and inhibition as deviations from a *resting potential*. A *leaky* model represents these perturbations as decaying toward the resting potential. A spike arises when the balance of input exceeds a

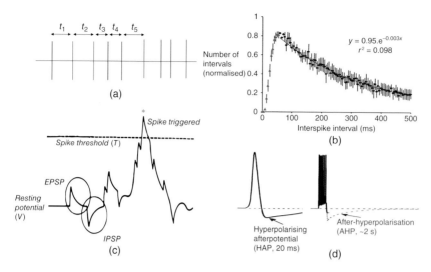

Figure 7.4   Spike activity in oxytocin cells. Under background conditions, oxytocin cells discharge spikes at 1–3 spikes/s. This spiking can be characterized by measuring interspike intervals (t1, t2, etc. as shown in (a)), and constructing an interspike interval histogram. (b) Such histograms have a characteristic distribution tails of the histogram (for intervals >50 ms) that can be well fitted by a single negative exponential (red line, fitted to average of 30 cells). From this, it appears that, after a spike, oxytocin cells have a relative refractory period of about 50 ms, after which spikes arise approximately randomly. In the model, (c) spikes arise in model cells when incoming random EPSPs and IPSPs cause a fluctuation in resting potential sufficient to exceed a spike threshold. The relative refractoriness of oxytocin cells is the result of two post-spike hyperpolarizing mechanisms and (d) a short but large HAP, and a smaller but longer acting AHP (which has a major effect only after bursts). In the model, these two mechanisms are modeled as transient changes in spike threshold that occur after each spike, rather than as changes in the membrane potential – this is equivalent to changes in the membrane potential, but computationally simpler to implement.

spike threshold. A *modified* model, or *spike-response model*, incorporates activity-dependent changes in excitability to mimic the effects of slow voltage and Ca^{2+}-dependent conductances; these may, for example, mimic hyperpolarizing- or depolarizing-after potentials that follow spikes.

In this model, every oxytocin cell receives its own, random synaptic input. This is modeled as stochastic excitatory and inhibitory postsynaptic potentials (EPSPs and IPSPs, with realistic reversal potentials); in the model, this input is (normally) balanced, reflecting an equal average mixture of EPSPs and IPSPs (the cells receive an approximately balanced synaptic input, mainly involving the neurotransmitters glutamate and GABA). The resting potential and spike threshold are fixed according to measurements made *in vitro*, and the size and time course of EPSPs and IPSPs also match observations made *in vitro*. In the model, these inputs are not directly affected by suckling; they simply ensure that, under basal conditions, each cell has a different, irregular, level of background spiking activity.

7.2.1   Activity-dependent effects on excitability

After every spike, oxytocin cells are refractory because of a hyperpolarizing afterpotential (HAP) that results from a Ca^{2+}-dependent K^+ conductance, and which follows spikes in oxytocin cells (because spikes activate high-threshold voltage-activated Ca^{2+} channels). This is modeled as a transient rise in spike threshold, and this alone is sufficient for reproducing the characteristic distribution of interspike intervals observed for oxytocin cells *in vivo.*

Another modification mimics, the effect of a slower activity-dependent afterhyperpolarization (AHP). This is another Ca^{2+}-dependent K^+ conductance; it mediates a prolonged reduction in excitability after intense activation, and it is enhanced in oxytocin cells during lactation. Including this mechanism enables the model to fully reproduce the *shape* of milk-ejection bursts.

7.2.2   Dendritic oxytocin release

Oxytocin secretion from the neurohypophysis is known to be facilitated at high spike frequencies. We assume that activity-dependent dendritic release is similarly nonlinear, and so allow that dendritic oxytocin release only occurs when spikes occur with an interspike interval that is less than a critical value.

How much oxytocin is released also depends on how much is *available* for release. In dendrites, only vesicles close to the plasma membrane (and hence close to voltage-gated Ca^{2+} channels) are released by spikes. This *readily releasable* pool of vesicles is depleted when oxytocin is released and is replenished during suckling – the *priming* effect.

7.2.3   Dendro-dendritic communication

Oxytocin cells communicate with each other via their dendrites. Each model cell is given two dendrites, each of which is part of a bundle that includes dendrites from other cells. Dendro-dendritic interactions are modeled by elements that mimic the excitatory effects of oxytocin. This is implemented as an activity-dependent reduction in the spike threshold that affects all of the oxytocin cells that have dendrites in the bundle where oxytocin is released. In the model, recognizing that receptor-mediated effects are subject to saturation, the depolarizing effect of oxytocin is limited to a maximum of 25 mV.

7.2.4   Endocannabinoid release

Oxytocin release is accompanied by the production of endocannabinoids which feed back to modulate synaptic input. Endocannabinoids are produced as a consequence of the mobilization of intracellular Ca^{2+}, and act via CB1 receptors on afferent nerve terminals. The rate of release of both EPSPs and IPSPs to all cells connected to a bundle is inhibited by the effects of endocannabinoids produced in that bundle.

7.3 Building the model

To model individual cells, we use a *leaky integrate-and-fire model* (Figure 7.4), which is modified to incorporate activity-dependent changes in excitability. Every cell receives an independent synaptic input that is a mixture of EPSPs and IPSPs, and these are represented by $N_{E,i}^{j}$, $N_{I,i}^{j}$, which are inhomogeneous Poisson processes of rates $\lambda_{E,i}^{j}(t)$ and $\lambda_{I,i}^{j}(t)$, respectively. $a_{E}(v_{E} - v_{\text{rest}})$ and $a_{I}(v_{\text{rest}} - v_{I})$ are the magnitude of single EPSPs and IPSPs at v_{rest}, and v_{E} and v_{I} are the excitatory and inhibitory reversal potentials.

7.3.1 Spike generation

The membrane potential v_{i} of cell i obeys

$$\frac{dv_{i}}{dt} = \frac{v_{\text{rest}} - v_{i}}{\tau} + \sum_{j=1}^{2}\left[a_{E}(v_{E} - v_{i})\frac{dN_{E,i}^{j}}{dt} - a_{I}(v_{i} - v_{I})\frac{dN_{I,i}^{j}}{dt}\right] \quad (7.1)$$

where τ is the membrane time constant, and v_{rest} is the resting potential.

A spike is produced in cell i at time $t = t_{i}^{s}, s = 1, 2, \ldots$, if $v_{i}(t_{i}^{s}) = T_{i}(t_{i}^{s})$, where $T_{i}(t)$ is the spike threshold at time t. After each spike, v_{i} is reset to v_{rest}. Activity-dependent changes in excitability and the effects of oxytocin are modeled by effects on spike threshold:

$$T_{i} = T_{0} + T_{\text{HAP},i} + T_{\text{AHP},i} - T_{\text{OT},i} \quad (7.2)$$

where T_{0} is a constant.

$T_{\text{HAP},i}$ models the effect of an HAP in cell i by

$$T_{\text{HAP},i} = k_{\text{HAP}}H(t - \hat{t}_{i})e^{-(t-\hat{t}_{i})/\tau_{\text{HAP}}} \quad (7.3)$$

where k_{HAP} and τ_{HAP} are constants, $\hat{t}_{i} = \max_{s}\{t_{i}^{s} : t_{i}^{s} \leq t\}$, and $H(x)$ is the *Heaviside step function*. This gives an increase in the spike threshold after each spike. Similarly, T_{AHP} models the AHP. The AHP builds up slowly, leading to a significant reduction of excitability only after intense activity. The variables $f_{i}, i = 1, \ldots, n$ represent the recent activity of each cell, and

$$\frac{df_{i}}{dt} = -\frac{f_{i}}{\tau_{\text{AHP}}} + \sum_{t_{i}^{s} < t} \delta(t - t_{i}^{s}) \quad (7.4)$$

where τ_{AHP} is the decay constant of the AHP, and $\delta(x)$ is the *Dirac delta function*. We set

$$T_{\text{AHP},i} = k_{\text{AHP}}\frac{f_{i}^{4}}{f_{i}^{4} + f_{\text{th}}^{4}} \quad (7.5)$$

where k_{AHP} and f_{th} are the constants adjusted to match the characteristics of spontaneous firing in oxytocin cells.

7.3.2 Effects of oxytocin

The network topology (Figure 7.5) – how the cells are interconnected – is represented by matrices $C_k = \{c_{ij}^k\}, k = 1, \ldots, n$, where $c_{ij}^k = 1$ if dendrite j of cell i is in bundle k, and zero otherwise. The increase in excitability due to oxytocin is T_{OT},

$$\frac{dT_{OT,i}}{dt} = -\frac{T_{OT,i}}{\tau_{OT}} + k_{OT} \sum_{k=1}^{n_b} \sum_{j=1}^{n} \sum_{l,\,m=1}^{2} c_{il}^k c_{jm}^k \rho_j^m(t) \tag{7.6}$$

where τ_{OT}, k_{OT} are constants, $\rho_j^m(t)$ is the release rate from dendrite m of cell j, and the sums pick up all the cells whose dendrites share the same

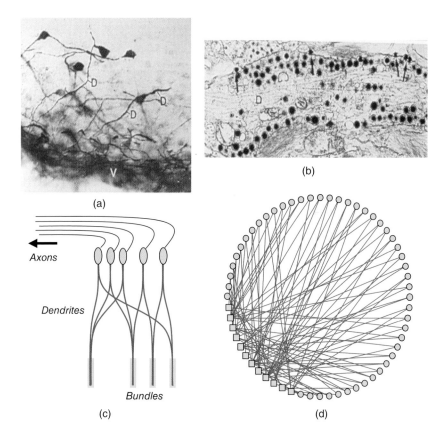

(a)

(b)

Axons

Dendrites

Bundles

(c)

(d)

Figure 7.5 Structure of the model network. Oxytocin cells in the supraoptic nucleus have 1–3 large dendrites, most of which project ventrally (shown by immunocytochemistry in (a). These dendrites contain large numbers of neurosecretory vesicles (shown by electron microscopy in (b)). In the model, cells (c, in blue) have two dendrites (in red) that are coupled within bundles (indicated in yellow). The organization of the oxytocin network is shown in (d); the yellow boxes represent dendritic bundles.

bundle as cell i. The oxytocin-dependent reduction of the spike threshold is limited to a maximum $(T_{\text{OT,max}})$ of 25 mV.

7.3.3 Oxytocin release from the dendrites

The readily releasable pool of oxytocin in dendrite j of cell i is r_i^j, where

$$\frac{dr_i^j}{dt} = -\frac{r_i^j}{\tau_r} + k_p(t) - \rho_i^j(t) \tag{7.7}$$

where τ_r is a time constant, $k_p(t)$ is the rate of priming due to suckling ($k_p(t)$ is a positive constant during suckling and zero otherwise), and ρ_i^j is the instantaneous release rate from dendrite j. Release from a dendrite is proportional to the size of the readily releasable pool of oxytocin in that dendrite, so

$$\rho_i^j(t) = k_r r_i^j(t) \sum_i \delta(t - t_i^s - \Delta) \tag{7.8}$$

where k_r is the maximum fraction of the pool that can be released by a spike, Δ is a fixed delay before release, and the summation extends over the set $\{t_i^s < t, t_i^s - t_i^{s-1} < \tau_{\text{rel}}\}$, with τ_{rel} a constant. Only spikes occurring at intervals of less than τ_{rel} induce any dendritic release. We set $\tau_{\text{rel}} = 50$ ms, but the exact value is not critical.

7.3.4 Endocannabinoids

The variables $\epsilon_k(t), k = 1, \ldots, n_b$ represent the concentration of endocannabinoids in each bundle, and evolve according to

$$\frac{d\epsilon_k}{dt} = -\frac{\epsilon_k}{\tau_{\text{EC}}} + k_{\text{EC}} \sum_{n=1}^{n} \sum_{j=1}^{2} c_{ij}^k \rho_i^j \tag{7.9}$$

where τ_{EC} is the decay time constant, and k_{EC} scales the amount of oxytocin released within the bundles into an increase of endocannabinoid concentration (i.e., oxytocin and endocannabinoids are assumed to be released in parallel). The rates of EPSPs and IPSPs are equally affected by endocannabinoids:

$$\lambda_{x,i}^j(t) = \left[1 - \alpha \sum_k c_{ij}^k F_{\text{att}}(\epsilon_k)\right] \overline{\lambda}_{x,i}^j(t) \tag{7.10}$$

where $\overline{\lambda}_{x,i}^j(t), x = E, i$ are the unmodified synaptic input rates for dendrite j of cell i, α is the maximal fractional attenuation of the input, and

$$F_{\text{att}}(\epsilon) = \frac{\epsilon^4}{\epsilon^4 + \epsilon_{\text{th}}^4} \tag{7.11}$$

where ϵ_{th} is a constant. The parameter values are given in Table 7.1 unless otherwise stated. The equations were integrated numerically by the Euler–Maruyama method with a time step of 0.1 ms. The MATLAB code for simulating the system is given in www.wiley.com/go/leng/computational.

7.3.5 Network topology

The network has n cells and n_b bundles, and each cell has two dendrites in different bundles (Figure 7.5). To assign dendrites to bundles, and for an integer $d > 0$, we start by considering a set of $n_b = (2n/d)$ empty bundles. For each cell, we choose two bundles as follows. The index of the first bundle (i_1) is selected at random from $\{1, 2, \dots, n_b\}$, the second index is selected at random from $\{1, 2, \dots, n_b\} - \{i_1\}$, ensuring that no cell has two dendrites in the same bundle. This, repeated for all cells, leads to a random allocation of dendrites into bundles.

7.4 Model behavior

In the model, in the absence of suckling, cells fire spikes independently at a rate that depends on the level of synaptic input, and with interspike interval distributions that are very similar to those of oxytocin cells recorded *in vivo* (Figures 7.6 and 7.7). When the suckling input (k_p) is switched on, there is (at first) little change in this activity, but there is a progressive priming of activity-dependent oxytocin release, and this is accompanied by the production of endocannabinoids. As these begin to take effect, faster firing cells tend to slow down and slower firing cells tend to speed up. After a delay, synchronized bursts arise throughout the network, and these recur every few minutes.

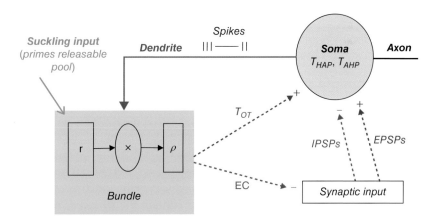

Figure 7.6 **The structure of a single model cell**. A single model cell receives random EPSPs and IPSPs, and its excitability is modeled as a dynamically changing spike threshold that is influenced by an HAP (parameter T_{HAP}), and a slower AHP (T_{AHP}). Each cell interacts with its neighbor via two neurons by dendrites (red) that are coupled within bundles (yellow), and its excitability is increased when oxytocin is released in these bundles (T_{OT}). Activity-dependent production of endocannabinoids (EC) feeds back to reduce synaptic input rates.

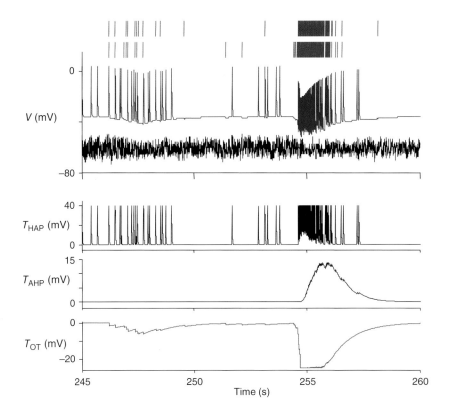

Figure 7.7   The behavior of one model cell during a burst. The upper two red traces show the times of occurrence of all oxytocin release events in the two dendritic bundles to which the cell is connected. Below this is the soma activity: the blue line shows the spike threshold, showing the effects of post-spike activity changes and of oxytocin; the black line *(V)* shows the impact of EPSPs and IPSPs. The bottom three traces show T_{HAP}, T_{AHP} and T_{OT}.

7.4.1   Example simulations

Figure 7.8 shows simulations from a network of 48 cells and 12 bundles (with a mean of 8 dendrites per bundle) with the topology as shown in Figure 7.6 (the results are similar in networks of up to 3000 cells). Bursts occur when, and only when, suckling is present, that is, priming of dendritic release is essential. The model parameters were tuned to match the interspike interval distributions of oxytocin cells and the temporal characteristics of bursts (Table 7.1). Bursts contain 50–70 spikes in 1–3 s (0.9–4.6 s *in vivo*), and recur at intervals of about 4 min, in close agreement with *in vivo* observations.

Interspike interval distributions (Figure 7.9) calculated from the activity of model cells between bursts match *in vivo* data indistinguishably, so the model describes the background activity of oxytocin cells well, as well as bursting activity. Normally, all cells participate in the reflex in the

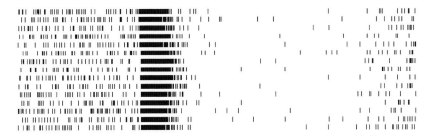

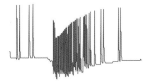

Figure 7.8 Synchronized bursting in model oxytocin cells. Each row of the raster shows the spike activity of just one of the 348 cells in a network model; each bar shows the timing of a spike. Bursts are approximately synchronized, while background activity is asynchronous. The red trace below shows how T changes during a burst in one of the cells; each spike causes a large transient rise in T. As oxytocin is released, it causes a fall in T that is offset by a slow rise caused by the AHP. Note how similar this profile is to the extracellularly recorded voltage trace of oxytocin cells in Figure 7.1.

model, and the mean variation in burst onset is about 200 ms, close to measurements *in vivo*. Model cells show a brief silence before many bursts; in the model, endocannabinoids released from the first cells that burst can suppress synaptic input enough to inhibit other oxytocin cells before they are activated by oxytocin release, and similar pre-burst silences occur *in vivo*.

7.4.2 Roles of the HAP and AHP

In the model, the shape of bursts is determined by the AHP, which reduces the peak firing rate and shortens the burst duration. Removing the AHP has little effect on the timing of bursts, as it activated relatively little at background firing rates.

The HAP parameters were fixed to provide a match to the interspike interval distribution between bursts. The choice of parameters affects the timing of bursts, as the HAP limits the occurrence of short interspike intervals; when there are more frequent short intervals, the readily releasable stores of dendritic oxytocin are more depleted, but there is also an increased incidence of events that can potentially trigger a burst.

7.4.3 Pacemaker activity

As observed *in vivo*, there are no fixed leader or follower cells in the network – the order in which cells start to burst varies randomly from burst to burst. Bursting in the model is, thus, an *emergent activity*, due to the interplay

Table 7.1 Model parameters (a.u., arbitrary units).

Name	Description	Value	Units
n	Number of cells	48	
n_b	Number of bundles	12	
τ	Membrane time constant	10.8	ms
v_{rest}	Resting potential	−62	mV
$a_E(v_E - v_{rest})$	EPSP amplitude	4	mV
$a_I(v_I - v_{rest})$	IPSP amplitude	4	mV
v_E	EPSP reversal potential	0	mV
v_I	IPSP reversal potential	−80	mV
$\bar{\lambda}_E$	Excitatory input rate	80	Hz
$\bar{\lambda}_I$	Inhibitory input rate	80	Hz
k_{HAP}	HAP, maximum amplitude	40	mV
τ_{HAP}	HAP, decay time constant	12.5	ms
k_{AHP}	AHP, maximum amplitude	40	mV
τ_{AHP}	AHP, time constant	2	s
f_{th}	AHP, half-activation constant	45	a.u.
τ_{OT}	Time decay of oxytocin-induced depolarization	1	s
k_{OT}	Depolarization for unitary oxytocin release	0.5	mV
Δ	Time delay for oxytocin release	5	ms
$T_{OT,max}$	Maximum oxytocin-induced depolarization	25	mV
k_p	Priming rate	0.5	s^{-1}
τ_r	Time constant for priming	400	s
k_r	Fraction of dendritic stores released per spike (max)	0.045	
τ_{EC}	Time constant for [EC] decay	6	s
k_{EC}	Endocannabinoid increase per unit oxytocin release	0.0025	a.u.
ϵ_{th}	[EC] threshold for synaptic attenuation	0.03	a.u.
τ_{rel}	Maximum interspike interval for release	50	ms
α	Fractional attenuation of synaptic input rate (max)	0.6	

between the single neuron dynamics and network dynamics. The lack of a marked leader/follower character is accentuated by the homogeneous arrangement of the network connections; because all bundles contain the same number of dendrites, all are equally possible sites of burst initiation. We considered a network with the same number of cells and bundles (and the same mean connectivity) but where the number of dendrites varied in each bundle; in this case, bursts are more likely to start in regions of the network where dendritic bundling is more pronounced.

7.4.4 Synchronization

Without any suckling input, the firing of oxytocin cells in the model is uncorrelated (as *in vivo*). Between bursts, spiking activity is characterized by a small but increasing cross-correlation of firing rates, a consequence of the strengthening interactions between cells. Activity becomes more irregular close to a burst, shown by a rising *index of dispersion* of the firing rate. These results conform to experimental findings *in vivo*. In the model, increased

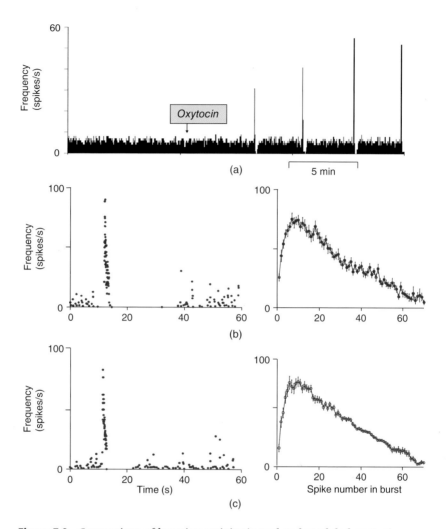

Figure 7.9   Comparison of bursting activity in real and modeled oxytocin cells. (a) Milk-ejection bursts triggered by i.c.v. injection of oxytocin in a urethane – anaesthetised (b) A milk-ejection burst in an oxytocin cell recorded *in vivo* (red) and a model cell (blue) plotted as instantaneous firing rate (each point is the reciprocal of the interval since the previous spike). This profile is indistinguishable to burst profiles observed *in vivo*. (c) Mean profiles of milk-ejection bursts from a living oxytocin cell (red) (Data file[g1]) and from a model cell (blue). Each profile is constructed from 17 bursts, and shows the mean ± S.E. instantaneous firing rate plotted for each interspike interval within the bursts.

variability arises because, toward a burst, activity produces both dendritic oxytocin release, with excitatory consequences, and endocannabinoid production, with inhibitory consequences. If endocannabinoid release is eliminated (by setting $\alpha = 0$), then there is no increase in variability.

In a network of 1000 cells with just two dendrites in each bundle, bursts are rare, propagate slowly, and involve only some cells. With more

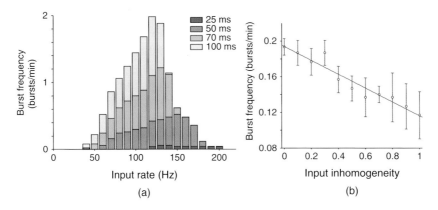

Figure 7.10   Dependence of bursting on synaptic input (a) In simulations of the model network, bursting behaviour is observed only within a range of values for the excitatory input. A minimum level of excitation is necessary to start the reflex. Increasing the input rate speeds up bursting until the excess of oxytocin release causes an abrupt breakdown. Bar colors correspond to varying the threshold for frequency-dependent release, defined as the maximum interspike interval allowed for dendritic release. (b) The effect of a spatially inhomogeneous input on bursting activity. Cells were subject to (balanced) inputs of rate $\lambda = \lambda_0(1 + \epsilon)$, with ϵ drawn from a normal distribution. Plotted is the bursting frequency (based upon 50 min of dynamics; average over five trials with independently distributed rates) vs the SD of ϵ. Bars are SD; the dashed line is a linear fit.

dendrites in each bundle, there is a faster propagation of bursts and better synchronization. Figure 7.10 shows how a burst is propagated between cells, and the effects of varying the degree of random connectivity. Large, randomly coupled networks can be rapidly synchronized even if the coupling is sparse, but if cells are coupled less randomly (i.e., more regularly), synchronization is poorer and "traveling waves" can arise.

7.4.5   Post-burst silences

Bursts are followed by silent periods of up to 20 s. *In vivo*, post-burst silences are variable in duration (7–56 s), indicating that they are not simply the deterministic consequence of an activity-dependent AHP. In the model, the post-burst silence is mainly a consequence of the prolonged suppression of afferent input by endocannabinoids. *In vivo*, it has been reported that a few otherwise typical oxytocin cells show no bursts at milk ejection but instead fall silent. A similar phenomenon can be replicated in the model by assuming that some cells do not express oxytocin receptors (by setting $k_{OT} = 0$ for these cells).

7.4.6   Dendritic stores

In the model, the dendritic stores of readily releasable vesicles are incremented by suckling. Their level tends to increase between bursts despite activity-dependent depletion, and bursts tend to occur when the stores are relatively large. At high store levels, dendritic release is reduced because of the suppression of synaptic input by endocannabinoids. This prevents dendritic release from becoming regenerative, and helps the stores to accumulate. In this phase, network activity becomes irregular because of the opposing feedbacks: excitation by oxytocin release, and suppression of afferent input by endocannabinoids. If just a few neighboring cells coincidentally show increased activity as a result of random fluctuations in their input rates, and if they have large enough stores, then enough oxytocin may be released to trigger a burst.

7.4.7 Paradoxical behaviors

Between bursts, spike activity causes the depletion of the readily releasable pool and hence too much of this activity can suppress bursting. Conversely, an increase in the rate of inhibitory input can promote the reflex in a system which fails to express bursting because of insufficient priming (Figure 7.10). Such "paradoxical" behaviors have been detailed *in vivo*; for example, injections of GABA into the supraoptic nucleus of a suckled rat can trigger milk-ejection bursts; conversely, many stimuli that activate oxytocin cells suppress the reflex. Occasionally, a burst occurs shortly *after* removing the suckling stimulus. This feature is also shared (occasionally) by the reflex *in vivo*, showing that suckling itself is not a strictly necessary trigger.

7.4.8 Network structures

In the model, during suckling, oxytocin cells that are strongly excited produce endocannabinoids that reduce the overall level of synaptic input. This protects the system from over-excitation and maintains the network in an optimal range for bursting. This is important, because bursting is possible only within a range of values of synaptic input. The precise range depends on the strength of the coupling between spike activity and dendritic secretion. At a low level of excitation, an increase in synaptic input favors bursting by increasing the frequency of release episodes which can trigger a burst, but above a critical level, such release events may be so frequent that stores are not replenished fast enough for the stores to reach the critical level required to trigger a burst. Bursts become rarer and less predictable, until eventually over-excitation disrupts the reflex. Spatial inhomogeneity in the stochastic input can also degrade the reflex. The system performs optimally when the activity is relatively homogeneous between oxytocin cells, a conclusion previously drawn from experimental studies.

7.5 Discussion

During lactation, oxytocin is released in pulses following quasi-synchronous bursts of spike activity in oxytocin cells. Here, computational modeling shows that such bursting can arise as an emergent property of a spiking neuronal network. The model does not incorporate all elements of the physiology of oxytocin cells, but is a minimalist representation to help identify the key processes.

7.5.1   Key assumptions

In formulating this model, we are hypothesizing that, during lactation, the oxytocin system is a network where cells interact by dendritic release of oxytocin, coupled nonlinearly to electrical activity. This requires a stimulus-dependent *priming* of the dendritic stores, whereby these are made available for activity-dependent release. Dendritic release of oxytocin occurs only when the cell's firing rate is sufficiently large, so interactions between cells are rare and erratic between bursts and in the absence of the suckling stimulus. Accordingly, spiking is asynchronous except during the bursts themselves; thus the network is essentially a *pulse-coupled network*.

7.5.2   Emergent behavior

In this model, bursting is an *emergent behavior* of a sparsely connected population of cells. Bursting can begin at any of many foci of neuronal interactions – within any of the dendritic bundles that link just a few of the cells, from where it will spread to the remaining bundles. Bursting arises by positive feedback resulting from activity-dependent oxytocin release, and this is diminished after a burst (by depletion of the pool of readily releasable vesicles). The core mechanism, positive feedback followed by synaptic depression, is similar to that used in some other models of bursting. However, the oxytocin cell network is sparsely connected compared to others, and the biological substrate is different – here the intercommunication is dendro-dendritic rather than synaptic.

7.5.3   Making biological inferences

Comparing the model with the living system can help us to understand the role of several biological mechanisms. For example, the AHP affects the burst profile, but contributes little to burst timing or to post-burst silences. Second, although the core burst mechanism is a positive feedback, negative feedbacks are also important. In fact, there are many negative feedbacks involving diverse signaling molecules; these are represented by just one, and this is an oversimplification. In the model, endocannabinoids are produced in parallel with oxytocin release, but the dynamics of their effects differ from those of oxytocin, and the competing effects promote increased variability in the firing rate as the system swings from excitation to inhibition. The "upswings" mean that, for a given mean firing rate, there are more short intervals toward the end of an interburst interval, and they are more likely to be correlated with cells, making them more potent as potential burst-triggering events. At the same time, the depressive effects on the mean firing rate means that, at high synaptic input rates, there is less depletion of the releasable pool of oxytocin. Together, these effects mean that the rate at which bursts arise is relatively independent of the synaptic input rate over a reasonably wide range.

7.5.4 New questions that arise

The model makes it possible to study how bursting behavior relates to network connectivity. Mathematically, the network can be described by a *bipartite graph* $G = \{N \cup B, E\}$, where N is the set of cells, B is the set of bundles, and E is the set of connections from cells to bundles such that, for cell a in N and bundle b in B, $(a, b) \in E$ if a has a dendrite in b (Figure 7.11). The network topology is specified by $O = \{o_{ij}\}, i = 1, \ldots, n, j = 1, \ldots, n_b$, where $o_{ij} = 1$ if cell i has a dendrite in bundle j, and $o_{ij} = 0$ otherwise. If dendro-dendritic connections are formed at random, then O is a

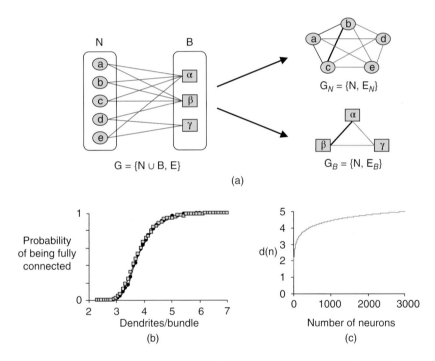

Figure 7.11 How bursting behavior relates to network connectivity. (a) The network can be described by a *bipartite graph*, where N is the set of cells, B is the set of bundles, and E is the set of connections from cells to bundles such that, for cell a in N and bundle b in B, if a has a dendrite in b. From these graphs, we can derive graphs G_N and G_B for connections between the cells and between the bundles. For the network to be collectively activated during a burst, it must be *connected*, that is, any two cells must be connected by some path. (b) Plots the probability that a network of 1000 cells, each with two dendrites, will be fully connected for different numbers of dendrites per bundle. Above a critical value of about 4.5, the network is almost certainly fully connected. (c) Shows how the critical value is affected by the number of cells in the network.

random binary matrix whose rows satisfy $\sum_{j=1}^{n_b} o_{ij} = 2$. From the graph $G = \{N \cup B, E\}$, we can derive the graphs $G_N = \{N, E_N\}$ and $G_B = \{B, E_B\}$ for connections between the cells and the bundles, respectively. The *edge set* of G_N, E_N contains all pairs of cells which share at least one bundle, while the edge set of G_B, E_B contains all pairs of bundles which are "bridged" by at least one cell. For G_B, the *node degrees* represent the number of dendrites in the corresponding bundles, that is, $d_j = \sum_{i=1}^{n} o_{ij}, j = 1, \ldots, n_b$. If the bundles are formed at random, the latter form a set of identically distributed random variables of mean $\bar{d} = 2n/n_b$. The average number of connections formed by each cell can then be estimated as $2(\bar{d} - 1)$.

For the network to be collectively activated during a burst, it must be *connected*, that is, any two cells must be connected by some path. The probability that the network is connected can be estimated by approximating G_N (or G_B) with a random graph of the same size and average degree; a random graph of n nodes is almost certainly connected if its average degree is $\geq \log n$, suggesting that a network of n cells will be connected if $\bar{d} \geq 1 + \frac{1}{2} \log n$. However, the oxytocin network has different topological properties, so we compared the fraction of connected networks in a sample of 1000 random networks and 1000 approximating random graphs, with varying $\bar{d}$. For each value of $\bar{d}$, we considered a set of n cells and $n_b^0 = 2n/\bar{d}$ bundles. Then, for each cell i, we chose (uniformly at random) two bundles of indices $(i_1, i_2), i_1, i_2 = 1, \ldots, 2N/\bar{d}, i_1 \neq i_2$, and set $o_{ij_1} = o_{ij_2} = 1$. Finally, bundles with no dendrites were removed from the bundle set. The result is a graph of n cells and $n_b = n_b^0 - n_b^{(e)}$ bundles, where $n_b^{(e)}$ is the number of empty bundles. The mean number of dendrites per bundle was then recomputed as $\bar{d} = 2n/n_b$. We calculated the average degree of the resulting network, and then generated a random graph with the same average degree. We confirmed the validity of the approximation with a network of 1000 cells (which is about as many as there are oxytocin cells in one supraoptic nucleus). Figure 7.11 plots the critical value of $\bar{d}$ for the random graph; the predicted value for $n = 1000$ is 4.45. When $\bar{d}$ is larger than this, more than 85% of the generated networks are fully connected. This result is in accord with the empirically observed connectivity of oxytocin cells (oxytocin cells have 1–3 dendrites in bundles of 3–8 dendrites).

7.5.5 Model topology and wave propagation

The topology of the oxytocin network is important for both the generation and the synchronization of bursts. The interconnections within bundles, combined with the excitatory effect of oxytocin, lead to a positive feedback which sustains burst generation. At the same time, random connections between bundles reduce the typical path length between any two cells of the network, enhancing synchronization. We studied a network of 384 cells with dendrites in 96 bundles using a different, ring topology. Here, cells are grouped in clusters, those in a given cluster project to the same two bundles, and each bundle receives dendrites only from two adjacent clusters, forming a chain-like structure. This is equivalent to assuming that cells preferentially contact their closest neighbors. In this network, bursting is not synchronized; two wave fronts travel along the network, and it takes ~5 s for a burst to propagate across the whole network. Figure 7.12 shows the results in networks with increasing probability of rewiring p.

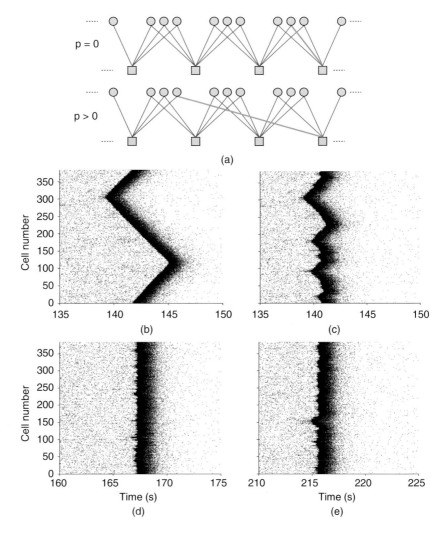

Figure 7.12 Impact of network topology on the propagation of bursting. The network topology is critical for whether bursting is synchronous, or occurs as a traveling wave. (a) Schematic diagram illustrating a network with a ring structure ($p = 0$, top) and with random rewiring ($p > 0$, bottom); blue circles indicate cells, yellow boxes indicate bundles. One dendrite (in green) is randomly chosen and re-assigned; this is shown for only one cell, but the rule was applied to all cells independently. (b–e) Raster plots of spikes generated in networks with increasing probability of rewiring: $p = 0$ (b) 0.05 (c) 0.5 (d), and 0.95 (e).

Starting from the ring topology, we randomly rewired one dendrite for each cell with probability p. As the probability of rewiring increases (i.e., with more random connectivity), bursts become progressively more synchronized. Thus, the bursting synchronization is sensitive to the network topology, and is observable with a *small-world*-type topology.

7.5.6   Bursting, spiking and multiscale dynamics

Whereas neurons exchange information mostly via spikes, endocrine cells rely on hormonal pulses to signal to their target tissues. For many neurons, clustered spike activity is optimally effective in inducing the required changes on the targets, but for endocrine cells to generate a signal large enough to be read at a distance, their secretory activity must not only be optimal for each cell, their activity must also be coordinated; hence, hormone signals are generally pulsatile. Many neurons in the brain produce a peptide as well as a conventional transmitter, and many peptides have effects on organismal behavior that are hormone-like in that they act at dispersed and distant targets to produce prolonged organizational changes. For a hormone-like, pulsatile signal to be produced reliably, the activity of peptide-secreting cells must be coordinated in a physiologically adaptable manner. In the present model, network interactions are mediated only by spikes that occur with interspike intervals less than τ_{rel}; similar spike doublets are thought to play a critical role in the synchronization of network activity in many neural systems.

7.5.7   Limitations of the model

The present model produces a very close match to electrophysiological data, and its strength is the simplicity of the core representation of a single cell; this makes it possible to explore how properties of the network affect the system's behavior. The simplifications that we made in modeling the reflex are mainly unlikely to have had any major influence, with two possible exceptions. First, we have not included intracellular $[Ca^{2+}]$ changes as a variable, although the mobilization of intracellular Ca^{2+} stores can trigger dendritic oxytocin release, and, therefore, probably contributes to oxytocin release during milk ejection. Implicitly, we assumed that this overlaps with activity-induced oxytocin release and, hence, can be neglected, but it seems very possible that in some circumstances, oxytocin release triggered by Ca^{2+} release from intracellular stores might precipitate a burst. Second, we modeled dendritic release as a relatively common deterministic event. In fact, dendritic release probably occurs as the relatively rare exocytosis of large vesicles that each contain a large amount of oxytocin (about 85000 molecules) – and the release process is likely to be stochastic, with interval length governing the probability of release rather than determining it. Whether this will affect the model behavior substantially remains to be tested.

7.6 **Perspectives**

The model described here is a "systems level model." It describes a complex system in a concise way; it does not include representations of the full level of detail that is known, but it tests our understanding of the ways in which particular qualitative behaviors arise. A system, in this sense, is just an arrangement of circumstances that makes things happen in a certain way. We look to model something that has a measurable input and a measurable output, which are connected by known or hypothesized rules. This could be a signaling pathway within a single cell, but often we apply the "systems" tag to things that involve higher level processing, with many components, some of which may be unknown. The purpose of such modeling is to generate hypotheses about the types of processing that take place, and about how it might be organized.

In this case, the *measurable output* is the spike activity of oxytocin cells during suckling. These derive from extracellular recordings, so while we know much about spike generation in oxytocin cells from *in vitro* studies, there is little to be gained by a fully biophysical model of oxytocin cells because we have no intracellular recordings of the bursting activity of oxytocin cells with which to compare the model performance. There is little point in generating predictions about things that cannot be measured, and which depend upon extrapolations from data derived under conditions that deviate in uncertain ways from the situation to be modeled.

Even the present model displays outcomes that would have been hard to predict and are correspondingly hard to explain; the more detailed a model, the harder to understand *why* it does what it does. If the aim of a model is to test the completeness and limitations of our understanding, it is important to build a model that can be understood and amenable to systematic investigation. The more parameters that a model has, the harder it is to systematically study its behavior. These difficulties increase exponentially with the number of free parameters; keeping models simple is essential for making them useful.

Dataset 1 Available at www.wiley.com/go/leng/computational

Excel file giving raw data of spike times from 13 successive milk-ejection bursts recorded from a single oxytocin cell in a urethane-anesthetized rat, from the experiments reported by Dyball and Leng (1987). Each cell entry is the instantaneous frequency (the reciprocal of the interspike interval for successive interspike intervals), and each column records a single burst. The yellow areas highlight preburst activity; the bursts are aligned to the first occurrence of an interspike interval of <100 ms in a long sequence of short intervals.

Bibliography

Essential references

First report of the milk-ejection burst model
Rossoni E, Feng J, Tirozzi B, Brown D, Leng G, Moos F (2008). Emergent synchronous bursting of oxytocin neuronal network. *PLoS Comput Biol.* **4**(7).

The integrate-and fire model applied to oxytocin cells
Leng G *et al.* (2001). Responses of magnocellular neurons to osmotic stimulation involves co-activation of excitatory and inhibitory input: an experimental and theoretical analysis. *J Neurosci.* **21**: 6967–6977.

First account of priming of dendritic release
Ludwig M *et al.* (2002). Intracellular calcium stores regulate activity-dependent neuropeptide release from dendrites. *Nature* **418**: 85–89.

Key paper on actions of endocannabinoids
Hirasawa M *et al.* (2004). Dendritically released transmitters cooperate via autocrine and retrograde actions to inhibit afferent excitation in rat brain. *J Physiol.* **59**: 611–624.

Key reviews of the biological background
Leng G, Brown D (1997). The origins and significance of pulsatility in hormone secretion from the pituitary. *J Neuroendocrinol.* **9**: 493–513.

Leng G, Brown CH, Russell JA (1999). Physiological pathways regulating the activity of magnocellular neurosecretory cells. *Prog Neurobiol.* **57**: 625–655.

Leng G, Ludwig M (2006). Information processing in the hypothalamus: peptides and analogue computation. *J Neuroendocrinol.* **18**: 379–392.

Ludwig M, Leng G (2006). Dendritic peptide release and peptide dependent behaviours. *Nat Neurosci Rev.* **7**: 126–136.

Russell JA, Leng G, Douglas AJ (2003). The magnocellular oxytocin system. The fount of maternity: adaptations in pregnancy. *Front Neuroendocrinol.* **24**: 27–61.

Theodosis DT (2002). Oxytocin-secreting neurons: a physiological model of morphological neuronal and glial plasticity in the adult hypothalamus. *Front Neuroendocrinol.* **23**: 101–135.

A detailed theoretical analysis based on bifurcation theory in the model
Wu Y *et al.* (2012). Bifurcations of emergent bursting in a neuronal network. *PLoS One* **7**(6): e38402.

Source papers for key biological data on the milk-ejection reflex

The two papers below, by Jonathan Wakerley and Dennis Lincoln, were the first descriptions of the milk-ejection reflex
Lincoln DW, Wakerley JB (1974). Electrophysiological evidence for the activation of supraoptic neurons during the release of oxytocin. *J Physiol.* **242**: 533–554.

Wakerley JB, Lincoln DW (1973). The milk-ejection reflex of the rat: a 20- to 40-fold acceleration in the firing of paraventricular neurones during oxytocin release. *J Endocrinol.* **57**: 477–493.

Quantitative aspects of milk-ejection bursts, from the laboratory of Françoise Moos

Belin V, Moos FC (1986). Paired recordings from supraoptic and paraventricular oxytocin cells in suckled rats: recruitment and synchronization *J Physiol.* **377**: 369–390.

Brown D, Fontanaud P, Moos FC (2000). The variability of basal action potential firing is positively correlated with bursting in hypothalamic oxytocin neurones. *J Neuroendocrinol.* **12**: 506–520.

Brown D, Moos FC (1997). Onset of bursting in oxytocin cells in suckled rats. *J Physiol.* **503**: 625–634.

Moos FC, Fontanaud P, Mekaouche M, Brown D (2004). Oxytocin neurones are recruited into co-ordinated fluctuations of firing before bursting in the rat. *Neuroscience.* **125**: 593–602.

Experimental studies displaying key features of the reflex

Dyball REJ, Leng G (1986). The regulation of the milk-ejection reflex in the rat *J Physiol.* **380**: 239–256.

Lambert RC, Dayanithi G, Moos FC, Richard P (1994). A rise in the intracellular Ca2+ concentration of isolated rat supraoptic cells in response to oxytocin *J Physiol.* **478**: 275–288.

Lambert RC, Moos FC, Richard P (1993). Action of endogenous oxytocin within the paraventricular or supraoptic nuclei: a powerful link in the regulation of the bursting pattern of oxytocin neurons during the milk-ejection reflex in rats *Neuroscience* **57**: 1027–1038.

Moos FC (1995). GABA-induced facilitation of the periodic bursting activity of oxytocin neurons in suckled rats *J Physiol.* **488**: 103–114.

Wang YF, Hatton GI (2004). Milk ejection burst-like electrical activity evoked in supraoptic oxytocin neurons in slices from lactating rats. *J Neurophysiol.* **91**: 2312–2321.

Related theoretical papers

Albert R, Barabsi AL (2002). Statistical mechanics of complex networks. *Rev Mod Phys.* **74**: 47–97.

Kopell N, Karbowski J (2000). Multispikes and synchronization in a large neural network with temporal delays. *Neural Comput.* **12**: 1537–606.

Leng G, MacGregor DJ (2008). Mathematical modeling in neuroendocrinology *J Neuroendocrinol.* **20**: 713–718.

Shao J, Tsao T, Butera RJ (2006). Bursting without slow kinetics: a role for a small world? *Neural Comput.* **18**: 2029–2035.

Whittington MA, Kopell N, Ermentrout GB (2000). Gamma rhythms and beta rhythms have different synchronization properties. *Proc Natl Acad Sci USA* **97**: 1867–1872.

CHAPTER 8

Dynamics of the HPA Axis: A Systems Modeling Approach

John R. Terry[1,2,], Jamie J. Walker[1,2,*], Francesca Spiga[2], and Stafford L. Lightman[2]*

[1]College of Engineering, Mathematics and Physical Sciences, University of Exeter, Exeter, UK
[2]Henry Wellcome Laboratories for Integrative Neuroscience and Endocrinology, University of Bristol, Whitson Street, Bristol, UK
*Denotes equal contribution.

8.1 Introduction

Physical or psychological stress activates autonomic and neuroendocrine pathways leading to downstream physiological processes that enable a rapid and effective response to the threat. This is known as the classic "fight or flight" response and puts the organism in an optimal situation to cope with any challenge to its internal or external environment. One of the most important systems controlling the stress response is the hypothalamic-pituitary-adrenal (HPA) axis, a vital neuroendocrine system that regulates the release of glucocorticoid hormones (cortisol in man, corticosterone in rodents – CORT) from the adrenal glands. Stress-induced changes in circulating CORT levels are a critical component of the body's response to internal or environmental stress, and are important for maintaining *homeostasis* within the body via regulation of neural, metabolic, immunological, and cardiovascular activity.

At the level of the brain, CORT secretion is controlled by the activity of a small cluster of neurons whose cell bodies lie within the paraventricular nucleus (PVN) of the hypothalamus (Figure 8.1). The PVN is a highly responsive structure that can detect cognitive or emotional stressors from limbic areas of the central nervous system, such as the amygdala and hippocampus, as well as more physical stressors, such as inflammation or hypotension from brain stem structures (Ulrich-Lai and Herman, 2009). The PVN also receives a major input from the *suprachiasmatic nucleus* (SCN) of the hypothalamus, which receives light/dark information from the retinohypothalamic tract and thereby coordinates the circadian (i.e., daily) activity of the organism (Reppert and Weaver, 2002).

Computational Neuroendocrinology, First Edition. Edited by Duncan J. MacGregor and Gareth Leng.
© 2016 John Wiley & Sons, Ltd. Published 2016 by John Wiley & Sons, Ltd.
Companion Website: www.wiley.com/go/Leng/Computational

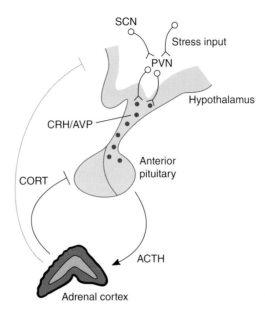

Figure 8.1   The hypothalamic–pituitary–adrenal (HPA) axis. The hypothalamic paraventricular nucleus (PVN) receives homeostatic/stress inputs from the brainstem and from regions of the limbic system such as the hippocampus and amygdala, as well as a circadian input from the suprachiasmatic nucleus (SCN). The PVN projects to the median eminence where it releases corticotrophin-releasing hormone (CRH) and arginine vasopressin (AVP) into the hypothalamic–pituitary portal circulation. CRH and AVP pass through this vascular route to access corticotroph cells in the anterior pituitary, which respond with the rapid release of adrenocorticotrophic hormone (ACTH) from pre-formed vesicles into the general circulation. In turn, ACTH reaches the adrenal cortex where it activates the synthesis and secretion of glucocorticoid hormones (CORT). CORT feeds back directly on the anterior pituitary to inhibit ACTH secretion, as well as acting at higher centres in the brain, including the hypothalamus and hippocampus.

A subpopulation of neurons within the PVN, the parvocellular neurosecretory cells, projects to the median eminence at the base of the hypothalamus from where they release the peptide hormones, corticotrophin-releasing hormone (CRH) and arginine vasopressin (AVP), into the *hypophyseal portal system* (Ixart *et al.*, 1991). CRH and AVP flow along this vascular route to reach the anterior lobes of the pituitary gland. The anterior pituitary contains a number of different specialized cell types that release specific hormones important for the regulation of many aspects of physiology, including reproduction, growth, metabolism, and the physiological response to stress. Approximately 10% of the anterior pituitary is made up of corticotroph cells, which respond to CRH and AVP by releasing the peptide adrenocorticotrophic hormone (ACTH) into the systemic circulation. This is an extremely rapid process – corticotroph cells store newly synthesized ACTH at high concentration in readily releasable *secretory vesicles* at the cell membrane, which are rapidly released in response to hypothalamic stimulation. When ACTH reaches the adrenal glands, it activates its specific receptor at the membrane of cells within the zona fasciculata of the adrenal cortex, which, in turn, leads to the synthesis and secretion of CORT. Like all steroid hormones, CORT is fat-soluble and can therefore freely exit the adrenocortical cells by diffusion across the plasma membrane (a phospholipid bilayer). In contrast to peptide hormones (e.g., CRH, AVP, and ACTH), this means that CORT cannot be pre-synthesized and stored within the cell, but requires *de novo* synthesis in response to ACTH stimulation.

Once released from the adrenal glands, CORT travels through the blood to access target tissues, such as the liver (to increase fuel release into the blood), the heart and vascular tissues (to increase blood supply to vital organs), and the brain (to promote cognitive processes necessary to cope with a threatening situation). CORT also regulates the activity of the HPA axis, and thus its own production, by feeding back in a negative manner, most significantly on the pituitary gland, but also on the PVN and other brain structures that influence the activity of the PVN, such as the hippocampus, where specific receptors responsive to CORT – glucocorticoid receptors (GR) and mineralocorticoid receptors (MR) – are expressed.

Besides the robust activation in response to stress, the HPA axis is also characterized by basal rhythms of activity. In man, levels of CORT are high in the early morning (increasing levels of glucose in the blood to prepare the body for daily activity), and low in the evening during the sleep period. In rodents, which are nocturnal animals, this daily or *circadian* rhythm of hormone secretion is reversed – CORT is high during the night (the rodent's active phase) and low in the morning when they are resting. Rather than following a circadian profile that varies smoothly over the course of the day, CORT actually displays a much more dynamic pattern of pulsatile hormone release that occurs with a characteristic *ultradian* frequency of approximately one pulse per hour (Figure 8.2). It is, in fact, the amplitude of the CORT pulses that varies in a circadian manner.

In mammals, pulses of CORT induce pulses of gene transcription in target tissues (Conway-Campbell *et al.*, 2010; Stavreva *et al.*, 2009), suggesting that systems have evolved to use ultradian CORT rhythms to optimize the body's response to its environmental influences and to maintain normal internal regulatory processes. The effect of these rhythms is profound at molecular, physiological, and behavioral levels. Indeed, in the rat, oscillating levels of CORT are necessary for normal neurochemical and behavioral responses to stress (Sarabdjitsingh *et al.*, 2010). Moreover, CORT oscillations become disrupted under a number of different physiological and pathological conditions (Lightman and

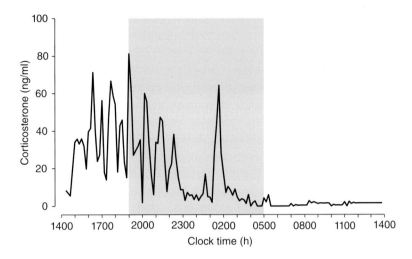

Figure 8.2   Circadian and ultradian CORT rhythms in the rat. CORT was measured in blood samples collected at 10 min intervals from a freely behaving male Sprague–Dawley rat. Shaded region indicates the dark phase. Data adapted from Walker *et al.* (2012).

Conway-Campbell, 2010). It is therefore vital to elucidate the mechanisms underlying these rhythms, not only to understand normal physiological function, but also to understand why they change in disease and how these changes cause or protect us from pathological consequences.

The origin of the circadian rhythm of CORT has been clearly associated with the SCN (Moore and Eichler, 1972), but the mechanisms governing the ultradian pulsatile dynamics of the system remain poorly understood. It has recently been shown that, while the circadian CORT rhythm disappears following lesioning of the SCN, the ultradian pulsatile pattern of CORT is maintained, suggesting that it is generated independently of SCN regulation (Waite *et al.*, 2012). Classically, it has been presumed that ultradian pulsatile CORT release is a consequence of neural signaling to the anterior pituitary encoding a dynamic pulsatile pattern of hypothalamic peptides (i.e., CRH and AVP) into the hypophyseal portal system. Although measuring levels of hypothalamic peptides in portal blood are extremely challenging, there have been a small number of studies in the freely behaving rat where, by using push–pull perfusion, it has been shown that CRH levels in the median eminence display irregular pulsatile dynamics with an approximate frequency of three pulses per hour (Ixart *et al.*, 1991). The frequency of CRH pulsing does not appear to vary significantly over the 24-hour period, but the mean levels of CRH secreted are significantly different – evening concentrations are nearly twice as high as those in the morning (Ixart *et al.*, 1993). The origin of this pulsatile activity in CRH is not known, but there is some *in vitro* data from the Macaque showing that hypothalamic explants release CRH in an episodic manner, suggesting that the anatomical basis for CRH pulse generation lies within the hypothalamus itself (Mershon *et al.*, 1992).

It may seem natural to assume that these pulses of CRH secretion are the primary mechanism driving the downstream ultradian oscillations in ACTH and CORT. If this was the case, we would expect the frequency of ACTH and CORT pulses to follow that of CRH. However, the available data show a slower temporal scale of near-hourly ACTH and CORT oscillations compared to the 20-min pulsing of CRH (Walker *et al.*, 2010b). In light of this mismatch in frequency, alternative mechanisms for these slower ultradian oscillations in ACTH and CORT clearly require further investigation, and the purpose of this chapter is to describe how integrative modeling and experimental studies have advanced our understanding of these mechanisms.

8.2 Mathematically modeling the HPA axis

Systems approaches to modeling hypothalamic–pituitary neuroendocrine pathways that incorporate negative feedback have been evolving since at least the early 1990s when Liu and Peng (1990) proposed a mathematical model of the hypothalamic–pituitary–thyroid (HPT) axis. Their initial model was based upon the principles of Michaelis–Menten kinetics (principles which govern most of the subsequently described approaches) and characterized the HPT axis at the steady state. This model was subsequently extended to incorporate the "auto regulation" of thyrotrophin-releasing hormone (TRH) (Li *et al.*, 1995), and this fast feedback process was shown to be sufficient to account for the pulsatile activity of the system observed experimentally. The group then extended this approach to study the HPA axis, where they included equations describing CRH, ACTH, and CORT (Liu *et al.*, 1999). The model included a negative feedback mechanism, mediated by levels of CORT on ACTH and CRH, which was shown to give rise to oscillatory behavior as a consequence of Hopf bifurcation.

An alternative model describing fluctuating levels of CRH, AVP, ACTH, and CORT, incorporating a logistic function to mimic the dose-responsive behavior of CORT feedback, has been proposed by Keenan *et al.* (2001). The authors hypothesize a hypothalamic pulse generator, whereby pulses of CRH and AVP (considered as a combined feedforward signal) drive the pulsatile secretion of ACTH and CORT following a short time delay. This model is significant as it considers the role of negative feedback mediated by CORT in regulating pulsatile hormone secretion in the HPA axis. However, the mechanism governing oscillatory behavior in this model is a hypothalamic pulse generator, rather than system-level CORT feedback.

More recent mathematical work has focused on building more biologically realistic models and using them to gain an insight into disease processes characterized by altered HPA dynamics. For example, Gupta *et al.* (2007) constructed a model of the HPA axis that takes into account the role of GR in mediating CORT negative feedback at the level of the pituitary. They found that this process results in the existence of two simultaneously stable concentrations of GR (low and high), which in turn result in two altered levels of CORT, and they discuss the possible relationship between these altered steady-state values and stress-related disease. This approach has in turn led to other studies that attempt to relate disruptions in HPA axis function to post-traumatic stress disorder (PTSD) (Ben-Zvi *et al.*, 2009, Sriram *et al.*, 2012). The first of these studies postulates that model-based control may be used to perturb the HPA axis from a state of abnormal CORT secretion back to a state corresponding to normal CORT levels. The more recent study by Sriram *et al.* (2012) discusses how positive feedback in the model developed by Gupta *et al.* (2007) leads to the previously described bistability. They proceed to describe the interplay between increases in negative feedback and transitions in a dynamic structure that they relate to clinical measurements of CORT in patients.

While both of the above studies incorporate increasing levels of biological plausibility in their models, they do not discuss the known ultradian pulsatility of both ACTH and CORT. In the models discussed above that *do* focus on ultradian activity in the HPA axis, the model output does not entirely concur with data – specifically, the output of these models shows CRH, ACTH, and CORT oscillations that are phase locked in all hormones and (in some cases) occur with a non physiological frequency. Thus, our objective for building a mathematical model is to identify candidate mechanisms that could underpin the emergence of ultradian activity in the system and that are consistent with the experimentally observed dynamics of CRH, ACTH, and CORT, as described above (Walker *et al.*, 2010a). Our starting point is the model of Gupta *et al.* (2007), a qualitative model that provides a reasonable balance between biological plausibility and analytical tractability. This model has four variables, the dynamics of which are described by four ordinary differential equations (ODEs):

$$\frac{dC}{dT} = \frac{K_c + F}{1 + B/K_{i1}} - K_{cd}C \tag{8.1}$$

$$\frac{dA}{dT} = \frac{K_a C}{1 + BR/K_{i2}} - K_{ad}A \tag{8.2}$$

$$\frac{dR}{dT} = \frac{K_r (BR)^2}{K + (BR)^2} + K_{cr} - K_{rd}R \qquad (8.3)$$

$$\frac{dB}{dT} = K_b A - K_{bd}B \qquad (8.4)$$

Based on reaction kinetics, these equations describe hormone signaling between the three anatomical components of the HPA axis. The variables C, A, and B represent concentration levels of CRH, ACTH, and CORT, respectively. The variable R represents a receptor for CORT in the anterior pituitary. Each equation expresses the rate of change in the concentration of a variable (C, A, R, B) as the difference between a synthesis/production term and a degradation/clearance term. Moreover, a constant independent basal production term is included for R in the anterior pituitary. K_c and F are time-varying parameters that represent circadian and stress inputs to stimulate CRH release from the hypothalamus. Parameters K_{cd}, K_{ad}, K_{rd}, and K_{bd} are the degradation parameters for C, A, R, and B, respectively. The model assumes that the degradation rate of each variable is not actively regulated by any other variable of the system, and that it is purely determined by its half-life, which in the case of ACTH and CORT can be estimated from experimental data. In this model developed by Gupta *et al.* (2007), the inhibition by circulating CORT acts at the level of both CRH production (first term of Equation (8.1)) and, via interactions with its receptor, ACTH production (first term of Equation (8.2)).

In light of experimental observations of a frequency mismatch between pulsatile CRH secretion (~3 pulses per hour) and ACTH/CORT (~1 pulse per hour), in deriving our model we make the key assumption that CORT negative feedback at the hypothalamus is not an important factor in regulating the basal dynamic activity of the system. That is, we assume that the primary regulator of the basal dynamics is CORT-mediated negative feedback at the level of the anterior pituitary, and we, therefore, treat hypothalamic CRH drive on the pituitary as a parameter of the system, rather than a variable. This assumption results in a system that is essentially an excitatory–inhibitory loop consisting of the pituitary and adrenal components, which undergoes external forcing from hypothalamic CRH (C):

$$\frac{dA}{dT} = \frac{K_a C}{1 + BR/K_{i2}} - K_{ad}A \qquad (8.5)$$

$$\frac{dR}{dT} = \frac{K_r (BR)^2}{K + (BR)^2} + K_{cr} - K_{rd}R \qquad (8.6)$$

$$\frac{dB}{dT} = K_b A - K_{bd}B \qquad (8.7)$$

We non dimensionalize this system of equations using a (non unique) coordinate transformation, which gives rise to the dimensionless form

$$\frac{da}{dt} = \frac{C_d}{1 + p_2 br} - p_3 a \qquad (8.8)$$

$$\frac{dr}{dt} = \frac{(br)^2}{p_4 + (br)^2} + p_5 - p_6 r \qquad (8.9)$$

$$\frac{db}{dt} = a - b \qquad (8.10)$$

Here, a, r, and b are dimensionless representations of the original variables A, R, and B, respectively, and the new parameters C_d and p_{2-6} are dimensionless combinations of the original parameters that are defined as follows:

$$C_d = K_{bd} K_r^{-1} C \qquad (8.11)$$

$$p_2 = K_r^2 K_a K_b K_{i2}^{-1} K_{bd}^{-4} \qquad (8.12)$$

$$p_3 = K_{ad} K_{bd}^{-1} \qquad (8.13)$$

$$p_4 = K K_{bd}^8 K_r^{-4} K_a^{-2} K_b^{-2} \qquad (8.14)$$

$$p_5 = K_{cr} K_r^{-1} \qquad (8.15)$$

$$p_6 = K_{rd} K_{bd}^{-1} \qquad (8.16)$$

The dimensionless parameter C_d represents the level of "hypothalamic drive" on the anterior pituitary – we do not attempt to distinguish between a gain mediated by CRH or AVP, and instead, without loss of generality, lump both of these together.

A further significant change from the model described by Gupta *et al.* (2007) reflects the disparate nature of the mechanisms of synthesis and release of ACTH and CORT. In corticotroph cells of the anterior pituitary, ACTH is pre-synthesized and stored at high concentration in secretory vesicles in readily releasable pools docked to the cell membrane (Kelly, 1985). Hence, ACTH is rapidly (i.e., within seconds) released from these pre-formed vesicles into the general circulation in response to CRH activation. In contrast, in adrenocortical cells, CORT is only synthesized following stimulation by ACTH, after which it is passively released into the general circulation (Stocco and Clark, 1996). Crucially, this steroid synthesis stage results in a time delay of a few minutes in ACTH-induced CORT secretion from the adrenal cortex (Papaikonomou, 1977). Within our model, we take this slow process in the adrenal cortex into account by including a delay term in the equation for CORT, which leads to the following system of delay differential equations (DDEs):

$$\frac{da}{dt} = \frac{C_d}{1 + p_2 br} - p_3 a \tag{8.17}$$

$$\frac{dr}{dt} = \frac{(br)^2}{p_4 + (br)^2} + p_5 - p_6 r \tag{8.18}$$

$$\frac{db}{dt} = a(t - \tau) - b \tag{8.19}$$

The final equation expresses the rate of change of CORT as a function of ACTH concentration at some fixed time $(t - \tau)$ earlier (dimensionless units). While incorporating a delay to account for the production time of CORT makes theoretical analysis more challenging, it does have the advantage of minimizing the number of additional equations and (unknown) parameters in the model that would be necessary to account explicitly for the multiple steps involved in steroidogenesis.

As a deterministic (i.e., nonstochastic) system, the dynamics of Equations (8.17)–(8.19) are governed entirely by the model parameters (and the time delay). For reproducibility, the dimensionless parameter values used in our analysis are provided in Table 8.1. Of these, only C_d may be thought of as a time-varying parameter as it corresponds to CRH drive on the anterior pituitary. The remaining parameters are assumed to remain constant (at least over the ultradian timescale of interest) for any individual, although there could quite conceivably be a degree of inter-individual variation. Whilst it is not possible to estimate all of the model parameters from data, good approximations are possible for some, which enables a more systematic analysis of model dynamics. In particular, the half-lives of ACTH and CORT in the blood have been reported in experimental studies. In the rat, the half-life of ACTH $(A_{1/2})$ has been estimated to be approximately 1 min (Sydnor and Sayers, 1953), and similarly, the half-life of CORT in the rat $(B_{1/2})$ has been estimated to lie in the range 7.2–10 min (Windle *et al.*, 1998a).

Table 8.1 Dimensionless parameter values for the model

Parameter	Value	Description
C_d	Free	CRH drive
p_2	15	Relates to inhibition of ACTH by CORT
p_3	7.2	Ratio of decay rates between ACTH and CORT
p_4	0.05	Relates to regulation of R by CORT
p_5	0.11	Basal production of R in anterior pituitary
p_6	2.9	Ratio of decay rates between R and CORT
τ	Free	Delay in ACTH-induced CORT release

Referring back to Equation (8.5), in the absence of hypothalamic drive (i.e., when $C = 0$), ACTH will decay exponentially at a rate determined by the parameter K_{ad}. This decay constant for ACTH is given by

$$K_{ad} = \frac{\ln(2)}{A_{1/2}} \tag{8.20}$$

Similarly, in the absence of ACTH (i.e., when $A = 0$), the decay constant for CORT is given by

$$K_{bd} = \frac{\ln(2)}{B_{1/2}} \tag{8.21}$$

Referring back to the relationship between parameters in their dimensional and non dimensional forms (Equations (8.11)–(8.16)), we can apply the following parameter constraint:

$$p_3 = \frac{K_{ad}}{K_{bd}} = \frac{B_{1/2}}{A_{1/2}} \tag{8.22}$$

$$\Rightarrow 7.2 \leq p_3 \leq 10 \tag{8.23}$$

and define the relationship between timescales as

$$t = K_{bd}T = \frac{\ln(2) \cdot T}{B_{1/2}} \tag{8.24}$$

In addition to the half-lives of ACTH and CORT, the delay in ACTH-induced CORT secretion from the adrenal gland of the rat has also been investigated experimentally (Papaikonomou, 1977). In our analysis of the model, we consider this delay to be in the dimensional range of 0–20 min. Using Equation (8.24), this results in a dimensionless delay in the range $\tau = $ 0–1.9254. However, for the convenience of the reader, in the results we subsequently present, time is shown in its dimensional form (i.e., minutes), whereas all other parameters are shown in a dimensionless form (with arbitrary units).

8.3 Unveiling the mechanism of ultradian pulsatility

Having defined the mathematical model (Equations (8.17)–(8.19)) and fixed some of the model parameters (as in Table 8.1), we proceed to understand the dynamical behavior of the model. Bifurcation analysis is a powerful mathematical approach that explains how the asymptotic dynamics of a model depends on the values of its parameters, and here we use this technique to explore how the level of hypothalamic drive on the anterior pituitary (C_d) and the delay in ACTH-induced CORT secretion

(τ) influence the dynamics of ACTH and CORT. We employ the numerical continuation package DDE-BIFTOOL (Engelborghs *et al.*, 2001) to track bifurcations of the system through parameter space. To begin with, we consider a one-parameter bifurcation analysis of the system, where we vary only C_d, for three fixed choices of adrenal delay T_{lag} = 5, 10, and 15 min, which shows how ACTH (not shown) and CORT dynamics vary as a function of the level of CRH stimulation (Figure 8.3).

For a small delay (T_{lag} = 5 min), the pituitary–adrenal system evolves toward a steady-state solution, regardless of the level of CRH drive (Figure 8.3a). However, for slightly larger delays (T_{lag} = 10 and 15 min), there is a qualitative change in the dynamics of the system as the level of CRH drive increases (Figure 8.3b and c). First, the steady-state destabilizes due to the Hopf bifurcation (H), and then subsequently restabilizes at a higher level of CRH via a second Hopf bifurcation point. In between these bifurcation points, sustained ACTH (not shown) and CORT oscillations occur. The two curves emanating from the Hopf bifurcations correspond to the maximum and minimum values of this oscillation in CORT. Significantly, in computing the period of the oscillation between the two Hopf points (Figure 8.3d and e), we find a range of values between 45 and 70 min, which is in good agreement with experimental observations of CORT pulse frequency in the rat (Windle *et al.*, 1998b,a).

From this initial analysis, it is clear that both the level of CRH drive and the adrenal delay play critical roles in regulating the dynamics of ACTH and CORT. We can gain a more comprehensive understanding of this relationship by computing a two-parameter bifurcation diagram in (T_{lag}, C_d)-space (Figure 8.4a). The diagram consists of bifurcation curves that separate the two-dimensional parameter space into regions of qualitatively different dynamics. The main features of the plot are defined by a curve of Hopf bifurcations (H). On one side of the curve, the pituitary–adrenal system remains in the steady state, whilst on the other side, the system oscillates. The three one-parameter bifurcation diagrams of Figure 8.3 are effectively vertical "slices" through this two-dimensional diagram at values of T_{lag} = 5, 10, and 15 min, respectively. The bifurcation diagram shows that the critical value of the delay, beyond which oscillatory dynamics are possible, is $T_{lag} \sim 6.5$ min. For all considered values of the delay beyond this, oscillations occur at a physiological frequency (the period is indicated by the color bar) for "intermediate" levels of CRH drive (Figure 8.4a and c). As the level of CRH drive increases or decreases from this intermediate range, the dynamics of the system return to the steady-state levels of ACTH and CORT (Figure 8.4a, b, and d).

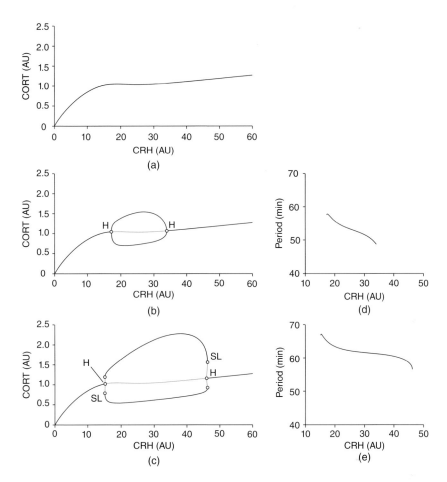

Figure 8.3   Influence of constant CRH drive on the dynamics of the pituitary–adrenal system. Computed one-parameter bifurcation diagrams showing the influence of different levels of *constant* CRH drive (C_d) on the dynamics of the pituitary–adrenal system for three different values of adrenal delay (T_{lag}). (a) For $T_{\text{lag}} = 5$ min, the system is always at a stable steady state, independent of the level of CRH stimulation. (b) For $T_{\text{lag}} = 10$ min, sustained oscillations occur for a range of CRH levels between two supercritical Hopf bifurcation points H. (c) For $T_{\text{lag}} = 15$ min, sustained oscillations occur for an even larger range of CRH levels. Both Hopf bifurcations H have become subcritical and there are now saddle–node bifurcations of limit cycles (SL) and two very narrow regions of bistability (the regions between H and SL). (d) Period of the oscillation between the two Hopf bifurcation points in (b) as a function of CRH. (e) Period of the oscillation between the two Hopf bifurcation points in (c) as a function of CRH. In panels (a–c), black curves indicate stable solutions (either steady state, or maximum and minimum of the oscillation); gray curves indicate unstable solutions (either steady state, or maximum and minimum of the oscillation). AU, arbitrary units.

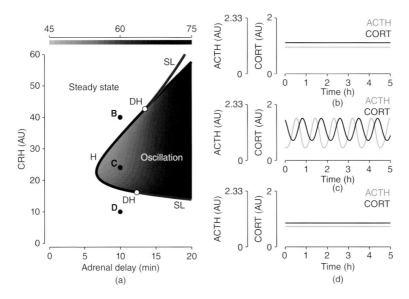

Figure 8.4   Influence of constant CRH drive and adrenal delay on the dynamics of the pituitary–adrenal system. (a) Computed two-parameter bifurcation diagram shows that different combinations of *constant* CRH drive (C_d) and adrenal delay (T_{lag}) result in qualitatively different dynamic responses from the pituitary–adrenal system. On one side of the Hopf curve (H), the pituitary–adrenal system responds to the steady-state levels of ACTH and CORT. On the other side of the bifurcation curve H, the pituitary–adrenal system responds to oscillations in ACTH and CORT. Within the region of oscillatory dynamics, the period of the oscillation is indicated by the color bar. (b–d) Numerical simulations for ACTH (gray) and CORT (black) corresponding to the points B, C, and D in panel (a). Simulations are shown for a 5-h period *after* transient dynamics have decayed. AU, arbitrary units.

Some further aspects of this bifurcation diagram are interesting from a theoretical perspective. On both the upper and lower branches of the Hopf curve, there is a degenerate Hopf point (DH), from which a curve of saddle–node bifurcations of limit cycles (SL) emerges (red curves in Figure 8.4a). The thin region bounded between H and SL is, therefore, bistable – a stable steady-state coexists with a stable periodic solution, separated in phase space by an unstable periodic orbit (the gray curves connecting H and SL in the one-parameter bifurcation diagram in Figure 8.3c). Bistable regions such as these provide a mechanism for rapidly switching between the steady state and oscillatory dynamics. However, these regions are relatively small, and only become significantly larger for much higher values of adrenal delay that are presumably nonphysiological. It remains an open question whether these regions could become enlarged and, therefore, significant as a consequence of pathological derangements to the axis.

It is important to note that bifurcation analysis provides us with an overall picture of what happens to the dynamics of the system in the *long term*; that is, the dynamical behavior to which the system eventually evolves over time. For example, within the oscillatory region, the system evolves toward a stable periodic solution (Figure 8.4a and c), independent of the choice of initial conditions. Likewise, outside of the oscillatory region, the system evolves toward a stable steady state (Figure 8.4a–c). However, if we are to explore the dynamics of the system experimentally (for example, the stimulation of the pituitary–adrenal system using synthetic CRH), it is not only the long-term response of the system that is of interest, but also the transient dynamic response of the system; that is, the dynamics during the short time period following the onset of the CRH stimulation. To consider this, we assume that the level of CRH is zero prior to infusion, and that following the start of the infusion, the rate of change of CRH concentration C_d in the blood of the animal can be represented by the difference between a CRH infusion rate term α, and a CRH degradation (i.e., metabolic clearance) rate term βC_d. The dynamics of the parameter C_d are now governed by the following differential equation and initial condition:

$$\frac{dC_d}{dt} = \alpha - \beta C_d \quad ; \quad C_d(0) = 0 \tag{8.25}$$

$$\Rightarrow C_d(t) = \frac{\alpha}{\beta}(1 - e^{-\beta t}) \tag{8.26}$$

We fix the parameter governing the decay rate $\beta = \ln(2)/C_{1/2}$, assuming a short half-life for CRH in plasma ($C_{1/2} = 0.7$ min). We consider four different values of the infusion rate term: $\alpha = 7.5\beta, 15\beta, 30\beta, 40\beta, 50\beta$. The adrenal delay is fixed at $T_{\text{lag}} = 10$ min and we fix all other model parameters to the values given in Table 8.1.

Numerical simulations of both the transient and long-term dynamics of the model show that, in addition to sustained oscillations observed within the region bounded by the Hopf curves (Figure 8.5a and d), the system still "wants" to oscillate at a near-hourly frequency in response to a monotonic increase in levels of CRH when the pituitary–adrenal system is in the steady-state region (Figure 8.5a–c, e, and f). This oscillatory tendency is stronger (i.e., the transient oscillations are larger) for levels of CRH above the oscillatory region than those below (e.g., compare Figure 8.5c with Figure 8.5e). This observation can be explained by computing the leading eigenvalue(s) along a steady-state branch for CRH = 0–60 and fixed $T_{\text{lag}} = 10$ min (Figure 8.6). Plotting the imaginary part of the leading eigenvalue(s) shows that the steady state is a focus (as opposed to a node) with complex leading eigenvalue(s) for levels of CRH > 2, which explains the transient oscillations observed in the steady-state region (both above and

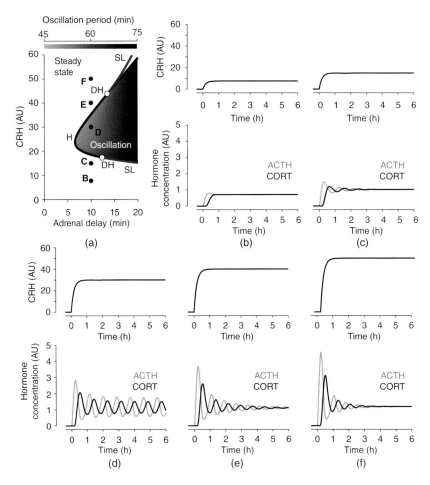

Figure 8.5   Transient pituitary–adrenal dynamics in response to constant CRH infusion. (a) Computed two-parameter bifurcation diagram showing how the qualitative dynamics of the pituitary–adrenal system depends on the level of *constant* CRH drive (C_d) and adrenal delay (T_{lag}). (b–f) Numerical simulations of the model corresponding to the points B, C, D, E, and F in panel (a). Simulations show both transient and long-term ACTH (gray) and CORT (black) dynamics in response to different CRH infusion rates: $\alpha = 7.5\beta$ (b), $\alpha = 15\beta$ (c), $\alpha = 30\beta$ (d), $\alpha = 40\beta$ (e), and $\alpha = 50\beta$ (f). AU, arbitrary units.

below the oscillatory region). The plot also reveals why the transients in the steady region are larger above the oscillatory region than below. The rate of convergence to the steady state is governed by the magnitude of the real part of the leading complex eigenvalue, and the real part is closer to zero for CRH levels in the upper steady-state region (i.e., beyond the second Hopf bifurcation) compared to the lower steady-state region.

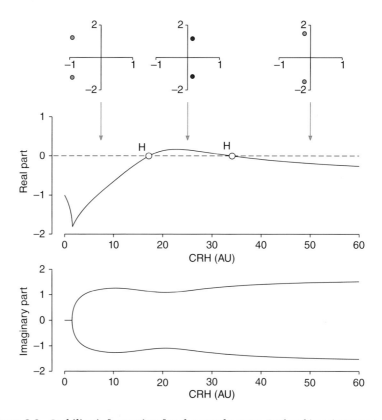

Figure 8.6 **Stability information for the steady state**. Real and imaginary parts of the leading eigenvalue(s) of a steady-state branch computed for CRH = 0–60 and T_{lag} = 10 min. At the points H, the real part of the leading pair of eigenvalues crosses through zero, corresponding to Hopf bifurcations (a transition between steady-state and oscillatory dynamics) (Kuznetsov, 2004). The three top panels show the leading pair of complex conjugate eigenvalues in the complex plane for three different values of CRH = 7.5, 25, and 50. AU, arbitrary units.

8.4   Exploring model predictions experimentally

The analysis of our model in the preceding section provides us with a number of theoretical predictions. The model predicts that oscillations in ACTH and CORT will be observed for "intermediate" constant levels of CRH, and that these oscillations should occur at a physiological frequency; that is, at the same frequency as endogenous CORT oscillations observed in the rat during the peak phase of the circadian cycle. This prediction is in stark contrast to the long-standing view that pulses of CRH are required for pulsatile ACTH and CORT secretion. Moreover, the model also suggests that these CORT oscillations will become "damped" for higher (or lower) levels of CRH.

These predictions from the model can be explored experimentally by controlling the level of CRH and simultaneously measuring levels of ACTH and CORT (Walker *et al.*, 2012). An ideal experimental model to test these predictions is the freely behaving male Sprague–Dawley rat, which has a distinct and prolonged nadir phase in the HPA circadian cycle (0700–1300 h), when endogenous CRH, ACTH, and CORT secretion are minimal (see Figure 8.2). This "quiescent period" provides a time window during which we can manipulate the system without interference from endogenous HPA hormone release.

Infusion of constant levels of CRH (during the circadian nadir) results in different temporal patterns of CORT secretion that are dependent on the level of CRH. In keeping with the predictions of our mathematical model, a constant infusion of CRH can induce sustained ultradian CORT oscillations with an amplitude that remains relatively constant throughout the infusion (Figure 8.7a). Note that these responses to constant CRH infusion reflect a direct action of CRH itself, and not a stress response to the procedure. This can clearly be seen in control rats constantly infused with vehicle (saline), where endogenous levels of CORT remain low throughout the infusion (Figure 8.7b).

It is important to explore whether the mechanism regulating CORT oscillations induced by constant infusion of exogenous CRH is the same mechanism that regulates ultradian CORT oscillations during the circadian peak. If this is the case, there should be good agreement between the characteristic frequencies of the CRH-induced and endogenous oscillations. To test this, we compute the dominant frequency component in the CRH-induced oscillations, and compare this with the dominant frequency component in endogenous CORT oscillations during the circadian peak.

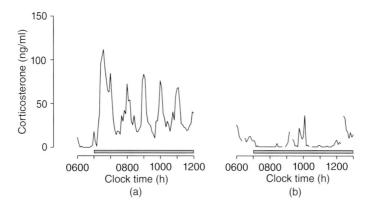

Figure 8.7 CORT oscillations induced by constant CRH infusion. (a) Exemplar CORT response to constant 0.5 µg/h CRH infusion. (b) Exemplar CORT response to constant saline infusion. Gray bars indicate the period of infusion.

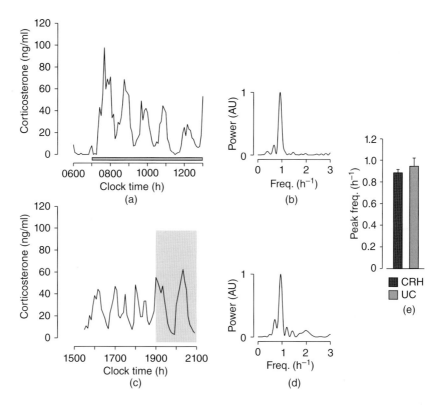

Figure 8.8 **Frequency comparison of CRH-induced and endogenous CORT oscillations**. (a and b) Normalized power spectra (b) of CORT oscillations (a) induced by constant CRH infusion (0.5 μg/h) in an exemplar rat. (c and d) Normalized power spectra (d) of endogenous CORT oscillations (c) during the circadian peak in an exemplar rat. (e) Mean peak frequency (i.e., frequency corresponding to the maximum power in the spectrum) of CORT oscillations in response to constant CRH infusion (0.5 μg/h; CRH; $n = 6$), and of CORT oscillations during the circadian peak in untreated control rats (UC; $n = 13$). Gray bar indicates the period of infusion. Shaded region indicates the dark phase. AU, arbitrary units. Error bars represent mean ± SEM.

In both the CRH-induced CORT oscillations and the endogenous CORT oscillations during the circadian peak, there is a peak frequency of approximately one pulse per hour (Figure 8.8), suggesting that constant CRH stimulation is indeed inducing CORT oscillations in a physiological way.

Another key prediction of our mathematical model is that CORT oscillations induced by constant CRH stimulation are driven by oscillations in ACTH, with a phase shift between ACTH and CORT. This prediction is in keeping with experimental observations – ultradian ACTH oscillations have previously been experimentally observed in the rat (Carnes *et al.*, 1989) and have been shown to be critical for regulating CORT secretion from the adrenal cortex (Spiga *et al.*, 2011). Moreover, coordinated phase-shifted

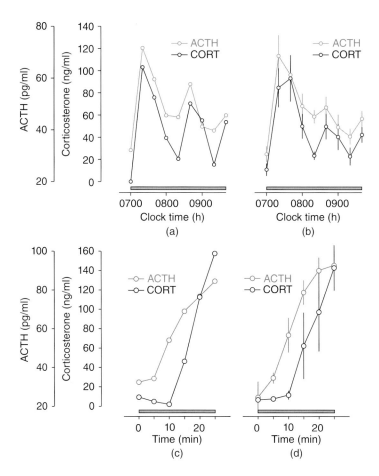

Figure 8.9 ACTH and CORT oscillations induced by constant CRH infusion. (a and b) Individual (a) and mean (b) ACTH and CORT oscillations in response to constant CRH infusion (0.5 µg/h) ($n = 6$). (c and d) Individual (c) and mean (d) time course of the ACTH and CORT response to constant CRH infusion (0.5 µg/h) during the initial activation phase (0–25 min) of the oscillation ($n = 4$). Gray bars indicate the period of infusion (starting at 0700 h); error bars represent mean ± SEM.

ACTH and CORT oscillations have been observed in human studies (Henley *et al.*, 2009). Measuring both ACTH and CORT during the constant CRH infusion shows that the CRH does indeed induce coordinated ultradian oscillations in both hormones (Figure 8.9a and b). Moreover, if we measure ACTH and CORT at a higher sampling frequency over the "activation phase" of the first pulse, we observe the phase shift between ACTH and CORT that the model predicts (Figure 8.9c and d).

The modeling work in the previous section suggests that the dynamic response of the pituitary–adrenal system to constant levels of CRH is dependent on the specific level of CRH; that is, the model suggests that

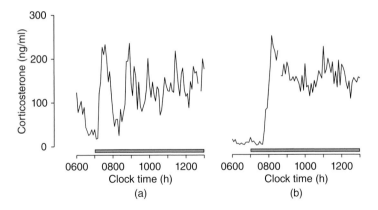

Figure 8.10   Damped oscillatory CORT responses to constant CRH infusion.
(a) Exemplar CORT response to constant 1.0 µg/h CRH infusion. (b) Exemplar CORT
response to constant 2.5 µg/h CRH infusion. Gray bars indicate the period of infusion.

"intermediate" CRH levels give rise to oscillatory responses (as investigated above), but "low" or "high" levels of CRH should result in a damped
oscillatory response that evolves toward a steady-state solution. As shown
in Figure 8.10, constant infusion of higher levels of CRH (two different
CRH doses are shown) results in a CORT response that does not show
sustained oscillations, but approaches a steady-state level throughout the
course of the infusion.

8.5   Significance of ultradian pulsatility for stress responsiveness

The previous section demonstrates the predictive power of mathematical
modeling. By carefully designing a model so that it can be linked directly
to the biological question of interest, new experiments can be carried out
to explore the predictions of the model. This reiterative process of model
development, experimental design and testing, followed by further model
development and further experiment, is the hallmark of successful mul-
tidisciplinary collaboration between mathematicians and biologists and is
becoming increasingly established within the biological community. In this
section, we reiterate this process once more and consider, both theoretically
and through comparison with experimental data, the significance of ultradian pulsatility for stress responsiveness, and in particular, the interplay
between the ultradian oscillation and acute stress.

So far, we have focused on the HPA axis as a generator of basal ACTH and
CORT oscillations that form the basis for an extremely rapid and sensitive
hormone signalling system. However, as discussed in the opening section of

this chapter, the HPA axis also provides a rapid hormonal response to stress that is vitally important for the homeostatic state of the organism. Acute stress (psychological or physical) leads to a rapid surge of CRH/AVP secretion into the hypophyseal portal system, which in turn stimulates the rapid release of ACTH and finally the secretion of CORT from the adrenal glands.

Pulsatile patterns of CORT encode an important biological signal that regulates receptor signaling throughout the central nervous system and in peripheral tissues. In light of this, it is important to understand how stressful stimuli interact and affect the pulsatile dynamics of the system. To address this question, we extend our mathematical model of the pituitary–adrenal system (Equations (8.17)–(8.19)) to incorporate the CRH response to an acute stress. We perturb the basal level of CRH with a "stress impulse" of the form $I = \Lambda \times t^2 e^{-t}$, where the amplitude Λ of the impulse is expressed as a multiple of the basal level of CRH (see Figure 8.11a) – note that we fix the basal level of CRH = 25 such that in the unperturbed state there is an approximately hourly oscillation in ACTH and CORT. This mathematical form for a CRH impulse neatly captures downstream changes in CORT levels following an acute stress (see Rankin *et al.* (2012) for further details).

We apply the CRH impulse following a peak in CORT with relative phase ϕ_C, scaled by the endogenous period P. For a range of discrete values of ϕ_C, we can compute two quantities from the pituitary–adrenal response: the amplitude response, and the phase shift of subsequent peaks in CORT relative to the endogenous case. Computing these quantities across one period of the endogenous oscillation allows us to calculate both the amplitude response curve and also the phase response curve (PRC). The PRC is useful for understanding the transient change in the cycle period of an oscillator as a result of a perturbation, and can be visualized by plotting the normalized phase ϕ_C of the oscillator against the resulting change in phase $\Delta\phi$. This approach has been widely applied in the study of biological rhythms over time frames ranging from rapid neural oscillations (Brown *et al.*, 2004) to circadian cycles (Winfree, 2001).

The CORT response to a 10 min acute noise stress has previously been investigated in different strains of freely behaving rats: female Sprague–Dawley (Windle *et al.*, 1998a), female Lewis (Windle *et al.*, 1998b), and male Piebald-Viral-Glaxo (PVG) with induced arthritis (Windle *et al.*, 2001). In each study, the timing of the stress relative to the phase of the underlying ultradian oscillation was seen to be crucial in determining the magnitude of the response of CORT to the stress. In particular, it was observed that when the acute stress was presented during the rising (secretory) phase of the ultradian oscillation, CORT concentrations rose markedly. In comparison, the same acute stress presented during the falling phase resulted in a greatly reduced CORT response.

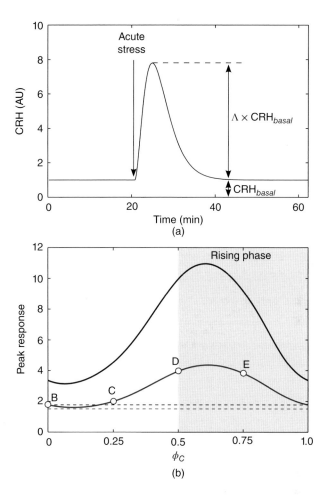

Figure 8.11 Timing of CRH stress impulse determines the magnitude of the CORT response. (a) Profile of CRH impulse where the amplitude Λ is scaled by the basal level of CRH. (b) Amplitude response curves of ACTH (solid blue) and CORT (solid red) computed for $\Lambda = 6.8$ with varying phase ϕ_C of the CRH impulse. As a reference, the maximum levels of basal oscillations in ACTH (dashed blue) and CORT (dashed red) are also plotted. The shaded region indicates values of ϕ_C that correspond to the rising phase. Markers on the CORT amplitude response curve correspond to the time histories plotted in Figure 8.12.

Due to the nature of these studies, the timing of the stress could only be determined retrospectively upon comparison with measured CORT levels and determined to the nearest 10 min (the sampling frequency used in the studies).

We use the experimental data from these studies to calibrate the parameters of the stress input of our model in terms of the amplitude of the CORT response to this incoming stress. For each of the three experimental groups, we compute the ratio between the maximum of the mean CORT response to a stress applied during the rising phase, and the maximum of the mean CORT response to a stress applied during the falling phase. The resulting ratios for the three different groups of animals are 2.48 (female Sprague–Dawley), 2.67 (female Lewis), and 1.90 (PVG), which we average to give a final ratio of 2.33. The amplitude Λ of the CRH impulse applied in the model is then tuned to match the ratio observed experimentally. Figure 8.11b shows the amplitude response curves of ACTH and CORT, where values of ϕ_C corresponding to the rising phase are indicated by the shaded region – as a reference, the maximum value of the basal oscillations for ACTH and CORT are also shown as dashed lines. Taking the mean CORT response during the rising phase as the area between the amplitude response curve (solid red) and the endogenous maximum line (dashed red), and similarly for the falling phase, we find that a value of $\Lambda = 6.8$ gives the correct ratio of 2.33 (Figure 8.11b).

For this chosen value of Λ, we simulate individual ACTH and CORT profiles for a CRH stress impulse applied at four different values of the phase ($\phi_C = 0$, 0.25, 0.5, and 0.75; Figure 8.12). The black arrows on the horizontal axes indicate the precise timing of the onset of the CRH impulse (i.e., ϕ_C), and black circles indicate peaks in CORT. The gray curve shows a time history of CORT for the endogenous unperturbed case (i.e., when no stress impulse is applied), and the vertical gray lines mark peaks of the endogenous CORT oscillation. In all cases, the CRH impulse is rapidly followed by a rise in ACTH secretion, which is in turn followed by a response in CORT. The most notable difference between the four cases is that, in agreement with the experimental studies, the magnitudes of the ACTH and CORT responses depend critically on the value of ϕ_C; that is, the *timing* of the stress relative to the phase of the intrinsic ultradian oscillation. The ACTH and CORT responses to a stress impulse applied at phase $\phi_C = 0$ are barely noticeable relative to peak levels of the endogenous oscillation, whereas the amplitude of the response is considerably larger for a stress impulse applied at phase $\phi_C = 0.75$, for example, both relative to a stress applied during the falling phase, and to the peak levels of the endogenous oscillation. Thinking about this from a dynamical systems perspective, when the stress perturbation coincides with the rising phase, the stress is acting in the same direction of motion as the endogenous oscillation, resulting in a pituitary–adrenal response that is significantly greater than the maximum of the basal oscillation. In contrast, when levels of hormone are decreasing, the stress perturbation acts against the direction of motion of the endogenous oscillation. Thus, even a large amplitude stress impulse applied during the falling phase may only result in a limited hormonal response from the pituitary–adrenal system.

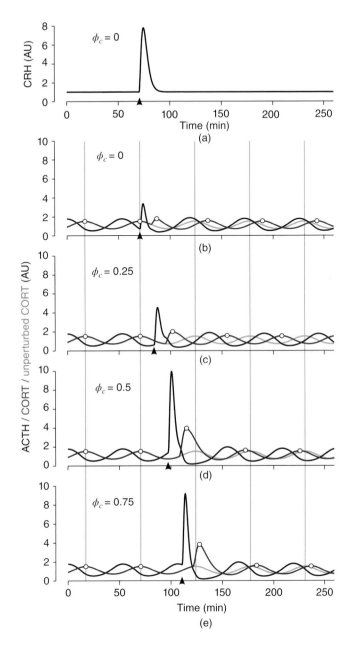

Figure 8.12   Computational illustrations of the timing relationship between a CRH stress impulse and the magnitude of the CORT response. (a) CRH impulse corresponding to $\phi_C = 0$ for $\Lambda = 6.8$. (b–e) Time histories showing levels of ACTH (blue) and CORT (red) for fixed $\Lambda = 6.8$ and values of ϕ_C as indicated in the panels. Vertical arrow in each panel indicates the timing of the applied CRH impulse. Levels of CORT in the absence of an impulse are shown in gray, with expected peaks indicated by vertical lines. The induced phase shift is the time separation between expected peaks (vertical lines) in the unperturbed case and the actual peak in CORT (black circles) for the perturbed case.

The model also predicts that stress impulses can induce phase shifts in the endogenous ultradian oscillation, as seen from examining the simulations in Figure 8.12 and comparing the timing of the last peak in CORT in both the perturbed (red) and unperturbed (vertical gray lines) cases. For example, for $\phi_C = 0$, the phase is delayed and the peak in CORT comes after the unperturbed peak, whereas for $\phi_C = 0.25$ and $\phi_C = 0.5$, the phase is advanced, and the peak in CORT is brought forward in time; for $\phi_C = 0.75$, there is almost no change in phase. Thus, depending on the *timing* of the stress, the phase of the ultradian oscillation can either be advanced or delayed. This phase shift behavior can be visualized in detail by plotting ϕ_C against the phase shift $\Delta\phi$, defined as the difference between the phase in CORT of the perturbed and unperturbed oscillatory solutions, where a positive value of $\Delta\phi$ represents a phase delay, and a negative value a phase advance (Figure 8.13a).

We can then use the model to understand how this PRC for the system depends on the magnitude of the acute stress, as defined by Λ (Figure 8.13a). To do this, we compute $\Delta\phi$ for 200 discrete values of ϕ_C in the interval $[0, 1]$ and for five different magnitudes of stressor ($\Lambda = \{1.2, 1.8, 2.4, 3, 6.8\}$). For $\Lambda = 1.2$ and 1.8 (red curves), the PRCs are smooth and continuous, and pass through $\Delta\phi = 0$ at $\phi_C \approx 0.2$. For $\Lambda = 2.4$, 3, and 6.8 (blue curves), the PRC has an apparent discontinuity where

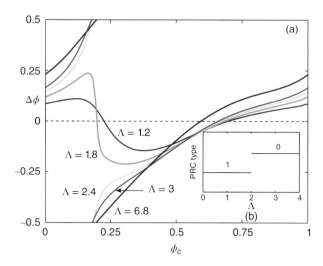

Figure 8.13   Parameter-dependent profiles of phase response curves. (a) Phase response curves (PRCs) for different values of the pulse amplitude Λ as indicated. For $\Lambda < 2$, the model exhibits Type-1 phase resetting (red shades) with a sharp change in phase near $\phi_C = 0.2$. For $\Lambda > 2$, the model exhibits Type-0 phase resetting (blue shades) with a discontinuous change in phase near $\phi_C = 0.2$. (b) Type of PRC curve plotted against Λ.

it passes through $\Delta\phi = 0.5$, which coincides with $\Delta\phi = -0.5$ due to the periodic nature of $\Delta\phi$. There is in fact a phase slip at $\phi_C \approx 0.2$ for these higher values of Λ. The continuous PRCs that pass through $\Delta\phi = 0$ are classically known as "Type 1," and the PRCs with a phase slip are known as "Type 0" (Winfree, 2001). This qualitative change in the type of PRC curve occurs in this system for $\Lambda \approx 2$ (Figure 8.13b, inset panel).

We now return to the experimental data to seek evidence for this phase-resetting mechanism predicted by the model. To do this, we estimate the period of the endogenous CORT oscillation in the data and determine the phase at which the 10 min noise stress is applied. We only consider data which satisfy the following conditions (see the exemplars in Figure 8.14):

1 At least two clear pulses after the application of the noise stress.

2 At least one clear pulse prior to the application of the noise stress.

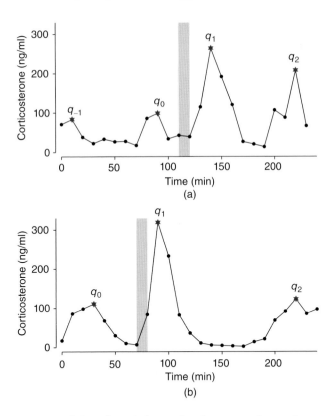

Figure 8.14 Determining phase information from experimental stress-response data. (a and b) Illustration of how peaks are selected in order to compute the phase information from experimental stress-response data. The time histories show levels of CORT sampled at 10-min intervals in exemplar female Sprague–Dawley (a) and female Lewis (b) rats. Shaded region indicates the period of the applied noise stress. Selected peaks (q) are marked red.

The first condition enables us to approximate the period P of the endogenous oscillation as the time interval between the two pulses. While there is inevitably some variability in this inter-pulse frequency, typically this is of the order $P \pm 10$ min. The second condition enables us to approximate the relative position (the phase) on the endogenous period P at which the noise stress is applied. For example, in Figure 8.14a, $P \sim 80$ min and the 10 min noise stress (shaded region) is applied approximately 20 min after the pulse q_0. This corresponds to a relative phase $\phi_C \sim 0.25$. Finally, we compute the magnitude of the phase shift by considering the time interval between q_0 (the prestress pulse) and q_1 (the first post-stress pulse) relative to the endogenous period P.

The phase resetting information for all individuals ($n = 19$) is shown in Figure 8.15. Where the points from more than one individual coincide, the point is circled in black. The PRC determined from our mathematical model for the experimentally determined stress impulse amplitude ($\Lambda = 6.8$) is also shown. Significantly, the data appear visually consistent with a Type-0 PRC with a phase slip close to 0.2, representing the "transition point" between an apparent phase advance and phase delay of the endogenous oscillation.

It is possible that this close agreement between the experimental data and the theoretical PRC could have occurred by chance. To consider the

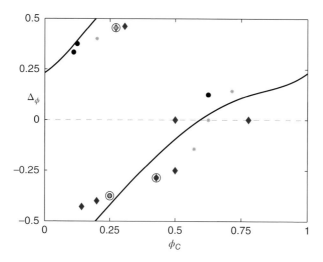

Figure 8.15 Comparison of theoretical PRC with experimental data confirms a Type-0 phase-resetting mechanism. The Type-0 phase response curve for $\Lambda = 6.8$ as computed with the model (black curve). The experimental data, plotted at discrete points, are shown for eight female Sprague–Dawley rats (black dots), five female Lewis rats (red diamonds), and six PVG rats (green stars). Points where two samples take the same value are circled.

likelihood of this, we calculate the goodness of fit between the theoretical PRC and the values extracted from the experimental study, using least squares to estimate the Euclidian distance between the theoretical curve and experimental data. We then employ bootstrap statistics whereby equivalent fits are calculated by choosing 19 randomly selected phase shifts with equivalent phase positions to those of the experimental data. This results in a p-value $< 10^{-6}$ when comparing the fit of the experimental data to those random fits, making our observations highly unlikely to have occurred by chance.

It is interesting that the HPA axis – a system that is classically known to be crucial for maintaining "physiological stability" in the body – is so dynamically variable. We can use our model to try to understand what, if any, advantages there are for this system to be so dynamically active in terms of its ability to respond to stress. To do this, we consider the amplitude response in CORT resulting from an acute stress applied when the system is either at a steady state or in an oscillating state (see Figure 8.4a). In the oscillatory case, we average the amplitude of the CORT response across all values of the phase ϕ_C in the interval $[0, 1]$. We then consider how these CORT responses vary for different amplitudes (Λ) of the acute stress. Note that, for the oscillating case, we fix the basal level of CRH $= 25$

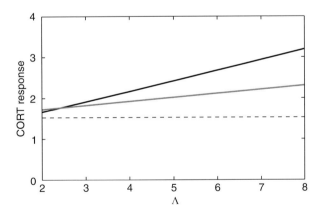

Figure 8.16 **Comparing the CORT response to an incoming stress between the oscillatory and steady-state regimes**. For the oscillating case, the basal level of CRH $= 25$, and for the steady-state case, the basal level of CRH is set such that the steady-state CORT level matches the maximum level of CORT in the oscillating case (dashed black). In the steady-state case, the response to a stress is independent of the timing of the stress (gray), whereas for the oscillatory case, we present the averaged response to an incoming stress applied at every point over the period of an oscillation (solid black). Λ represents the magnitude of the stress. For small stressors, the response in both cases is comparable, whilst for larger stressors, the response in the oscillatory case is significantly greater.

(as above), and for the steady-state case we fix the basal level of CRH such that the steady-state CORT level matches the maximum level of CORT in the oscillating case.

As shown in Figure 8.16, for a stress amplitude of $\Lambda = 6.8$ (which we estimated from experimental noise stress data above), the average CORT response in the oscillating case is approximately 50% greater than in the steady-state case. Moreover, in the oscillating case, as the value of Λ decreases (corresponding to a stress of smaller amplitude), the average value of the CORT response drops toward the maximum value of the basal oscillation in CORT (dashed line in Figure 8.16). This shows that the system can effectively filter out lower-amplitude perturbations from the internal or external environment, but remain markedly responsive to more significant perturbations, such as an acute stress. In other words, small perturbations can be safely ignored as the system will naturally return to its basal state, but a larger perturbation will result in a swift response to ensure the internal environment does not become a threat to life.

8.6 Discussion

We have developed a mathematical model describing a mechanism for the generation of ultradian oscillations in the HPA axis. We have tested the predictions of our model *in vivo* and our results support our hypothesis that ACTH and CORT oscillations are generated by a feedforward–feedback mechanism between the pituitary and adrenal glands. Furthermore, we have used our mathematical model and experimental data to show that the hormonal response to acute stress depends not only on the magnitude of the stress, but also on the *timing* of exposure to the stress relative to the phase of the endogenous ultradian oscillation.

We have shown that oscillations in ACTH and CORT are possible even for constant levels of CRH, which challenges the long-standing hypothesis that pulsatile CRH is required for generating pulsatile secretion of ACTH and CORT. However, although we believe this pituitary–adrenal interaction to be the primary oscillating mechanism governing the ultradian rhythm of ACTH and CORT, we are not discounting the potential significance of the pulsatile patterns of CRH that have been observed experimentally. It is quite possible that pulsatile CRH release is important for maintaining responsiveness of the pituitary–adrenal system. This is consistent with findings that sustained levels of CRH can result in a down regulation and desensitization of CRH receptors (Aguilera, 1994; Aguilera *et al.*, 2004). Moreover, it remains to be seen how the pulsatile pattern of CRH modulates and interacts with the endogenously rhythmic pituitary–adrenal system.

The model we have described in this chapter is a "systems-level" mathematical model in the sense that it does not incorporate microscale processes, such as the cellular regulation of the synthesis, storage and release of ACTH from corticotroph cells, or the synthesis and secretion of CORT from cells of the adrenal cortex. There are, of course, many levels of regulation in this system, including the rhythmic activity of clock genes, local feedback pathways, and autonomic innervation of components of the axis. At present, however, there is insufficient data on these processes to enable us to mathematically investigate their influence on the emergent dynamics of the system. Incorporating cellular-level processes may well be an important factor to consider in the future in order to further our understanding of how and why the dynamics of this system changes in both health and disease.

8.7 Perspectives

Nothing in biology is static – everything is in a state of oscillation, whether it is the stochastic binding of transcription factors to DNA, the electrophysiological firing of neurons, or the daily, monthly, or even yearly cycles of reproductive function. At the level of the neuroendocrine HPA axis, we have shown that an approximate hourly oscillation emerges as a function of a feedforward–feedback relationship between the anterior pituitary and the adrenal glands, providing a remarkably effective and responsive control mechanism for the maintenance of mammalian homeostasis.

References

Aguilera G (1994). Regulation of pituitary ACTH secretion during chronic stress. *Front. Neuroendocrinol.* **15**, 321–350.

Aguilera G, Nikodemova M, Wynn PC, Catt KJ (2004). Corticotropin releasing hormone receptors: two decades later. *Peptides* **25**, 319–329.

Ben-Zvi A, Vernon SD, Broderick G (2009). Model-based therapeutic correction of hypothalamic–pituitary–adrenal axis dysfunction. *PLoS Comput Biol.* **5**(1), e1000273.

Brown E, Moehlis J, Holmes P (2004). On the phase reduction and the response dynamics of neural oscillator populations. *Neural Comput.* **16**, 673–715.

Carnes M, Lent S, Feyzi J, Hazel D (1989). Plasma adrenocorticotropic hormone in the rat demonstrates three different rhythms within 24 h. *Neuroendocrinology* **50**, 17–25.

Conway-Campbell BL, Sarabdjitsingh RA, McKenna MA, Pooley JR, Kershaw YM, Meijer OC, de Kloet ER, Lightman SL (2010). Glucocorticoid ultradian rhythmicity directs cyclical gene pulsing of the clock gene period 1 in rat hippocampus. *J Neuroendocrinol.* **22**, 1093–1100.

Engelborghs K, Luzyanina T, Samaey G (2001). DDE-BIFTOOL v. 2.00: a Matlab package for bifurcation analysis of delay differential equations. Technical Report TW-330, Department of Computer Science, K.U. Leuven, Leuven, Belgium.

Gupta S, Aslakson E, Gurbaxani BM, Vernon SD (2007). Inclusion of the glucocorticoid receptor in a hypothalamic pituitary adrenal axis model reveals bistability. *Theor Biol Med Model.* **4**, 8.

Henley DE, Leendertz JA, Russell GM, Wood SA, Taheri S, Woltersdorf WW, Lightman SL (2009). Development of an automated blood sampling system for use in humans. *J Med Eng Technol.* **33**, 199–208.

Ixart G, Barbanel G, Nouguier-Soulé J, Assenmacher I (1991). A quantitative study of the pulsatile parameters of CRH-41 secretion in unanesthetized free-moving rats. *Exp Brain Res.* **87**, 153–158.

Ixart G, Siaud P, Barbanel G, Mekaouche M, Givalois L, Assenmacher I (1993). Circadian variations in the amplitude of corticotropin-releasing hormone 41 (CRH41) episodic release measured in vivo in male rats: correlations with diurnal fluctuations in hypothalamic and median eminence CRH41 contents. *J Biol Rhythms* **8**, 297–309.

Keenan DM, Licinio J, Veldhuis JD (2001). A feedback-controlled ensemble model of the stress-responsive hypothalamo-pituitary-adrenal axis. *Proc Natl Acad Sci U.S.A.* **98**, 4028–4033.

Kelly RB (1985). Pathways of protein secretion in eukaryotes. *Science* **230**, 25–32.

Kuznetsov YA (2004). *Element of Applied Bifurcation Theory (3rd edition)*. Springer-Verlag, Berlin, Germany.

Li G, Liu B, Liu Y (1995). A dynamical model of the pulsatile secretion of the hypothalmo-pituitary-thyroid axis. *BioSystems* **35**, 83–92.

Lightman SL, Conway-Campbell BL (2010). The crucial role of pulsatile activity of the HPA axis for continuous dynamic equilibration. *Nat Rev Neurosci.* **11**, 710–718.

Liu YW, Hu ZH, Peng JH, Liu BZ (1999). A dynamical model for the pulsatile secretion of the hypothalamus-pituitary-adrenal axis. *Math Comput Model.* **29**, 103–110.

Liu BZ, Peng JH (1990). A mathematical model of hypothalamo-pituitary-thyroid axis. *Acta Biochimica et Biophysica Sinica* **6**, 431–437.

Mershon JL, Sehlhorst CS, Rebar RW, Liu JH (1992). Evidence of a corticotropin-releasing hormone pulse generator in the macaque hypothalamus. *Endocrinology* **130**, 2991–2996.

Moore RY, Eichler VB (1972). Loss of a circadian adrenal corticosterone rhythm following suprachiasmatic lesions in the rat. *Brain Res.* **42**, 201–206.

Papaikonomou E (1977). Rat adrenocortical dynamics. *J Physiol.* **265**, 119–131.

Rankin J, Walker JJ, Windle R, Lightman SL, Terry JR (2012). Characterizing dynamic interactions between ultradian glucocorticoid rhythmicity and acute stress using the phase response curve. *PLoS One* **7**(2), e30978.

Reppert SM, Weaver DR (2002). Coordination of circadian timing in mammals. *Nature* **418**, 935–941.

Sarabdjitsingh RA, Conway-Campbell BL, Leggett JD, Waite EJ, Meijer OC, de Kloet ER, Lightman SL (2010). Stress responsiveness varies over the ultradian glucocorticoid cycle in a brain-region-specific manner. *Endocrinology* **151**, 5369–5379.

Spiga F, Waite EJ, Liu Y, Kershaw YM, Aguilera G, Lightman SL (2011). ACTH-dependent ultradian rhythm of corticosterone secretion. *Endocrinology* **152**, 1448–1457.

Sriram K, Rodriguez-Fernandez M, Doyle FJ III (2012). Modeling cortisol dynamics in the neuro-endocrine axis distinguishes normal, depression, and post-traumatic stress disorder (PTSD) in humans. *PLoS Computational Biol.* **8**(2), e1002379.

Stavreva DA, Wiench M, John S, Conway-Campbell BL, McKenna MA, Pooley JR, Johnson TA, Voss TC, Lightman SL, Hager GL (2009). Ultradian hormone stimulation induces glucocorticoid receptor-mediated pulses of gene transcription. *Nat Cell Biol.* **11**, 1093–1102.

Stocco DM, Clark BJ (1996). Regulation of the acute production of steroids in steroido-genic cells. *Endocr Rev.* **17**, 221–244.

Sydnor KL, Sayers G (1953). Biological half-life of endogenous ACTH. *Proc Soc Exp Biol Med.* **83**, 729–733.

Ulrich-Lai YM, Herman JP (2009). Neural regulation of endocrine and autonomic stress responses. *Nat Rev Neurosci.* **10**, 397–409.

Waite EJ, McKenna M, Kershaw Y, Walker JJ, Cho K, Piggins HD, Lightman SL (2012). Ultradian corticosterone secretion is maintained in the absence of circadian cues. *Eur J Neurosci.* **36**, 3142–3150.

Walker JJ, Spiga F, Waite E, Zhao Z, Kershaw Y, Terry JR, Lightman SL (2012). The origin of glucocorticoid hormone oscillations. *PLoS Biology.* **10**(6), e1001341.

Walker JJ, Terry JR, Lightman SL (2010a). Origin of ultradian pulsatility in the hypothalamic–pituitary-adrenal axis. *Proc R Soc B.* **277**, 1627–1633.

Walker JJ, Terry JR, Tsaneva-Atanasova K, Armstrong SP, McArdle CA, Lightman SL (2010b). Encoding and decoding mechanisms of pulsatile hormone secretion. *J Neuroendocrinol.* **22**, 1226–1238.

Windle RJ, Wood SA, Lightman SL, Ingram CD (1998b). The pulsatile characteristics of hypothalamo-pituitary-adrenal activity in female Lewis and Fischer 344 rats and its relationship to differential stress responses. *Endocrinology* **139**, 4044–4052.

Windle RJ, Wood SA, Kershaw YM, Lightman SL, Ingram CD, Harbuz MS (2001). Increased corticosterone pulse frequency during adjuvant-induced arthritis and its relationship to alterations in stress responsiveness. *J Neuroendocrinol.* **13**, 905–911.

Windle RJ, Wood SA, Shanks N, Lightman SL, Ingram CD (1998a). Ultradian rhythm of basal corticosterone release in the female rat: Dynamic interaction with the response to acute stress. *Endocrinology* **139**, 443–450.

Winfree AT (2001). *The Geometry of Biological Time.* Springer-Verlag, Berlin, Germany.

CHAPTER 9

Modeling the Dynamics of Gonadotropin-Releasing Hormone (GnRH) Secretion in the Course of an Ovarian Cycle

Frédérique Clément[1] and Alexandre Vidal[2]

[1]INRIA Paris-Rocquencourt Research Centre, Domaine de Voluceau, Le Chesnay, France
[2]Laboratoire de Mathématiques et Modélisation d'Évry (LaMME), Université d'Évry-Val-d'Essonne, Évry, France

9.1 Introduction

9.1.1 GnRH surge and the triggering of ovulation

In mammals, ovulation is a key limiting step of reproductive success. Ovulation is the process by which a fertilizable oocyte is released from a fully mature (ovulatory) ovarian follicle and collected into a fallopian tube. Depending on the species, either one (in mono-ovulating species) or several (in poly-ovulating species) oocytes are ovulated within an ovarian cycle. The triggering of ovulation is controlled by the central nervous system, first on the hypothalamic level, and then on the pituitary level (Figure 9.1).

In every mammalian species investigated so far in a physiological setting, ovulation is triggered by the so-called GnRH surge, which corresponds to a dramatic and quite sudden increase in GnRH secretion from the usual pulsatile secretion regime and which brings about a surge in the secretion of luteinizing hormone (LH) (Christian and Moenter, 2010). In spontaneous ovulators (such as human, sheep, or cattle, for instance), the GnRH surge is triggered in response to the ever higher levels of estradiol secreted by the ovaries in the follicular phase of the ovarian cycle, without any other driving force than the neuroendocrine feedback loops within the hypothalamo-pituitary-ovarian axis. In some spontaneous ovulators (such as rat), the GnRH surge is, nevertheless, subject to a circadian control and can only occur during a specific time of the day (this circadian control ultimately explains the distribution of the rat ovarian cycles between 4-day or

Computational Neuroendocrinology, First Edition. Edited by Duncan J. MacGregor and Gareth Leng.
© 2016 John Wiley & Sons, Ltd. Published 2016 by John Wiley & Sons, Ltd.
Companion Website: www.wiley.com/go/Leng/Computational

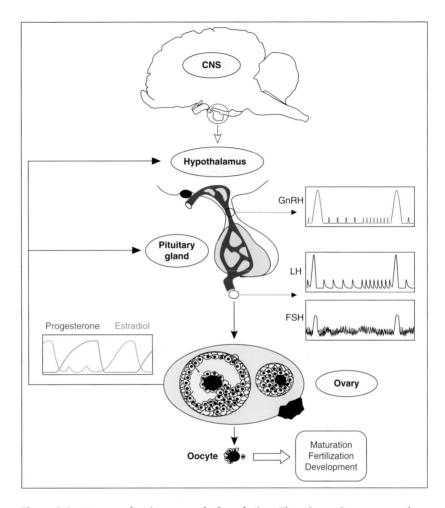

Figure 9.1   Neuroendocrine control of ovulation. The release of one or several oocyte(s) is a cyclic event that results from the endocrine dialogue between the hypothalamus, pituitary gland, and ovaries. The hypothalamic hormone GnRH (gonadotropin-releasing hormone) is the master neurohormone controlling reproduction. During most of the ovarian cycle, the pattern of GnRH secretion is pulsatile. The release of GnRH into the hypothalamo-pituitary portal blood induces the secretion from the pituitary gland of luteinizing hormone (LH), which also follows a clear pulsatile pattern, and follicle-stimulating hormone (FSH). LH and FSH control the development of ovarian follicles and their secretory activity. In turn, hormones released by the ovaries (steroid hormones such as progesterone and estradiol or peptide hormones such as inhibin) modulate the secretion of GnRH, LH, and FSH within entangled feedback loops. In females, the GnRH secretion pattern dramatically alters once per ovarian cycle, in response to the time-varying levels of ovarian steroids, and switches to the GnRH surge characterized by a massive release of GnRH (surges in two successive cycles are shown in red). In turn, the GnRH surge triggers the LH surge, whose duration is shorter. The GnRH-induced LH surge finally brings about ovulation – the release of fertilizable oocytes from ovarian follicles.

5-day cycles). In induced ovulators (such as cat and rabbit, but also llama and camel, for instance), the GnRH surge is triggered by mating. Yet, the mating-induced GnRH surge can only occur in a steroid-favorable environment of high estradiol levels, so that the endocrine dialogue between the ovaries and hypothalamus is still a master-piece of the ovulatory process.

9.1.2   GnRH secretion regimes

GnRH neurons are space-specific and scarce (of the order of 1 to a few thousands) neurons located in different hypothalamic areas (mostly in the preoptic area). Like the other neuroendocrine neurons that regulate the anterior pituitary, they are endowed with a very long secretory process that reaches the median eminence, where GnRH is released. The usual pattern of GnRH secretion in both males and females is pulsatile; each GnRH pulse results from at least partial synchronization within the GnRH neural network. How this very slow (on the order of the hour) network behavior emerges from fast individual neuronal dynamics is a fascinating question that is still unsolved and that we will not deal with in this chapter; we will take for granted that the default regime of GnRH secretion is pulsatile. We will rather focus on the equally fascinating question of how the GnRH secretion pattern switches from a pulsatile background regime to a surge regime back and forth. We will see that this question raises other corollary ones, and especially: how is the alternation between pulses and surge connected with the ovarian dynamics, and how is the frequency of pulses altered along an ovarian cycle (Figure 9.2).

9.1.3   Steroid control of GnRH secretion

The question of the effects of ovarian steroids (estradiol and progesterone) on GnRH neurons can be investigated from different angles according to the species. The most precise neuroanatomical studies have been performed in rodents (mice and rats) and have enabled investigators to draw a quite detailed picture of the circuitry of connections linking the neurons directly targeted by ovarian steroids to the GnRH neurons via possible other regulatory neurons. However, physiological studies intending to dissect in time the effects of ovarian steroids have mostly been undertaken in domestic species, especially in the ewe. This species is particularly useful for studying GnRH secretion rhythms, since (i) it has a large body size allowing repeated sampling of pituitary portal blood and cerebrospinal fluid allowing further analysis of GnRH time series, (ii) the duration of its ovarian cycle (around 21 days) makes it easier to dissect the different steps in the temporal sequence of steroid action, and (iii) it is closer to human ovarian physiology compared to rodents.

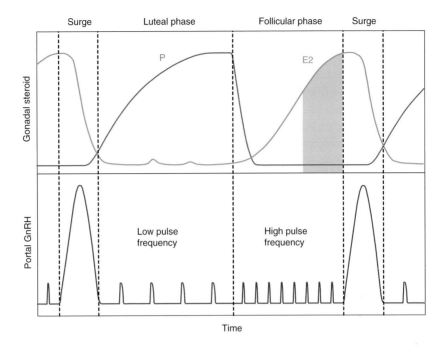

Figure 9.2   Schematic patterns of estradiol (E2) and progesterone (P) plasma levels and GnRH levels in portal blood through the course of an ovarian cycle in female mammals. The pulsatile secretion of GnRH is periodically interrupted by the ovulatory surge that involves a massive release of GnRH. Each surge is triggered by a prolonged exposure to high estradiol levels in a background environment of low progesterone. Between two surges, the pulsatile phase is split into two successive phases: the progesterone-dominated luteal phase, characterized by a low GnRH pulse frequency, and the estradiol-dominated follicular phase, characterized by a high GnRH pulse frequency. The gray area corresponds to the cumulated level of estradiol at surge onset.

In almost all studies dedicated so far to the study of the expression of steroid (nuclear) receptors in GnRH neurons (Rønnekleiv and Kelly, 2005), it has been shown that they do not express progesterone receptor, or type α estradiol receptor (ER α), yet they do express the type-β estradiol receptor (ER β) (Hrabovszky *et al.*, 2001; Skinner and Dufourny, 2005). This means that, except for possible acute direct effects of estradiol mediated through ER β (Abraham *et al.*, 2003), the effects of ovarian steroids on GnRH neurons are mostly indirect and involve intermediary neural relays that themselves project onto GnRH neurons.

9.1.4   Experimental setups for portal GnRH withdrawal

Access to kinetic and quantitative GnRH data has been made possible by two original experimental setups (Moenter *et al.*, 1990, 1991, 1992). First, a tricky surgical technique was developed to implant a dedicated apparatus for pituitary portal blood withdrawal; this technique involves drilling a tunnel in the sphenoid bone between the olfactory bulbs and under the optic chiasma before reaching the pituitary stalk. Second, an experimental protocol inducing an artificial ovarian cycle was designed. This rests on the general principles underlying the studies of endocrine feedback loops, that consist of "cutting" one of the loop branches to decouple the endocrine dialogue between the different organic levels involved in the loop. In the present case, we would like to get rid of the endogenous ovarian steroids and to administer (chemically similar) exogenous steroids in a way controlled both in time and dose. Thus, ewes are ovariectomized and then exposed to a regime of steroid mimicking the natural hormone release by the ovaries along an ovarian cycle. They are first given a progesterone implant, to reproduce a luteal-like phase. When the implant is removed, mimicking the occurrence of luteolysis, the ewes are exposed to increasing levels of estradiol, up to the species- and strain-dependent threshold needed to trigger the GnRH surge. Those combined technical and functional protocols have provided most of the information on the control exerted by ovarian steroids on the qualitative sequence of GnRH secretion events and on their quantitative properties, both during the pulsatile and surge regime, that will be detailed in the framework of our dynamical model in the next sections.

9.1.5 The GnRH generator: secreting and regulatory neurons

The whole set of all neuronal (and also glial) cell types involved in the control of GnRH secretion is commonly known as the "GnRH pulse generator." This includes the GnRH neurons themselves, as well as the regulatory neurons that process the steroids signals and relay them to GnRH neurons. A great variety of neural inputs, either excitatory (e.g., glutamate and norepinephrine), or inhibitory (e.g., GABA – gamma-aminobutyric acid—and endogenous opioids), have been characterized in afferents projecting onto GnRH neurons (Herbison, 1998). However, in the past 15 years, one particular regulatory system has come to the forefront of attention; several lines of evidence have combined to highlight the key role of kisspeptin producing neurons in mediating the steroid feedback control of GnRH secretion, through signaling via the GPR54 receptor (Pinilla *et al.*, 2012). Different subsets of kisspeptin neurons can, at least in rodents, be associated with hypothalamic areas involved differentially in the ovarian feedback exerted either on the pulse frequency in the pulsatile regime (arcuate nucleus, where the expression of kisspeptin is associated with that of neurokinin B and dynorphin that appear to act in a paracrine and/or autocrine way) or on the surge triggering (antero-ventral periventricular nucleus).

9.2   A single dynamical framework for the control of the GnRH pulse and surge generator by ovarian steroids

9.2.1   GnRH secreting system

In the absence of steroid input from the gonads, as in the case in adult ovariectomized ewes not supplemented with exogenous steroids, GnRH secretion consists of regular pulses which occur at a high frequency. Considering the network of GnRH neurons involved in the pulse regime as a single average neuron, we can use the classical FitzHugh–Nagumo (Fitzhugh, 1961; Nagumo *et al.*, 1962) system to represent this default secretion regime concisely:

$$\delta\frac{dx}{dt} = -y + f(x) \tag{9.1a}$$

$$\frac{dy}{dt} = a_0 x + a_1 y + I \tag{9.1b}$$

$$y_{\text{out}}(t) = y(t)\chi_{\{y(t)>y_{\text{th}}\}} \tag{9.1c}$$

where

$$f : x \to \lambda_3 x^3 + \lambda_1 x, \quad \lambda_3 < 0, \quad \lambda_1 > 0$$

Parameter δ is assumed to be positive and small. System (9.1a) and (9.1b) is therefore a "slow–fast system": x is the so-called fast variable and y is the "slow variable." Hence, away from the cubic x-nullcline (represented in Figure 9.3a and c), the trajectories are almost horizontal and fast (slow variable y remains almost constant since its dynamics is much slower than the x dynamics). However, trajectories near the x-nullcline are slow since the x dynamics is almost zero and the whole system is under the control of the slow dynamics.

GnRH secretion is represented by the output variable y_{out}, that is obtained after thresholding y. In some sense, the y_{th} threshold can be associated with the critical intracellular calcium concentration that is needed for the secretory vesicles to undergo exocytosis from the neuronal terminals.

9.2.2   Different dynamical regimes of secretion: pulse regime versus surge regime

If we now consider that the default secretion regime can be perturbed by dynamical inputs (entered as I in Equation (9.1b)), we can switch the secreting system from a pulsatile regime to a surge-like regime. For a given interval of values of I, the system (9.1a) and (9.1b) admits an unstable singular point lying on the middle branch of the cubic x-nullcline $y = f(x)$. In this case, the singular point is surrounded by a limit cycle of relaxation type (Figure 9.3a) with slow parts along the left and right branches of the cubic x-nullcline and fast parts corresponding to back and forth jumps between

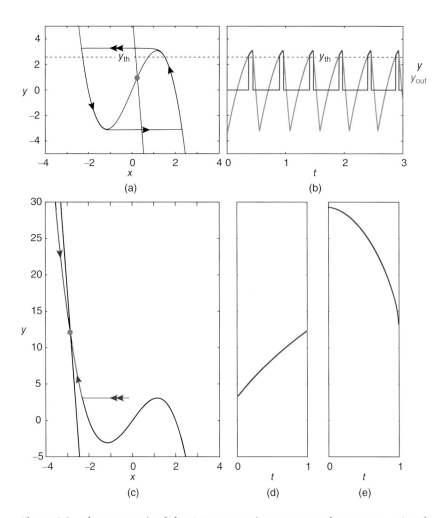

Figure 9.3 **Phase portrait of the GnRH secreting system and output y_{out} signal in the pulse regime (a and b) and surge regime (c, d, and e).** In each panel (a) and (b), the cubic curve and the straight line represent the x- and y-nullcline, respectively. The orange point corresponding to their intersection represents a singular point of the GnRH secreting system. For I in an interval of values defined by the other parameters, the GnRH secreting system admits an unstable singular point surrounded by an attractive limit cycle of relaxation type (a). Along this orbit, the generated y signal (gray pattern in panel (b)) is serrated and the thresholded y_{out} signal (blue pattern in (b)) is pulsatile. For greater values of I, a stable singular point lies on the left branch of the cubic x-nullcline. Due to the slow–fast property of the GnRH secreting system, the orbits first reach the x-nullcline quickly, and then follow it while tending to the singular point (c). (d) and (e) show the time trace of y along the lower and upper orbits displayed in (c), respectively.

the right and left branches. Hence, the value of y along the orbit oscillates around 0 and the generated y signal is serrated. It follows that the model output y_{out}, obtained after thresholding y, is a pulsatile signal (Figure 9.3b).

For higher values of I, the singular point lies high up on the left branch of the cubic x-nullcline and is attracting. Therefore, all the trajectories of the system (9.1a) and (9.1b) first reach quickly the left branch of the cubic x-nullcline (under the influence of the fast dynamics), follow this branch to reach the vicinity of the singular point, and then keep tracking this point as long as it lies on the cubic left branch (i.e., remains stable). Such trajectories are represented in Figure 9.3c. The corresponding time traces of variable y are displayed in Figure 9.3d and e: depending on the initial condition, (x, y) may go up or down along the cubic left branch to track the singular point and, consequently, y may either increase or decrease.

9.2.3 Recurrent periodic alternation between the pulse and surge regimes

Through the ovarian cycle, the dynamical inputs received by GnRH neurons account for the steroid-mediating control exerted by the regulatory neurons. To reproduce both the pulse and surge regimes, we use the following regulating system of FitzHugh–Nagumo type:

$$\epsilon \frac{dX}{dt} = -Y + g(X) \tag{9.2a}$$

$$\frac{dY}{dt} = X + b_1 Y + b_2 \tag{9.2b}$$

Parameter ϵ is assumed to be positive and small, and parameters b_1 and b_2 are chosen so that the system (9.2) admits a relaxation limit cycle (Figure 9.4a). The X signal (time trace of variable X) along the limit cycle displays two regimes separated by fast transitions (Figure 9.4b): a slow decrease from X_{max} to γ ($X > 0$) and a slow increase from X_{min} to $-\gamma$ ($X < 0$).

We model the control exerted by the regulating system onto the GnRH secreting system by introducing the linear dynamical input $I = cX$ and coupling the two systems on different time scales (Clément and Françoise, 2007). This yields the global model:

$$\epsilon \delta \frac{dx}{dt} = -y + f(x) \tag{9.3a}$$

$$\epsilon \frac{dy}{dt} = a_0 x + a_1 y + a_2 + cX \tag{9.3b}$$

$$\epsilon \frac{dX}{dt} = -Y + g(X) \tag{9.3c}$$

$$\frac{dY}{dt} = X + b_1 Y + b_2 \tag{9.3d}$$

$$y_{out}(t) = y(t) \chi_{\{y(t) > y_{th}\}} \tag{9.3e}$$

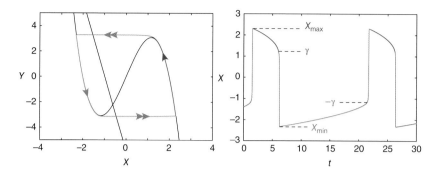

Figure 9.4   Limit cycle of the regulating system and the corresponding time trace of variable X. The values of parameters b_1 and b_2 are chosen so that the regulating system admits an unstable singular point lying on the middle branch of the cubic X-nullcline surrounded by a limit cycle (a). Due to the slow–fast property of the regulating system, the limit cycle is of relaxation type and the periodic X time trace is characterized by fast transitions between two main regimes: slow increase from X_{min} to $-\gamma$ and slow decrease from X_{max} to γ (b).

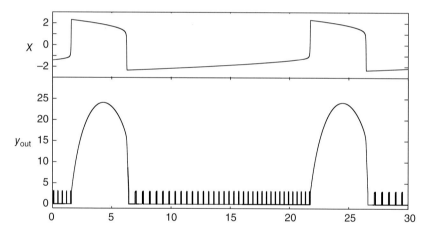

Figure 9.5   Output of the model: alternation of pulsatile and surge phases along time. The top panel shows the relaxation-type signal generated by variable X along the regulating system limit cycle. The bottom panel shows the corresponding y_{out} signal generated by the whole model. While X increases slowly from X_{min} to $-\gamma$, the GnRH secreting system remains in the pulsatile regime. While X decreases slowly between X_{max} and γ, the GnRH secreting system is shifted into the surge regime. The back-and-forth transitions from one regime to another are fast compared to the durations of both the pulsatile and surge phases.

An appropriate choice of c and a_2 values ensures that the output y_{out} of this model displays the following pattern (Figure 9.5) driven by the periodic oscillation of X along the relaxation limit cycle of the regulating system (9.3c) and (9.3d). During the slow increase of X from X_{min} to $-\gamma$ ($X < 0$), the GnRH secreting system (9.3a) and (9.3b) remains in the pulsatility regime. Since the coupling between the two systems is slow–fast, the GnRH secreting system produces many pulses in this time interval. When X jumps to positive values, the GnRH secreting system switches to the surge regime: (x, y) reaches the vicinity of the stable singular point and y (as well as y_{out}) undergoes a great increase. Once X returns to negative values, the GnRH secreting system switches back to the pulse regime, y (as well as y_{out}) decreases quickly, and the whole process starts again. Hence, the pattern of the model output reproduces the alternation between the pulse and surge regime shown in the bottom panel of Figure 9.5. Note that, since the GnRH secreting system is faster than the regulating system and the (X, Y) limit cycle is of relaxation type, the pulse regime coincides almost exactly with the phase $X < 0$, and the surge regime with $X > 0$.

9.3   GnRH secretion pattern along an ovarian cycle

9.3.1   Qualitative sequence of secretory events leading up to the surge

Transmission and activation phases

In sheep, as in many spontaneous ovulating species, the increase in estradiol levels during the follicular phase of the ovarian cycle leads to the GnRH surge (Figure 9.2). Estradiol levels do not remain elevated throughout the surge, but start to decline shortly after the surge onset (Moenter *et al.,* 1991). In experimentally induced follicular phases, the GnRH surge can be brought about by estradiol as soon as a minimal cumulated threshold (high enough estradiol levels lasting long enough) is satisfied (Moenter *et al.,* 1990). Estradiol need not be maintained throughout the whole presurge period (Evans *et al.,* 1997). The sequence of neuroendocrine events finishing with the surge itself can thus be split into an estradiol-dependent step (the activation phase) and an estradiol-independent step (the transmission phase). In agreement with these biological observations, we can consider that the regulatory neurons first proceed as time-moving integrators of prolonged and raised estradiol levels and then generate a (slightly delayed) surge-triggering signal to GnRH neurons.

Concomitant changes in plasma steroid levels and portal blood GnRH level

The pattern of GnRH secretion through an ovarian cycle corresponds, in the model, to the evolution of the output variable y_{out} over one period of the regulating system limit cycle (Vidal and Clément, 2010). It can be paralleled to the changes in plasma steroid (estradiol and progesterone) levels in the course of an ovarian cycle. Starting from the time of luteolysis, the GnRH secreting system first oscillates and generates a pulsatile y_{out}

output. When the cumulated dose of estradiol reaches a threshold (after 3 days in the ewe), the GnRH secreting system enters the surge mode and the magnitude of y_{out} increases greatly. At the time of the estradiol peak, the GnRH secreting system returns to an oscillatory mode: y_{out} decreases (surge decline) before pulsing again. For the following 13 days, progesterone levels are high, whereas estradiol levels are low, and the GnRH secreting system remains in an oscillatory mode. When progesterone levels fall and estradiol levels rise again (around $t = 16.5$d in the ewe), the whole sequence of alternation between the surge and pulse regime repeats itself.

Dynamical encoding of the GnRH pulses

Immediately after the surge, the pulse frequency is low (less than 1 pulse per 3 h in ewe). Afterward, during the estradiol rise and progesterone fall, the pulse frequency increases (up to 1 pulse per 75 min in the ewe). As a consequence, the interpulse interval (IPI) decreases during the whole duration of the pulse regime. The inflection point in the IPI time series marks the transition between the luteal phase and the follicular phase. In the course of the follicular phase, the pulse frequency exceeds a critical value, where the GnRH secreting system enters the route to the surge.

In ovariectomized ewes, estradiol affects the shape of GnRH pulses in a dose-dependent manner. More precisely, the durations of both the plateau and declining phase are shorter after estradiol administration (Evans *et al.*, 1995). Accordingly, the GnRH pulses reproduced by the model last longer in the luteal, progesterone-dominated phase than in the follicular, estradiol-dominated phase. The lower frequency and longer pulse duration after the surge can be explained concomitantly in the dynamical framework of the model (Figure 9.6). With each point (x_i, y_i) on the (x, y) phase plane, we can associate the magnitude of the instantaneous velocity vector (whose horizontal and vertical components are, respectively, dx/dt and dy/dt assessed at (x_i, y_i)). The speed of the current (x, y) point is slowed down each time it passes through the zone close to the right knee of the cubic function $y = f(x)$, leading to a low pulsatile frequency, and a quite great pulse duration. However, when the singular point is near the origin, the velocity of the current point along the limit cycle remains medium to very strong. Hence, the period of the limit cycle is much smaller (i.e., the generated pulse frequency is greater) and the generated pulse duration is smaller. In the course of an entire pulsatile phase, the pulse frequency is driven as follows. During the luteal phase, X remains near X_{min} and the pulse frequency is low. Then, as X increases, the singular point of the GnRH secreting system goes away from the right knee vicinity and the pulse frequency increases; this corresponds to the luteal to follicular phase transition. At the end of the follicular phase (for a value of X near $-\gamma$), the

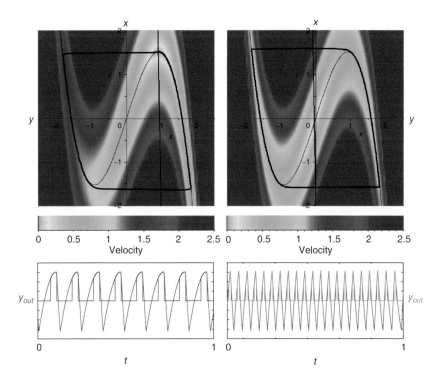

Figure 9.6 **Changes in the GnRH pulse frequency according to the value of** X **from** X_{min} **(left panels) to** $-\gamma$ **(right panels).** In each case, the upper panel displays the vector field magnitude (velocity of the current point) associated with the GnRH secreting system in the color code as well as the relaxation limit cycle (black line). The bottom panel displays the generated y_{out} signal. In the left panel case (X close to X_{min}), the limit cycle passes through the vicinity of the singular point, where the vector field is very weak (less than 0.1 in the orange region). However, in the right panel case, the vector field magnitude along the limit cycle remains everywhere higher than 0.5. Consequently, the period of the limit cycle in the left panel case is greater than in the right panel case, so that the pulse frequency is lower for X near X_{min} (beginning of the luteal phase) than for X near $-\gamma$ (end of the follicular phase).

pulse frequency hits its maximum value, which is much greater than the luteal phase frequency.

9.3.2 Quantitative specifications on the secretory events

Once the correct sequence of secretory events has been obtained qualitatively, the GnRH output can then be further constrained with respect to physiologically relevant quantitative specifications (Figure 9.7). These specifications deal with the durations of the luteal and follicular phases of the ovarian cycle and the ratios of (i) the surge duration to the whole

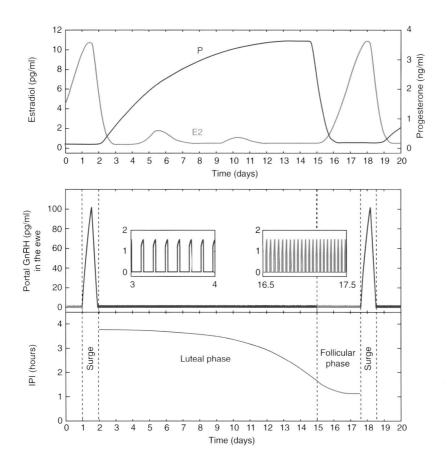

Figure 9.7 GnRH secretion pattern through an entire ovarian cycle. The GnRH output of the model (y_{out}) shown in the middle panel meets every qualitative and quantitative specifications available in the ewe (Global cycle duration: 16.5d; Surge phase duration: 1d; Luteal phase duration: 13d; Follicular phase duration: 2.5d; Pulse-to-surge amplitude ratio: 60; Pulse frequency increase ratio: 3.5). The bottom panel displays the corresponding series of InterPulse Interval (IPI) which illustrates the time-varying period of GnRH pulses. The top panel is a temporal guideline to draw a parallel between the changes in the estradiol and progesterone plasma levels, which are easily accessible experimentally (by jugular blood sampling), on the one hand, and the GnRH portal blood levels predicted by the model, on the other hand.

cycle duration, (ii) the pulse amplitude to the surge amplitude, and (iii) the pulse frequency in the mid-luteal phase to the pulse frequency in the end-follicular phase.

Building the specification list

We had to assemble the sparse information retrieved from GnRH portal blood time series with a high sampling rate (up to one measurement every minute) to derive quantitative specifications for the GnRH secretion pattern in the ewe. As there is good agreement between GnRH levels in cerebrospinal fluid compared to pituitary portal blood at the time of the GnRH surge (Skinner *et al.*, 1997), we also used cerebrospinal GnRH time series to adapt the specification list to another species, the rhesus monkey (Xia *et al.*, 1992). The algorithm procedure designed to tune the model parameters and based on pure dynamical considerations (Fenichel, 1979) has been described elsewhere (Clément and Vidal, 2009). We just discuss here the role of the parameters impacting most significantly the GnRH secretion pattern and underlying the differences observed between the ewe and the rhesus monkey.

Constraining the model parameters to meet the specifications

The ratio of the surge to whole cycle duration is ruled by the (b_1, b_2) pair; for any value of b_1, there exists a suitable value of b_2 fulfilling a given duration ratio. Moreover, parameter b_1 has an effect on the follicular phase duration in itself. When b_1 decreases, the dynamics is slowed down along the part of the regulating system limit cycle that corresponds to the follicular phase. For instance, with $b_1 = 0.246$, we get the 2.5-day follicular phase of the ewe, while with $b_1 = 0.187$, we get the 13-day follicular phase of the rhesus monkey.

The specification chosen for the surge amplitude corresponds to the physiological situation of a natural ovarian cycle, where the luteal phase precedes the follicular phase and subsequent surge. Changes in the surge amplitude without affecting its duration can be obtained through alteration in the a_0 parameter of the GnRH secreting system. The smaller the a_0, the steeper the ascendant slope of the surge. For instance, the surge amplitude is drastically different with $a_0 = 0.52$ (case of the ewe) than with $a_0 = 0.7$ (case of the rhesus monkey). The surges also differ in shape according to the species; the surge in the rhesus monkey is plateau shaped, while the ewe surge is spike shaped.

Embedding the progesterone priming effect on surge amplitude

As explained earlier, the effect of the time-varying amounts of steroids originating from the ovaries is directly embedded in the regulating system output. The choice of the nominal parameter values centers the field of the possible model behaviors on the physiological case. The model embeds not only the surge-inducing effect of estradiol, but also the enhancing effect on surge amplitude of progesterone priming during the preceding luteal phase (Caraty and Skinner, 1999). Progesterone priming can be explained by two concurrent explanations: the increase in the GnRH peptide store in GnRH neurons, due to the decreased release during the low-frequency luteal phase, and the progesterone-induced increased sensitivity to estrogen feedback in regulatory neurons. In the model, the effects of progesterone exposure on both the pulse frequency during the luteal phase and the amplitude of the following surge are linked via the symmetry between the extremum coupling term values. During the luteal phase (X near X_{min}), the progesterone priming is translated into a low pulse frequency via the cX_{min} term, while at the end of the follicular phase (X near X_{max}), the surge amplitude depends on the strength of the coupling term cX_{max} (with $X_{min} \simeq -X_{max}$).

9.4 Reproducing known effects of ovarian steroids on the surge

9.4.1 Luteal deficiency

We can first ask what would happen if progesterone is missing during the expected time for the luteal phase. Such luteal deficiency-like situation is observed, for example, during the first cycle at the onset of the breeding season in the ewe. The lack of progesterone exposure is expected to be accompanied by a greater than normal pulse frequency during the luteal phase and by a decreased sensitivity of the regulatory neurons toward the surge-triggering effect of estrogen. Accordingly, we reproduce the long-term effect of a lack of progesterone exposure during the luteal phase by simultaneously altering parameter c and the parameters of the regulating system. As a result, there is a significant decrease in the surge amplitude, as well as a higher pulse frequency in the period corresponding to the luteal phase (Figure 9.8).

9.4.2 Progesterone-induced surge blockade

Experimental progesterone blockade

A series of experimental studies have investigated experimental blockade of the estradiol-induced GnRH surge by progesterone (Evans *et al.*, 2002; Harris *et al.*, 1999; Kasa-Vubu *et al.*, 1992; Richter *et al.*, 2001a,b). It was first shown that progesterone acts centrally, on the hypothalamic level. Maintaining a mid-luteal progesterone environment (instead of removing progesterone implants) in face of a surge-triggering estradiol environment results in a complete block of the GnRH surge. When progesterone is not administered throughout, its effect depends on the time and pattern of exposure, relative to the different phases of the estradiol surge-inducing period. The ability of progesterone to block the surge is limited to the activation phase and to the earlier part of the transmission phase. Furthermore, even within these delimited periods, escape from the blocking effect of progesterone has been observed in some ewes. Since differences in the

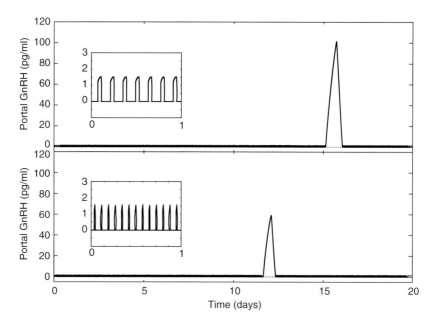

Figure 9.8   Limited surge amplitude in the case of luteal deficiency. The top
panel displays the physiological GnRH release in the ewe, obtained with the nominal
parameter values. The bottom panel illustrates the effect of a lack of progesterone
during the luteal phase. Compared to the top panel, the bottom panel displays both a
higher pulse frequency (highlighted by the inserts) during the luteal phase and a lower
surge (less than 0.6 times the surge amplitude in the physiological case).

progesterone levels induced by the experimental protocol have been carefully ruled out by the authors, this escape can be attributed to individual
differences in the sensitivity to progesterone.

Numerical progesterone blockade

The different effects of administering progesterone during the follicular
phase can be mimicked by starting to decrease the value of b_1 at a given
time t_{b_1} from the beginning of the follicular phase (that we take as initial
time), so that it reaches a lower value, b_1^{min}, with a given delay Δ_{b_1}. Δ_{b_1} is
inversely proportional to the slope of decrease in b_1. The progressive decay
in b_1 value is consistent with the delay needed by the regulatory neurons
to process and relay the progesterone signal.

First, it is worth noting that the surge cannot be blocked if b_1^{min}, which is
related to the dose of progesterone administered, is lower than a threshold
value b_1^h. If $b_1^{min} > b_1^h$, the effect depends on the time of progesterone
administration (t_{b_1}) with respect to the transmission phase. When this
time is close to the beginning of the transmission phase, the surge onset is
blocked, as expected (Figure 9.9b). If we now start to decrease the value

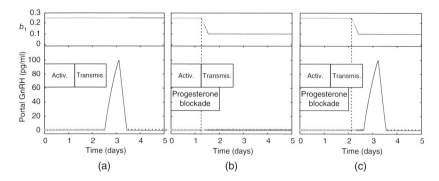

Figure 9.9 Progesterone-induced surge blockade. (a) displays the GnRH secretion pattern in the ewe from the beginning of the follicular phase in the physiological case, that is, when b_1 is kept constant equal to its nominal value (0.246). (b) and (c) The administration of progesterone is reproduced by a linear decrease in b_1 from 0.246 to 0.1. (b) Progesterone is administered early in the follicular phase which results in the surge blockade. (c) The late administration of progesterone fails to block the surge that is just delayed by a few hours compared to A.

of b_1 later in the transmission phase, progesterone fails to block the surge, which nevertheless occurs later than in the control situation (without any progesterone treatment), after a delay corresponding to the duration of progesterone administration (Figure 9.9c). A similar tendency of delayed surge onset has been observed experimentally after progesterone treatments that were insufficient to block the surge.

To delineate precisely the time window during which progesterone surge blockade can occur, we can investigate further the effect of the administration time. When considering a constant Δ_{b_1}, the limit time for surge blockade lies in a narrow range of less than 1 hr. However, small changes in Δ_{b_1} at around the limit time have a great impact, with a drastic surge-restoring effect of lengthening Δ_{b_1}. Δ_{b_1} appears to be an appropriate parameter to represent the individual differences in sensitivity to progesterone, that are thought to explain, at least in part, the different responses of different animals to the same experimental treatment.

Although similar studies of the effects of progesterone on the surge have not been performed in the rhesus monkey, we can speculate about differences predicted to arise from the specification lists corresponding to either the ewe or the monkey. The greatest difference is in the duration of the follicular phase, which is much longer in the rhesus monkey than in the ewe. This corresponds to a lower value of b_1, which is much closer to the dose threshold b_1^h than in the case of the ewe. However, the limit time when progesterone fails to block the surge occurs sooner (i.e., the delay between the limit time and surge onset is greater).

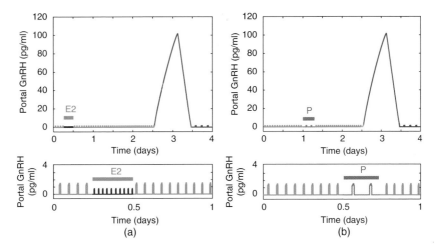

Figure 9.10 Steroid bolus challenges. (a) and (b) illustrate the impact of estradiol and progesterone administered as a bolus during the early and mid follicular phase, respectively. In each case, the top panel displays a global view of the follicular phase and surge, while the bottom panel provides a magnified view of the period corresponding to the bolus to highlight its effects on GnRH pulse frequency and/or amplitude.

9.5   Steroid challenges in the pulsatile regime

We will now examine how estradiol and progesterone control GnRH pulse patterns during the ovarian cycle. In the numerical simulations, the acute effects of either estradiol or progesterone administered as a bolus during the follicular phase are mimicked by changes in the parameters controlling the pulse frequency and amplitude during a time interval I_{bol} of relatively short duration, Δt_{bol} (typically less than half a day), and starting at time t_{bol} from the beginning of the follicular phase: $I_{bol} = [t_{bol}, t_{bol} + \Delta t_{bol}]$.

9.5.1   Estradiol bolus challenge

In the absence of progesterone, estradiol has a double action on GnRH, as it both decreases GnRH pulse amplitude with a concomitant shape modification and increases GnRH pulse frequency (Evans *et al.*, 1994, 1995). The net effect is a slight suppression of the cumulated secretion of GnRH, as the faster frequency does not exactly compensate for the lower amplitude.

In silico administration of end-follicular estradiol levels during the early follicular phase results in the pulse frequency being faster and the amplitude lower during the bolus than outside (Figure 9.10a). Despite the apparent balance between frequency increase and amplitude decrease, the cumulated GnRH amount secreted during the bolus is less than that secreted in the same amount of time before or after the bolus window.

This is due to a shortening of the pulse duration, which is dynamically related to the frequency increase. After bolus termination, the cycle resumes its endogenous dynamics and the surge onset occurs at the expected time.

9.5.2 Progesterone bolus challenge

Progesterone inhibits GnRH pulse frequency and the central inhibitory effects of progesterone on pulsatile GnRH secretion are temporally acute (Goodman *et al.*, 2002; Skinner *et al.*, 1998). Depending on the experimental conditions, the effects of progesterone on pulse amplitude can be stimulatory, inhibitory, or nonexistent. Because the effects of progesterone on amplitude are not consistent between experiments, we have chosen to account only for a frequency effect in our simulations.

In silico administration of luteal phase progesterone levels during the mid-follicular phase, results in the pulse frequency being slower during the bolus than outside. The pulse amplitude is unchanged. After bolus termination, the cycle resumes its endogenous dynamics, but the surge onset is slightly delayed (Figure 9.10b).

9.6 Conclusion

Our modeling goal was to account in a concise way for the qualitative and quantitative dynamical features of GnRH secretion and to manage to embed the changing steroid environment in the control of GnRH dynamics during an ovarian cycle. The model describes the macroscopic secretion activity on the GnRH neuronal network level (rather than on the individual neuron level). Our working hypothesis, based on biological knowledge, is that GnRH secretory rhythms arise from the interaction of the proper dynamics of GnRH neurons with that of regulatory neurons integrating the gonadal steroid feedback. The model can be considered as the most parsimonious explanation for the GnRH (qualitative and quantitative) secretory patterns consistent with data from a variety of experimental conditions.

Further exploration of the model has revealed other possible secretion regimes. In particular, during the transition from a surge back to a pulsatile phase, a *pause* consisting of small oscillations superimposed on a long-duration pulse may occur (Krupa *et al.*, 2012) for some parameter values. As most experimental protocols have focused on the transition corresponding to the GnRH surge triggering rather than the reverse transition corresponding to the resumption of the pulsatile regime, the biological mechanisms underlying the transition from the surge mode back to the pulsatile mode are still poorly understood, and the possible existence of a *pause* in the model is quite an intriguing observation.

References

Abraham IM, Han SK, Todman MG, Korach KS and Herbison AE (2003). Estrogen receptor β mediates rapid estrogen actions on gonadotropin-releasing hormone neurons in vivo. *J. Neurosci.* **17**, 5771–5777.

Caraty A and Skinner DC (1999). Progesterone priming is essential for the full expression of the positive feedback effect of estradiol in inducing the preovulatory gonadotropin-releasing hormone surge in the ewe. *Endocrinology* **140**, 165–170.

Christian CA and Moenter SM (2010). The neurobiology of preovulatory and estradiol-induced gonadotropin-releasing hormone surges. *Endocr Rev.* **31**, 544–577.

Clément F and Françoise JP (2007). Mathematical modeling of the GnRH-pulse and surge generator. *SIAM J Appl Dyn Syst.* **6**, 441–456.

Clément F and Vidal A (2009). Foliation-based parameter tuning in a model of the GnRH pulse and surge generator. *SIAM J Appl Dyn Syst.* **8**, 1591–1631.

Evans NP, Dahl GE, Glover BH and Karsch FJ (1994). Central regulation of pulsatile gonadotropin-releasing hormone (GnRH) secretion by estradiol during the period leading up to the preovulatory GnRH surge in the ewe. *Endocrinology* **134**, 1806–1811.

Evans NP, Dahl GE, Mauger DT and Karsch FJ (1995). Estradiol induces both qualitative and quantitative changes in the pattern of gonadotropin-releasing hormone secretion during the presurge period in the ewe. *Endocrinology* **136**, 1603–1609.

Evans NP, Dahl GE, Padmanabhan V, Thrun LA and Karsch FJ (1997). Estradiol requirements for induction and maintenance of the gonadotropin-releasing hormone surge: implications for neuroendocrine processing of the estradiol signal. *Endocrinology* **138**, 5408–5414.

Evans NP, Richter TA, Skinner DC and Robinson JE (2002). Neuroendocrine mechanisms underlying the effects of progesterone on the oestradiol-induced GnRH/LH surge. *Reprod Suppl.* **59**, 57–66.

Fenichel N (1979). Geometric singular perturbation theory for ordinary differential equations. *J. Differential Equations.* **31**, 53–98.

Fitzhugh R (1961). Impulses and physiological states in theoretical models of nerve membrane. *Biophys J.* **1**, 445–466.

Goodman RL, Gibson M, Skinner DC and Lehman MN (2002). Neuroendocrine control of pulsatile GnRH/LH secretion during the ovarian cycle: evidence from the ewe. *Reprod Suppl.* **59**, 41–56.

Harris TG, Dye S, Robinson JE, Skinner DC and Evans NP (1999). Progesterone can block transmission of the estradiol-induced signal for luteinizing hormone surge generation during a specific period of time immediatly after activation of the gonadotropin-releasing hormone surge-generating system. *Endocrinology* **140**, 827–834.

Herbison AE (1998). Multimodal influence of estrogen upon gonadotropin-releasing hormone neurons. *Endocr Rev.* **19**, 302–330.

Hodgkin AL and Huxley AF (1952). A quantitative description of membrane current and its application to conduction and excitation in nerve. *J Physiol.* **117**, 500–544.

Hrabovszky E, Steinhauser A, Barabas K, Shughrue P, Petersen S, Merchenthaler I and Liposits Z (2001). Estrogen receptor-β immunoreactivity in luteinizing hormone-releasing hormone neurons of the rat brain. *Endocrinology* **142**, 3261–3264.

Kasa-Vubu JZ, Dahl GE, Evans NP, Thrun LA, Moenter SM, Padmanabhan V and Karsch FJ (1992). Progesterone blocks the estradiol-induced gonadotropin discharge in the ewe by inhibiting the surge of gonadotropin-releasing hormone. *Endocrinology* **131**, 208–212.

Krupa M, Vidal A, Desroches M and Clément F (2012). Mixed-mode oscillations in a multiple time scale phantom bursting system. *SIAM J Appl Dyn Syst.* **11**, 1458–1498.

Moenter SM, Brand RC and Karsch FJ (1992). Dynamics of gonadotropin-releasing hormone (GnRH) secretion during the GnRH surge: insights into the mechanism of GnRH surge induction. *Endocrinology* **130**, 2978–2984.

Moenter SM, Caraty A and Karsch FJ (1990). The estradiol-induced surge of gonadotropin-releasing hormone in the ewe. *Endocrinology* **127**, 1375–1384.

Moenter SM, Caraty A, Locatelli A and Karsch FJ (1991). Pattern of gonadotropin-releasing hormone (GnRH) secretion leading up to ovulation in the ewe: existence of a preovulatory GnRH surge. *Endocrinology* **129**, 1175–1182.

Nagumo J, Animoto S and Yoshizawa S (1962). An active pulse transmission line simulating nerve axon. *Proc Inst Radio Engineers* **50**, 2061–2070.

Pinilla L, Aguilar E, Dieguez C, Millar RP and Tena-Sempere M (2012). Kisspeptins and reproduction: physiological roles and regulatory mechanisms. *Physiol Rev.* **92**, 1235–1316.

Richter TA, Robinson JE and Evans NP (2001a). Progesterone treatment that either blocks or augments the estradiol-induced gonadotropin-releasing hormone surge is associated with different patterns of hypothalamic neural activation. *Neuroendocrinology* **73**, 378–386.

Richter TA, Spackman DS, Robinson JE, Dye S, Harris TG, Skinner DC and Evans NP (2001b). Role of endogenous opioid peptides in mediating progesterone-induced disruption of the activation and transmission stages of the GnRH surge induction process. *Endocrinology* **142**, 5212–5219.

Rønnekleiv OK and Kelly MJ (2005). Diversity of ovarian steroid signaling in the hypothalamus. *Front Neuroendocrinol.* **26**, 65–84.

Skinner DC, Caraty A, Malpaux B and Evans NP (1997). Simultaneous measurement of gonadotropin-releasing hormone in the third ventricular cerebrospinal fluid and hypophyseal portal blood of the ewe. *Endocrinology* **138**, 4699–4704.

Skinner D and Dufourny L (2005). Oestrogen receptor beta-immunoreactive neurones in the ovine hypothalamus: distribution and colocalisation with gonadotropin-releasing hormone. *J Neuroendocrinol.* **17**, 29–39.

Skinner DC, Evans NP, Delaleu B, Goodman RL, Bouchard P and Caraty A (1998). The negative feedback actions of progesterone on gonadotropin releasing hormone secretion are transduced by the classical progesterone receptor. *Proc Natl Acad Sci USA* **95**, 10978–10983.

Vidal A and Clément F (2010). A dynamical model for the control of the GnRH neurosecretory system. *J Neuroendocrinol.* **22**, 1251–1266.

Xia L, VanVugt D, Alston EJ, Luckhaus J and Ferin M (1992). A surge of gonadotropin-releasing hormone accompanies the estradiol-induced gonadotropin surge in the rhesus monkey. *Endocrinology* **131**, 2812–2820.

Glossary

Activator–inhibitor system A dynamical system with positive feedback from an activator variable and negative feedback from an inhibitory variable. Generally, the inhibitor acts much more slowly than the activator, allowing large excursions from rest and in many cases oscillations. In the mathematical literature, this is sometimes called a fast–slow system to abstract from biochemical connotations.

Activation variable This takes on values from 0 to 1 and typically increases with increasing voltage.

Adenohypophysis The portion of the pituitary gland that contains hormone-secreting melanotrophs, somatotrophs, corticotrophs, lactotrophs, thyrotrophs, and gonadotrophs.

Arcuate nucleus An aggregation of neurons in the mediobasal hypothalamus immediately adjacent to the median eminence. The arcuate nucleus contains many different cell types, including GHRH neurons, neuroendocrine dopamine neurons that regulate *prolactin* secretion, *kisspeptin* neurons, neurons, which make *beta-endorphin* and alpha MSH, and neurons involved in the regulation of energy balance.

Afterhyperpolarizing potential (AHP) A small magnitude, long-time course hyperpolarization that results from the opening of Ca^{2+}-dependent K^+ channels, and so follows Ca^{2+}-channel-dependent action potentials. Because of its slow time course, it accumulates in a manner that reflects the clustering of spikes.

Antidromic stimulation When electrical stimuli are applied to an axon, action potentials are triggered that propagate both orthodromically (toward the axonal nerve endings) and antidromically (toward the soma and dendrites). Used in tandem with recording from the cell body, this is useful for identifying recorded cells, and for injecting exogenous action potentials to perturb ongoing activity.

Assortativity A similarity metric that describes the preference of nodes to connect to nodes with similar properties (e.g., degree).

Attractor A stable state (either an *equilibrium* or a *limit cycle*) toward which trajectories are attracted.

Basin of attraction The range of phase space in which trajectories are drawn to a particular *attractor*.

Computational Neuroendocrinology, First Edition. Edited by Duncan J. MacGregor and Gareth Leng.
© 2016 John Wiley & Sons, Ltd. Published 2016 by John Wiley & Sons, Ltd.
Companion Website: www.wiley.com/go/Leng/Computational

Bifurcation   A qualitative change in the behavior of a dynamical system caused when a parameter crosses a critical value. This generally changes the system from *stable* to *unstable*, or vice versa, and can act as a threshold for oscillations.

Bifurcation point   The point at which some input parameter changes the qualitative behavior of a system by changing the state of the equilibria. A *bifurcation diagram* plots the state of the equilibria (measured by a dimension from the phase plane, e.g., V) against the changing parameter (the bifurcation parameter).

Bipartite graph   One whose vertices can be divided into two disjoint sets such that every edge connects a vertex in one of the sets to a vertex in the other.

Bistability   A dynamical system is bistable when it has two stable equilibrium states. If the system is perturbed, it can, thus, abruptly "flip" from one state to the other, for example, in the case of the *vasopressin neuron*, from electrical silence to repetitive spiking. A bistable oscillator is a dynamic system that spontaneously switches repeatedly between two stable states.

Boltzmann function   A standard function for producing or fitting a sigmoid curve given by the following equation:

$$y = \frac{1}{1 + e^{(x-a)/b}}$$

where y is normalized to values between 0 and 1, a is the half-maximal, inflection value, and b gives the slope. Commonly used to fit channel activation variables in the Hodgkin–Huxley-type models to voltage clamp data.

Bursting   Oscillations composed of an active phase of spiking alternating with a silent phase without spiking. A ubiquitous type of fast–slow system.

Calcium (Ca^{2+})   A universal intracellular messenger involved in mediating electrical activity, *exocytosis*, transcription, apoptosis, and cell–cell communication.

Circadian rhythm   A biological oscillation with an intrinsic period of approximately 24 h (e.g., the daily cycle in *glucocorticoid* levels).

Channel open (closed) state   Ion channels are formed by proteins in the plasma membrane of a cell that, depending on the conformation of the protein, may form a pore that allows the passage of ions of a given size and polarity (open state), or may be impermeable to ions (closed state).

Chay-Keizer model   An early model for bursting in pancreatic β cells in which burst termination is driven by a rise in cytosolic Ca^{2+} acting on a Ca^{2+}-activated K^+ channel. It plays an important role in triggering the development of the mathematical analysis of bursting.

Corticotropin releasing hormone (CRH)   Also called the corticotropin releasing factor (CRF). See *corticotropes*.

Corticotropes (or corticotrophs)   These endocrine cells make up 10–15% of anterior pituitary cells and secrete *adrenocorticotropic hormone* (ACTH). ACTH acts on the *adrenal glands* to promote the production of glucocorticoids (cortisol in humans and corticosterone in rodents).

Depolarising afterpotential (DAP)   In many neuronal types, spikes are followed by a sequence of hyperpolarization and depolarization that reflects the opening of voltage-gated channels that allow the entry and egress of various ions. Typically, spikes are followed by an HAP that hyperpolarizes the cell by opening K^+ channels, but often this HAP is followed by a DAP making the cell transiently hyperexcitable. A DAP can arise through several different mechanisms, and its size and time course may be very different between cell types.

Dirac delta $\delta(x)$ Mathematical function used to model a tall narrow "spike" function; its value is zero everywhere except at $x = 0$ where its value is infinitely large so that its total integral is 1. It can be viewed as the derivative of the *Heaviside step function*.

Dynamic clamp (DClamp) technique   A method for injecting a current computed from a mathematical model directly into a cell through a patch electrode. The calculation of the model current is based on the cell's membrane potential.

Dynamical system   A dynamical system comprises a set of variables that collectively describe the system, and a set of rules (such as differential equations) that collectively determine how the state of the system (the values of all the variables at a given time) evolves over time. A *stable state* is one in which the values of the variables do not change (or change only very slowly) unless there is a large perturbation to the system (a large forced change in one of the variables). An *attractor* of a dynamical system is a stable state or a set of states, such as a closed loop (*limit cycle*), toward which a system tends to evolve for a wide range of starting conditions.

Dynorphin   An endogenous *opioid peptide* that acts on kappa opioid receptors. Dynorphin is made in many different cell types, including oxytocin neurons, vasopressin neurons, and kisspeptin neurons. Its actions are uniformly inhibitory.

Endocannabinoids   "Endogenous cannabinoids." Molecules that act at specific cannabinoid receptors (in this case CB1 receptors). CB1 receptors are widely expressed in the brain, mainly on nerve endings. Cannabinoids are produced in some neuronal populations in response to raised intracellular Ca^{2+}, and act on afferent nerve endings that express these CB1 receptors to inhibit transmitter release; cannabinoids are, thus, *retrograde transmitters*.

Endoplasmic reticulum (ER)   An internal compartment in the cell in which proteins undergo a number of forms of post-translational processing, including folding and attachment of localization signals, such as secreted proteins that are targeted to the exocytotic vesicles. For us, however, it is mainly a Ca^{2+} store that maintains a concentration much higher than the cytosol and comparable to the external environment.

Equilibrium   A point on the *phase plane* where both dimensions have a zero derivative, that is, where the nullclines intersect. If trajectories on either side tend to approach (are attracted to) this equilibrium, then it will be stable (an *attractor*), for example, resting potential; otherwise, it will be unstable.

Estradiol   A potent estrogen, estradiol is a steroid hormone produced by the ovaries and placenta in mammals. Estrogen acts at the uterus to prepare it for the implantation of the fertilized ovum and promotes the maturation of and maintenance of the female accessory reproductive organs and secondary sexual characteristics. It acts via nuclear estrogen receptors to influence gene expression in target cells, and estrogen receptors are expressed in many populations of neurons in the hypothalamus (and indeed at many other brain sites), and in cells of the *adenohypophysis*.

Estrogen   Female sex *steroid hormones*, in women comprising estrone, *estradiol* and estriol.

Exocytosis Usually Ca^{2+} triggered secretion from a cell membrane, which involves the docking of vesicles with the membrane, which then open up and release their contents into the extracellular space; used to secrete both neurotransmitters and peptides.

FitzHugh–Nagumo system This system was introduced by FitzHugh as a two-dimensional reduction of the Hodgkin–Huxley model of spike generation in squid giant axons.

Functional magnetic resonance imaging (fMRI) Measurement of brain activity relying on the changes in blood contrast which occur in response to energy consumption.

Folliculostellate cell A nonendocrine cell believed to be involved in long-distance intrapituitary communication through electrical propagation of signals.

Follicle stimulating hormone (FSH) See gonadotropes.

Fura-2 A ratiometric calcium indicator excited at 340 and 380 nm, which emits at 510 nm. The ratio between the respective emissions correlates with free cytosolic Ca^{2+}. For two-photon imaging, fura-2 is used in nonratiometric mode with recordings made past the isosbestic point (i.e., emission intensity decreases with increased $[Ca^{2+}]$).

Glial cell More abundant in the brain than neurons, glial cells are nonexcitable cells that play diverse supporting functions in the nervous system: they include many different cell types with diverse specialized roles.

GABA (gamma-aminobutyric acid) The most common inhibitory neurotransmitter in the mammalian brain, GABA is released from small synaptic vesicles at nerve endings, binds to $GABA_A$ receptors at the post-synaptic membrane to open membrane Cl^- channels. Generally, this results in a hyperpolarization, because in most neurons, the intracellular Cl^- concentration is so low that opening Cl^- channels means that Cl^- will enter the cell when these channels are open. However, this depends on cell type and developmental state, reflecting the level of expression of Cl^- transporters. GABA also acts on $GABA_B$ metabotropic receptors that promote the opening of K^+ channels.

Glucocorticoid hormones (principally *cortisol* in humans, *corticosterone* in rodents) Glucocorticoids are the end product of the HPA axis, released from the adrenal gland in response to ACTH. ACTH is released from the pituitary in response to acute stress as a result of the stimulation of corticotropes by *CRH*, a peptide hormone synthesized by a population of neuroendocrine neurons in the *paraventricular nucleus* of the hypothalamus and released from nerve endings at the *median eminence*.

Gonadotropes (or gonadotrophs) Endocrine cells of the adenohypophysis, which secrete *luteinising hormone* (LH) and *follicle stimulating hormone* (FSH), which play important roles in the reproductive cycle. In females, a midcycle surge in LH secretion is an essential trigger for ovulation, while at other times of the ovarian cycle, pulsatile secretion of LH maintains secretion of the ovarian steroids. In males, it controls the secretion of testosterone from the testes, and is essential for spermatogenesis. FSH stimulates the maturation of ovarian follicles. In males, FSH is important for sperm production. FSH and LH are both synthesized by and secreted from gonadotrophs, but the synthesis and secretion of the two hormones are independently regulated.

Gonadotropins follicle-stimulating hormone (FSH) and luteinizing hormone (LH) These are glycoprotein hormones secreted by the pituitary gland, which support the double gametogenic and endocrine function of the gonads. They signal on somatic gonadal cells through G-protein-coupled receptors and are involved in the control of the terminal development of ovarian follicles, ovulation triggering, and stimulation of the corpus luteum.

Gonadotropin releasing hormone (GnRH; also known as LHRH, LH-releasing hormone)   This peptide is synthesized by a small population of neurons in the anterior hypothalamus which project their axons to the median eminence. There, GnRH is secreted in an activity-dependent manner into the portal blood vessels that transport it to the adenohypophysis, where it acts on *gonadotropes* to stimulate the secretion of *LH* and *FSH*.

Granger causality   A regression-based correlation analysis that can forecast causality without *a priori* knowledge of the causal mechanisms.

Graph theory   The modeling of relations or connections between two objects which together form the graph.

Hyperpolarising after potential (HAP)   After an action potential, neurons typically display a large, brief hyperpolarization that results from the activation of voltage and Ca^{2+}-dependent K^+ channels. The magnitude and time course of the HAP vary between cell types. The effect of the HAP is to introduce a relative refractory period after a spike, limiting the frequency at which the cell can fire.

Heaviside step function *H*   It has a value of zero for a negative argument and one for a positive argument. It is used to represent a signal that switches on at a specified time and stays on indefinitely.

Heterotrimeric G proteins   Signaling molecules composed of α, β, and γ subunits. They are activated when a ligand binds to a G-protein-coupled receptor in the plasma membrane, which replaces the GDP molecule bound to the α subunit with GTP, and liberates the $\beta\gamma$ heterodimer. Both α-GTP and $\beta\gamma$ act on downstream targets. When the GTP is hydrolyzed to GDP, the α-GDP molecule binds to a free $\beta\gamma$ heterodimer, deactivating both.

Hill function   A sigmoidal function of the form

$$\frac{x^n}{K_d^n + x^n}$$

where x is usually the concentration of some ligand of a receptor or an enzyme, K_d is the half-maximal concentration, and n, which determines the steepness of the curve, is called the Hill coefficient.

Homeostasis   A term that refers to "physiological stability" within the body, and stress is any response to internal or external environmental challenges (i.e., stressors) that disturbs the homeostatic state of the body. In mammals, hallmarks of the stress response include the activation of the autonomic nervous system (resulting in the release of catecholamines such as adrenaline) and the hypothalamic–pituitary–adrenal (HPA) axis (resulting in the release of glucocorticoid hormones).

Hopf bifurcation   A *bifurcation* where a new *limit cycle* appears due to change in the stability of an equilibrium.

Hypophyseal portal system   A network of blood vessels that connects the anterior pituitary to the hypothalamus at the median eminence, at the base of the brain.

Inactivation variable   It takes on values from 0 to 1 and typically decreases with increasing voltage.

Index of dispersion   A convenient, normalized measure of the variability of firing rate. For a given bin width, it is defined as the standard deviation of the number of spikes per bin divided by the mean number of spikes. For spikes generated by a random process, the index has the value 1; the index is lower when spikes occur more regularly and can be higher than 1 when there is a bursting structure to the spike times.

Interspike interval The interval between successive action potentials in a neuron. For any given neuron, the statistical distribution of interspike intervals is determined by its intrinsic membrane properties and the nature of the network within which it is embedded, and hence input activity it receives. Different neuronal cell types often display characteristic interspike interval distributions by which they can be identified.

IP3, IP3 Receptor Inositol tris-phosphate and its receptor, a ligand-gated Ca^{2+} channel on the ER membrane. It releases Ca^{2+} from the ER when IP3 is elevated due to the action of one or more G-protein-coupled receptors acting through the G-protein G_q.

Kisspeptins GnRH neurons are controlled by a variety of afferent inputs. Besides classical neurotransmitters, other players participate in the complex neural network connected to GnRH neurons. Amongst them, kisspeptins are a family of structurally related peptides, encoded by the KISS1 gene, which act through the G-protein-coupled receptor GPR54. Their role in reproduction has first been discovered from genetic studies in patients suffering from familial or sporadic infertility of hypothalamic origin, and since then, kisspeptins have been shown to be involved in many reproductive processes (puberty onset, surge triggering, metabolic and seasonal control of reproduction, etc.)

Lactotropes (or lactotrophs) Endocrine cells that constitute 10–25% of anterior pituitary cells and secrete the peptide hormone *prolactin*. Prolactin has diverse actions at peripheral sites, but its major physiological role in all mammals is to sustain lactogenesis (milk production by the mammary gland).

Law of mass action It describes in terms of differential equations how two quantities change over time when their interaction is based on a reaction scheme. In chemistry, it states that the rate of a chemical reaction is directly proportional to the molecular concentrations of the reacting species. This concept extends to ion channel kinetics by thinking of the activation or inactivation variable as the concentration of a reacting species, and the reaction is gate opening or closing.

Leak current A simplified current used in a Hodgkin–Huxley-type (ionic current based) model to represent the combined effect of currents not explicitly included in the model.

Limit cycle When a system changes (e.g., by applying an input current) so that a stable equilibrium becomes unstable, a *limit cycle* can be generated, where the trajectory is propelled away from the now unstable equilibrium before returning toward it (after crossing a *nullcline*), overshooting, to be repelled again before another return, effectively orbiting the unstable equilibrium. Tonic spiking is an example of a limit cycle. If the gradients of the limit cycle are sufficient to maintain the momentum of the orbiting trajectory, then it will be stable; otherwise, it will be unstable, and the orbit will decay toward the equilibrium.

Li–Rinzel model A simplified model for Ca^{2+} for ER-driven oscillations in which the positive feedback comes from the activation of IP3R by cytosolic Ca^{2+} and negative feedback by the slow inactivation of IP3R by cytosolic Ca^{2+}.

Luteinising hormone (LH) See gonadotropes.

Median eminence A specialized site at the base of the hypothalamus containing the neurosecretory nerve endings of many neuroendocrine neurons and a network of convoluted small blood vessels, which have "fenestrations" that allow molecules to pass freely between the extracellular fluid and the blood. These vessels (the hypothalamo-hypophyseal portal vessels) transport hypothalamic hormones to the anterior pituitary gland.

Melanotropes (or melanotrophs) Endocrine cells that make up 95% of the cells in the intermediate lobe of the pituitary gland and secrete melanocyte-stimulating hormone (MSH).

Monte Carlo simulation A stochastic model that generates a probability distribution by iteratively sampling the input data or repeatedly substituting values with pseudorandom variables (i.e., measures the predictability of a system).

Nernst potential The value of the membrane potential at which the concentration gradient of an ion across the membrane is balanced with the electric gradient for that type of ion.

Neuroendocrine cells They are required to rapidly release proteins (e.g., peptide hormones, such as CRH, AVP, and ACTH) via exocytosis in response to specific signals. They are able to achieve this by packaging pre-synthesized hormones into readily releasable secretory vesicles. In response to a specific signal, the hormone-containing secretory vesicles fuse with the cell membrane and release their contents into the extracellular space.

Neurosecretory vesicles These are (relatively) large-membrane-bound vesicles tightly packed with oxytocin (and other fragments of the precursor protein from which oxytocin is cleaved). Each contains about 85,000 molecules of oxytocin. The tight packing of the peptides means that under the electron microscope, these vesicles have an electron-dense core, and so these are often referred to as "large dense-cored vesicles" to distinguish them from the small clear synaptic vesicles in which conventional neurotransmitters, such as glutamate and GABA, are packaged.

Nullcline Each axis (variable) of a phase plane has an associated *nullcline*, a line which connects all the points where trajectories change the direction on that axis, that is, points where the derivative of that variable equals zero.

Nyquist sampling theorem States that a periodic analog waveform can be reconstructed if the sampling rate is twice the highest frequency.

Opioid peptide Endogenous peptides that act in an "opiate-like" manner. There are three major classes of opioid peptides dynorphins, which act at kappa opioid receptors, enkephalins, which act at μ and δ opioid receptors, and endorphins (particularly β-endorphin), which act at μ receptors. At a cellular level, all opioids have inhibitory effects. Naloxone is a competitive antagonist at all opioid receptor types, though it has the highest affinity for μ receptors.

Osmotic pressure The pressure that needs to be applied to a solution to prevent the inward flow of water across a semipermeable membrane. In a biological context, the osmotic pressure of a biological fluid reflects the concentration of salts and other small molecules that do not freely cross biological membranes. The osmotic pressure of plasma or extracellular fluid thus is predominantly determined by the concentration of dissolved NaCl.

Oxytocin Peptide hormone, synthesized by neuroendocrine neurons of the *supraoptic nucleus* and *paraventricular nucleus,* and secreted into the systemic circulation from neuroendocrine nerve endings in the posterior pituitary gland. By its actions at the mammary gland, oxytocin is essential for milk let-down in response to suckling and by its actions on the uterus, it is important in regulating the progress of parturition.

Ovarian cycle   It is an almost-periodic process characterized by coordinated changes in the secretion of reproductive hormones on each level of the hypothalamo–pituitary–gonadal axis. It is composed of the *follicular phase*, during which a cohort of ovarian follicles undergo their final developmental stage up to ovulation, when they released an oocyte, followed by a *luteal phase*, during which the corpus luteum (the remnant of an ovulatory follicle) supports the preparation of the endometrium for a possible nidation. If no fecundation has occurred, the corpus luteum regresses at the time of luteolysis and a new follicular phase resumes.

Paraventricular nucleus (PVN)   An aggregation of neurons in the dorsal hypothalamus adjacent to the third ventricle. The PVN contains many different cell types, including magnocellular *oxytocin* and *vasopressin* neurons like those present in the *supraoptic nucleus,* but also parvocellular oxytocin and vasopressin neurons that project to central sites and neuroendocrine CRF neurons and TRH neurons.

Phase plane   A two-dimensional plot where each of the axes represents a dependent variable; used to study the behavior of a system of equations, in particular the form of the dependence between the two variables, for example, V (membrane potential) plotted against W (K^+ channel activation) for the Morris–Lecar model. The form of the plot (the *trajectory*) will depend on the initial values used for the two variables. Plotting multiple trajectories gives the *phase portrait,* showing a range of possible behaviors for the system.

Progesterone   A steroid hormone produced (mainly) by the corpus luteum; in pregnant animals, very high levels are secreted by the placenta and ovaries. Progesterone acts on many tissues in the body including on many different neuronal populations in the hypothalamus. It acts mainly via nuclear receptors to regulate gene expression, and can also affect neuronal membrane properties.

Plasma membrane (PM)   The lipid bilayer that demarcates the outer boundary of the cell and mediates interchange with the external environment. For us, mainly the site of ion channels and PMCA.

Plateau potential   A sustained depolarization of a neuron's membrane potential.

Plasma membrane calcium ATPase (PMCA)   The pump that maintains cytosolic Ca^{2+} at a concentration several orders of magnitude lower than the external environment.

Prolactin   See lactotropes.

Rapid equilibrium approximation   A way to reduce the dimensionality of a mathematical model. It treats a variable that changes much more rapidly than other variables as if its changes were instantaneous, allowing one to remove the differential equation for that variable and replace the variable with its equilibrium function.

Resting potential   For a neuron, the resting potential is the value of the membrane potential that will be sustained in the absence of external perturbations, and reflects the intracellular and extracellular concentrations of ions and the permeability of the cell membrane to those ions. The main determinant of the resting potential is K^+ permeability in conjunction with the actions of ion pumps in the plasma membrane that maintain a high intracellular concentration of K^+.

Ryanodine receptor   An *ER* Ca^{2+} channel that is activated by the plant alkaloid ryanodine.

Saddle   An unstable equilibrium where one *nullcline* tends to attract and the other tends to repel from the equilibrium so that trajectories can be initially attracted before being deflected away. The dividing lines of influence between the two nullclines are called the *manifolds*. One *manifold* goes directly toward the equilibrium, and the other directly away.

Saddle–node bifurcation (of equilibria)   A *bifurcation* where a node (either stable or unstable) and a *saddle* meet and disappear. This is the type referred to when just the term *saddle–node bifurcation* is used.

Saddle–node bifurcation (of limit cycles)   A *bifurcation* where two converging limit cycles meet and disappear.

Sarco-endoplasmic reticulum calcium ATPase (SERCA)   The ATP-consuming pump that maintains the gradient of Ca^{2+} between the *ER* and the cytosol.

Set point   The target value for a homeostatic process.

Sex-determining region Y-box 2 (SRY2/SOX2)   Progenitor population thought to give rise to most pituitary cell types.

Slow–fast systems   A slow–fast system is a system of ordinary differential equations involving two types of dynamical variables that evolve with different time scales.

Small-world network   A graph in which most nodes are not neighbors of each another, yet most nodes can be reached from any other node by a small number of steps (i.e., via a short chain of mutual acquaintances).

Somatostatin   See somatotropes.

GHRH   See somatotropes.

Somatotropes (or somatotrophs)   Endocrine cells that make up 50% of anterior pituitary cells and secrete growth hormone (GH), responsible for regulating body-wide growth and metabolism. Somatotrophs are stimulated by growth-hormone releasing hormone (GHRH), a hypothalamic peptide released at the median eminence from the nerve endings of neuroendocrine GHRH cells of the arcuate nucleus, and are inhibited by *somatostatin*, released by neuroendocrine cells in the periventricular nucleus of the hypothalamus.

Spike train analysis   A technique that examines a series of *interspike intervals* looking for any correlation between interval length and the length of intervals which have occurred immediately before; a positive or negative correlation indicating that excitability is dependent on previous spike activity as well as current input activity.

Stable node   This is a stable *equilibrium* where trajectories are swung toward the equilibrium by one *nullcline* and then follow a second *nullcline* into the equilibrium so that all trajectories approach from two opposite directions along the second *nullcline*. If trajectories overshoot the second *nullcline* before swinging back in, then it becomes a *stable spiral*.

Steroid hormones   The two main groups of steroid hormones are the gonadal hormones (*testosterone* in males, *estrogen* and *progesterone* in females) and the adrenal hormones (*glucocorticoid hormones* and the mineralocorticoid hormone aldosterone). Steroids cross lipid membranes freely, so they cannot be stored but must be produced on demand when required. Steroids mainly act at nuclear receptors to regulate gene expression but can also have direct effects on cell membranes.

Supraoptic nucleus   An aggregation of magnocellular neurosecretory neurons that, on both the left and right sides of the brain, is located at the ventral surface of the brain directly adjacent to the rostrolateral edge of the optic chiasm. The nucleus contains just two types of neuron, oxytocin cells and vasopressin cells, all of which project a single axon to the posterior pituitary gland.

Suprachiasmatic nucleus (SCN)   A small region of the hypothalamus that coordinates circadian (i.e., daily) rhythms in the body. It is an endogenous oscillator – even isolated SCN tissue kept under constant conditions *in vitro* displays approximately 24-h rhythms in electrical activity and gene expression. The SCN receives light information from photosensitive cells in the retina via the retinohypothalamic tract, which enables it to synchronize the body's circadian processes precisely to environmental time.

Thapsigargin   A plant toxin that blocks the SERCA pump.

Thyrotropes (or thyrotrophs)   Make up about 10% of anterior pituitary cells and secrete thyroid-stimulating hormone (TSH).

Two-photon imaging   A method that involves rapidly bombarding a fluorophore with two half-energy photons, resulting in the same excitation state as that achieved with a single photon of half-wavelength. Since the two-photon effect decreases quadratically as a function of distance from the excited plane, out-of-focus excitement is avoided, improving image quality. Moreover, infrared wavelengths required for two-photon excitation are scattered less in biological tissue, increasing penetration depth while reducing phototoxicity.

Ultradian rhythm   A biological oscillation with an intrinsic period of much less than 24 h (e.g., the near-hourly oscillation in *glucocorticoid* levels).

Unstable node   The reverse version of a *stable node*, an unstable *equilibrium* where trajectories are deflected along one *nullcline* before being bent toward the other *nullcine* and sent on an outwards path.

Vasopressin   Peptide hormone, synthesized by neuroendocrine neurons of the supraoptic nucleus and paraventricular nucleus, and secreted into the systemic circulation from neuroendocrine nerve endings in the posterior pituitary gland. Vasopressin is an antidiuretic hormone, stimulating water reabsorption by the kidney and, hence, concentrating the urine; it also has vasopressor actions (hence its name), constricting peripheral blood vessels.

Voltage clamp   A technique in electrophysiology using a stimulating and a recording electrode. The recording electrode measures the membrane potential. The stimulating electrode is used to apply a current sufficient to maintain the membrane potential at a fixed voltage. The actual measurement is the changes in the applied current which are required. The clamped voltage can also be used to test the voltage sensitivity of the cell, testing at a range of clamp voltages.

Index

Note: page numbers in *italics* refer to figures and those in **bold** to tables; figures and tables are only indicated when they are separated from their text references.

ACTH *see* adrenocorticotropic hormone
action potentials 3–8
  endocrine pituitary cells 80–82, 93–95
  Morris–Lecar model 24–29
  natural variability *5*, 7–8
  phase-plane analysis *25*, 29–38
  shape and timing 4–6
  voltage clamp data 6, *7*
activation functions
  Ca_v channels 85–86
  HCN channels 92
  K channels 87, *88*, 89, 90, 91
  Na_v channels 84, *85*
activation variables
  BK channels 91
  Ca_v channels 85, 86
  K_v channels 87, 88
  Na_v channels 84
activator–inhibitor systems 120, 137
activity-dependent excitation 170, 232
activity-dependent inhibition 170
adenohypophysis (anterior pituitary) 82–83, 253
adjacency matrix 210
adrenocortical cells, glucocorticoid secretion 259–260
adrenocorticotropic hormone (ACTH) 253–254
  experimental studies of model predictions 267–271
  mechanism of ultradian pulsatility 261–266
  modeling ultradian pulsatility 256–261
  stress response 271–280
  ultradian oscillations 256, 280–281
afterhyperpolarization (AHP) 8–9, 158
  oxytocin neurons *231*, 232, 234, *237*, 238–239, 244
  vasopressin neurons 173–174, 178–179, 189
2-aminoethoxydiphenyl borate (2-APB) *144*, 145, 149, 157, 159, 160
anterior pituitary (adenohypophysis) 82–83, 253

antidromic stimulation, vasopressin neurons 168, 189–191, *193*
apamin *144*, 145, 149, 157, 158
arginine vasopressin (AVP) *see* vasopressin
asynchronous behavior, vasopressin neurons 168, 170–171
attraction, sign of k determining 70
attractors 34, 48
A-type K^+ channels 87–88, 97–99
autonomous systems 19, 33
average path length (L) 211

backwards Hopf bifurcation 47
barnacle muscle *5*, 7, 8
basin of attraction 48–49
Berkeley Madonna 20
β cells, pancreatic 129–130, 132
bifurcation diagrams (BD) 43–50
  blockade of BK channels 133–134
  bursting 63, *64*, 68
  closed-cell Li–Rinzel model 121
  homoclinic bifurcation 58, *59*, 62
  HPA axis dynamics 262–264, *266*
  plateau bursting 127, 128–129, *130*
  plotting 49
  pseudo-plateau bursting 131, 132
  SNIC bifurcation *54*, 55, 62
bifurcation parameter 43–44
bifurcations 38, 43–62
  bursting and 49, 63, 68
  HPA axis dynamics 261–266
  locating 75–76
  spiking characteristics 49–50, 62
bipartite graph 245–246
bistability *43*, 45, 48–49
  asynchronous, vasopressin cells 170–171
  Ca^{2+} oscillations 128, 132
  emergent, vasopressin cells 183, *192*
  explicit, vasopressin cells 182–183
  HPA axis dynamics 257, *263*, 264

Computational Neuroendocrinology, First Edition. Edited by Duncan J. MacGregor and Gareth Leng.
© 2016 John Wiley & Sons, Ltd. Published 2016 by John Wiley & Sons, Ltd.
Companion Website: www.wiley.com/go/Leng/Computational

BK channels 90–91
  blockade 132–133
  dynamic clamp technique 104–105, *106*
  role in spontaneous bursting 95–97, 99
blue sky bifurcation 47
Boltzmann functions 13, 84, 85–86, 91
burst frequency
  extended Morris–Lecar model 66
  GnRH neurons, external [Ca²⁺] and 149, 159
bursting 63–68
  bifurcations and 49, 63, 68
  detection 179–180
  endocrine pituitary cells 80, *81*, 95–99
  endoplasmic reticulum-driven 123–125
  GnRH neurons/models 142–161
  network topology and 246–247
  oxytocin neurons *167*, *168*, 227–228,
    237–242, 244–248
  phasic *see* phasic bursting
  plasma membrane-driven 126–134
  plateau 80, 126–130
  pseudo-plateau 80, 130–132
  subthreshold channels modulating 97–99
  time-scale separation and 58

calcium (Ca²⁺)
  external ([Ca²⁺]), GnRH neuron activity and
    149, 159
  intracellular *see* intracellular calcium
calcium ATPases
  GnRH model 145, *150*, 157, 159
  plasma membrane (PMCA) 114, 115,
    122–123, *159*
  sarco-endoplasmic reticulum *see*
    sarco-endoplasmic reticulum calcium
    ATPase
calcium (Ca²⁺) balance equations 112–116
calcium (Ca²⁺) channels 3–4
  endocrine pituitary cells 94–95, 96–97,
    98–99, 100, 103–104
  GnRH model 152
  high-voltage activated 85
  low-voltage activated 85
  model action potentials 28
  Morris–Lecar model 8, 10, 12–13, *14*, 17, 22
  vasopressin secretion model 195, 196–197
  voltage-gated 84–87
calcium-controlled potassium (K_Ca) channels
  endocrine pituitary cells 90–91, 95–97
  ER–plasma membrane communication
    125–126, 130, 131–132
  GnRH model (I_AHP–UCL) 149, 152–153,
    156–158, 160, 161
  high conductance *see* BK channels
  intermediate conductance (IK) 90, *91*
  small conductance *see* SK channels
calcium (Ca²⁺) imaging 207, 215–216, 221, *222*
calcium (Ca²⁺) indicators 215, 218–219
calcium-induced calcium release (CICR)
  116–117, 135, 145, 152
calcium (Ca²⁺) oscillations 111–137

combined ER–PM model 123–134, **138**
  endoplasmic reticulum (ER)-driven 111,
    116–123
  plasma membrane (PM)-driven 111
calcium (Ca²⁺) transients
  GnRH model 148–149, *152*, 153–154, 157,
    158, 159
  GnRH neurons 143–144, 145
Chay–Keizer model 129–130
chloride channels, voltage-gated 83
chromaffin cells, adrenal 5
circadian rhythms
  glucocorticoid hormones 254, 255
  GnRH surge 284–286
closeness centrality (CC) 211
clustering coefficient (C) 211
complex biological systems 208–209
corticotropin-releasing hormone (CRH) 82,
    253–254
  experimental studies of model predictions
    267–271
  infusions, HPA axis responses 265–266, *267*,
    268–271
  mechanism of ultradian pulsatility 261–266
  modeling ultradian pulsatility 256–261
  pulsatile release 255–256, 280
  stress response 272, *273*, 274, *275*, 279–280
corticotropes, pituitary 82
  ACTH release 253–254, 259
  electrical activity 5, 93, 101, 102, 104
  network organization 206, 209
cortisol/corticosterone *see* glucocorticoid
  hormones
CRH *see* corticotropin-releasing hormone
current (applied)
  Dclamp technique 104–105
  Morris–Lecar model 9, 22, 24, *25*
  sustained injection 38–62
  voltage clamp 6
  voltage-dependent slowly varying 63–65
cyclic AMP (cAMP) 91–92, 100–102
cyclic GMP (cGMP) 91–92
cyclopiazonic acid (CPA) *144*, 145, 157, *159*

deactivation 4
degree centrality (D) 211
degree distribution (P(k)) 210, *223*
deinactivation 4
dendrites
  communication between 233
  oxytocin neurons 228, *229*, 235
  oxytocin release 232–233, 234–235
  priming of oxytocin stores 229–230, 242,
    244
  vasopressin release 171, 181
depolarization 3
depolarizing afterpotential (DAP) 173
  conductance-based model 186, 187
  spike-response model 174, 180–182,
    183–186, 187
derivative 11

Desmos 1, 14–17
DeYoung–Keizer model 117–122
differential equations 10–13
  one-dimensional linear 68–70
dihydropyridine-sensitive Ca^{2+} channels 85
Dirac delta function 234
direction field 32, 34
dopamine 82, 100
dynamical systems 1, 9–10, 19–29
dynamic clamp (DClamp) technique 104–105, *106*
dynorphin 181–182, 184, 189, *192*, 288

edges 209
eigendirections 71–72
eigenvalues 68–76
  calculating 74–75
  Hopf bifurcation 74
  at nodes 73
  at a saddle 72
  spiral equilibria 73–74
emergent behavior
  oxytocin neurons 239, 244
  vasopressin cells 183, *192*
empirical mode decomposition (EMD) 216, *217*
endocannabinoids 230
  milk-ejection reflex model 236, 237, 238, 240, 242, 243, 244
  release 233
endoplasmic reticulum (ER)
  bursting driven by 123–125
  Ca^{2+} balance equations 112–116
  Ca^{2+} oscillations driven by 111, 116–123
  regulation of Ca^{2+} entry 125–126
endothelins 100
equilibrium
  at intersection of nullclines 34
  saddle node bifurcation of 53
  SNIC parameter set 51–53, *54*
  stability 34–35, 41–42, 52–53
ER *see* endoplasmic reticulum
estradiol 286, *287*
  bolus challenge in GnRH pulse regime 301–302
  control of GnRH surge 293–294
  during ovarian cycle 294
estradiol receptors, type β (ER β) 287
excitability 1–77
  modeling 6–77
  natural variability *5*, 7–8
excitatory post-synaptic potentials (EPSP)
  oxytocin neurons *176*, *177*, 232, 233, 236, *237*
  vasopressin neurons 171–172
exocytosis
  oxytocin vesicles 227, 248
  vasopressin vesicles 170, 195, 196

facilitation, frequency, vasopressin secretion 195, 198, *199*, *200*
fast-slow systems 57–58, 127, 135–136, 196

fatigue, vasopressin secretion 183, 195, 196, 198, *199*
Fitzhugh–Nagumo (FHN) model 29, 154–155, 160, 289, 291
flow *25*, 31
fold bifurcation of limit cycles 47, 61
follicle-stimulating hormone (FSH) 142, *285*
folliculostellate cells 206
functional connectivity maps 220, *221*, *223*
functional magnetic resonance imaging (fMRI) 207
functional multi-cellular imaging (fMCI) 215–216, 221, *222*
fura-2 215–216, 221, *222*

GABA (gamma-aminobutyric acid) 100
  GnRH neurons *144*, 145–146, 161, 288
  oxytocin neurons 232, 243
GENESIS 147
glucocorticoid hormones (CORT) 252, *253*, 254
  circadian rhythms 254, 255
  experimental studies of model predictions 267–271
  mechanism of ultradian pulsatility 261–266
  modeling ultradian pulsatility 256–261
  stress response 271–280
  ultradian pulsatility 254–256, 280–281
glucocorticoid receptors (GR) 254, 257, 258
glutamate *144*, 145–146, 232
gonadotropin-releasing hormone (GnRH) 83, 142
gonadotropin-releasing hormone (GnRH) model (of spiking) 134, 142–163
  Ca^{2+} sub-model 150, 151, 155, 157, 163
  equations and parameters 161–163
  experimental data 143–146
  full model 150–154
  hypothalamic slices 148–149
  previous models 146–148
  results 157–160
  simplified 154–157
  V sub-model 150–151, 155–157, 161–163
gonadotropin-releasing hormone (GnRH) neurons 286, 288
  electrical activity 142–146
  neural inputs 145–146, 161, 288
  spiking model *see* gonadotropin-releasing hormone model
gonadotropin-releasing hormone (GnRH) pulse generator 288
gonadotropin-releasing hormone (GnRH) pulses 286, *287*
  dynamical encoding 294, *295*
  modeling 289–293, *296*
  ovarian steroid challenges 301–302
gonadotropin-releasing hormone (GnRH) secretion 284–302
  control by ovarian steroids 286–287, 289–293
  control of ovulation 284–286
  experimental methods 287–288, 296–297

gonadotropin-releasing hormone (GnRH)
   secretion (*continued*)
  modeling dynamics of 289–302
  during ovarian cycle *287*, 293–295
  regimes 286, *287*
gonadotropin-releasing hormone (GnRH)
   surge 284–286, *287*
  luteal deficiency 298, *299*
  modeling 289–294, *296*, 297–300
  progesterone-induced blockade 298–300
  progesterone priming effect 297–298
  secretory events preceding 293–294
gonadotropes, pituitary 83
  Ca^{2+} oscillations 122–125
  electrical activity 80–82, 93, 95, 103
  ion channels 84
  network organization 206, 209
GPR54 receptor 288
G-protein-coupled receptors (GPCR) 93,
   99–104, 117
G proteins 99–100
Granger causality 210, 220
graph theory 208
growth hormone (GH) networks *207*, 209
growth hormone-releasing hormone (GHRH)
   82–83, 102
GT1 cells 146, 149

hazard function 175–176, 180, *181*
HCN channels *see* hyperpolarization-activated
   cyclic nucleotide-gated channels
Heaviside step function 234
heteroclinic connection 53
Hilbert–Huant empirical mode decomposition
   (EMD) 216, *217*
Hill functions 90, 114
Hodgkin–Huxley model 6, 29, 120, 143, 146
  simplification 154–155
  vasopressin neurons 186, *187*
Hodgkin's Class I (integrator) neurons 49–50,
   54, 55
Hodgkin's Class II (resonator) neurons 49, *54*,
   55
Hodgkin's classification of neurons 55
homoclinic bifurcation (HC) 50, 58–62
  Ca^{2+} oscillations 127–128, 133
homoclinic loop 60
homoclinic parameter set **18**
  sustained current injection 55–56, 58, *59*, 60
  voltage-dependent slowly varying current
   63–65
Hopf bifurcation (HB) *43*, 44–45, 46
  backwards 47
  Ca^{2+} oscillations 127, 128, 131–132
  eigenvalues 74
  HPA axis dynamics 262, *263*
  subcritical 47, 131
  supercritical 47, 48
Hopf parameter set **18**, 38–39, *40*
HPA axis *see* hypothalamic–pituitary–adrenal
  axis

hyperpolarization-activated cyclic
   nucleotide-gated (HCN) channels 90,
   91–92, 101–102
hyperpolarized state 3
hyperpolarizing afterpotential (HAP)
  oxytocin neurons *231*, 232, 234, *237*,
   238–239
  vasopressin neurons 173, 174, 176–177,
   180, *181*
hypophyseal portal system 253
  CRH measurement 255–256
  GnRH levels 286, *287*, 293–294, 296–297
  sampling techniques 287–288
hypothalamic–pituitary–adrenal (HPA) axis
   252–281
  experimental studies of model predictions
   267–271
  modeling 256–261
  stress responsiveness 271–280
  ultradian oscillations *see* ultradian HPA axis
   oscillations
hypothalamic–pituitary–ovarian axis 284–286
hypothalamic–pituitary–thyroid (HPT) axis
   256
hypothalamic slices 148–149, 168–169

inactivation 4
inactivation functions
  Ca_v channels 86–87
  K_v channels *88*
  Na_v channels 84, *85*
inactivation variables
  Ca_v channels 86
  K_v channels 88
  Na_v channels 84
index of dispersion 240
inhibitory post-synaptic potentials (IPSP)
  oxytocin neurons *177*, 232, 233, 236, *237*
  vasopressin neurons 171–172
inositol 1,4,5-trisphosphate (IP_3) 103,
   117–122, 134–135
inositol 1,4,5-trisphosphate receptors (IP3R)
   90, 92–93, 103
  Ca^{2+} oscillations 117–118, *119*, 134–135
  GnRH model 145, 148, 152, 157
integrate-and-fire (spike-response) model 172,
   173, 174
  bursting in vasopressin cells 179–193, *194*
  modified leaky, oxytocin cells 231–232,
   233–243
  vasopressin secretion and 197, 198
interpulse interval (IPI) 294, *296*
interspike intervals (ISI)
  oxytocin neurons *231*, 236, 237
  vasopressin neurons 175–176, 178–179, 182
intracellular calcium (Ca^{2+}) 111
  balance equations 112–116
  bursting vasopressin cells 173, 187, 189, 191,
   192
  endocrine network dynamics 207
  endocrine pituitary cells *81*, 82, 93–104
  oxytocin release 228, 229–230

intrinsic mode functions (IMFs) 216, *217*
invariant circle 53
invariant sets 75
ion channels
    ligand-gated 89–93
    non-selective cation 89
    voltage-gated 83–89
ionic currents
    endocrine pituitary cells 93–99
    model action potentials *25*, *26*–28
    Morris–Lecar model 7, 11–13, *14*
    subthreshold 97–99
    voltage clamp 6, *7*
IP$_3$ *see* inositol 1,4,5-trisphosphate

kisspeptin neurons 288

lactotropes 82, 93
    ion channels 84, 91, 95
    network organization 206, 209, 220–223
    pseudo-plateau bursting 130–131
    regulation of bursting 100, 101, 102,
        103–104
    spontaneous bursting 80, *81*, 95
law of mass action 84
leak, Ca^{2+} from ER 114, 126, 129, 134
leak current 12, 187
    K$^+$ 187, 189, **191**
least-squares linear regression 218
LeBeau model of GnRH neurons 146, 147, 149
Liapunov exponents 76
ligand-gated ion channels 89–93
limit cycles 39–42, *43*
    fold bifurcation 47, 61
    saddle-node bifurcation 46–47, 62
    stable 42, 45
    three-dimensional *64*, 67–68
    unstable 44–46, 47
linearization
    eigenvalues and 68–70, 74
    vasopressin secretion 201, *202*
Li–Rinzel model
    closed cell 118–122
    open cell 122–123
L-type Ca^{2+} channels 85–86, 94–95, 100
luteal deficiency 298, *299*
luteinizing hormone (LH) 142, 284, *285*

magnocellular vasopressin neurons *see*
    vasopressin neurons
manifold
    stable 52, 53
    unstable 53
Mathematica 20
Matlab 20, 157, 236
median eminence 253, 286
melanotropes 82, 100, 101, 102, 104
membrane potential 172
milk-ejection reflex 168, 227–249
    modeling 231–249
    priming 229–230

model reduction (simplification)
    GnRH model 154–157
    time-scale separation and 58
Monte Carlo-based simulation 219, *222*
Morris–Lecar model 7, 8–19
    action potentials in phase plane 29–38
    bursting 63–68
    characteristics 9–19
    eigenvalues and stability 68–76
    extended 65–68
    modeling action potentials 19–29
    rationale 8–9
    sustained current injection 38–62

Nernst potential 12, 84, 85, 87
networks 208–214
    criteria 208–209
    jargon 209–210
    metrics 210–211
    oxytocin neurons 234, *235*, 236, 243–248
    pituitary endocrine cell 206–224
    undirected and directed 210, 220
network science 208
network topologies 210, 211–214
    oxytocin neurons 234, *235*, 236, 246–247
    pituitary lactotropes 220–223
    plotting 220, *221*
neurohypophysis (posterior pituitary) 170, 227
neuropeptide Y 100
neurosecretory vesicles *see* vesicles,
    neurosecretory
node association 210, 219
node degree 210
nodes
    eigenvalues 73
    network 209, 219
    stable *see* stable node
    unstable 52, 73
noise, synaptic 169
noise stress, HPA axis dynamics 272–274,
    277–278
non-selective cation channels 89
nullclines *25*, 30, 33–37
    SNIC parameter set 51–52, *54*
    tonic spiking 39–41
numerical simulation 11
Nyquist sampling theorem 215

ode files 20, 21–22
Ohm's law 83
one-dimensional linear differential equation
    68–70
osmotic pressure, vasopressin secretion and
    188, 198
ovarian cycle 284–286, *287*
    experimental manipulation 288
    modeling GnRH secretion 293–302
ovulation 284–286
oxytocin neurons 227–249
    dendro-dendritic communication 233
    endocannabinoid release 230, 233

oxytocin neurons (*continued*)
  modeling milk-ejection reflex 231–249
  modeling spiking behavior *175*, 176–179
  priming of dendritic stores 229–230, 242, 244
  spiking patterns *167*, 168, 227–228
  supraoptic nuclei 228, *229*
  vasopressin neurons vs 166, 180, *181*
oxytocin release
  modeling 232–233, 234–235, 243, 244
  suckling-induced 168, 227, 229–230

pacemaker activity, oxytocin neurons 239
paraventricular nucleus (PVN) 227, *229*, 252, 253, 254
parvocellular neurosecretory cells 253
periodic orbit *see* limit cycle
phase line, one-dimensional 69–70
phase planes 9, 26
  action potentials *25*, 29–38
  equilibrium point 30–31
  ER-driven Ca^{2+} oscillations 119–121
  plasma membrane-driven Ca^{2+} oscillations 128–129
  trajectories *25*, 29–30, 32
phase portrait 31
phase response curves (PRC), HPA axis 272, 276–279
phase space 37–38, *64*, 65, 67
phasic bursting 180
  mechanism 180–182
  modeling 179–193, *194*
  vasopressin neurons 166, *167*, 168, 170–171
  vasopressin secretion 192–193, *194*, 198, *200*
phospholipase C 103–104
pituitary endocrine cell networks 206–224
  analytical methods 208–214
  defining contributions to hormone release 207–208
  experimental and analytical protocol 214–220
  free cytosolic calcium and 207
  worked example 220–223
pituitary endocrine cells 80–106
  bursting 80, *81*, 95–99, 132–133
  G-protein-coupled receptors 93, 99–104
  ion channels 83–93
  pseudo-plateau bursting 80, 130–131, 132
  resting membrane potential 93
  spontaneous electrical activity 80–82, 93–106
  types 82–83
pituitary slices, preparation 214–215
PKA (protein kinase A) 101, 102–103
plasma membrane (PM)
  bursting driven by 126–134
  Ca^{2+} flux across 112–116
  driving Ca^{2+} oscillations 111, 123–134
plasma membrane calcium ATPase (PMCA) 114, 115, 122–123, *159*
plateau bursting 80, 126–130

plateau potential 180–181, 186
Poisson distribution 175
post-burst silences, oxytocin neurons 241–242
posterior pituitary (neurohypophysis) 170, 227
post-spike potentials
  oxytocin neurons *231*
  vasopressin neurons 173–174
post-synaptic potentials (PSP) 171–172, *173*, 177, 232
post-traumatic stress disorder (PTSD) 257
potassium (K$^+$) channels 4, 87–89
  A-type 87–88, 97–99
  calcium-controlled *see* calcium-controlled potassium channels
  effects of different parameter sets 51, *54*, 55–57
  endocrine pituitary cells 93, 94–99, 100, 102, 103
  ether-a-go-go-gene-related (ERG) 87
  GnRH model 152, 154
  high conductance *see* BK channels
  inwardly rectifying (K$_{ir}$) 88–89, 93, 100, *101*, 102–103
  kinetics of gating 16–17
  model action potentials 26–28, 35–36
  Morris–Lecar model 8, 10, 12–13, *14*, 16–17, 22
  rapidly activating delayed rectifier 87
  slow delayed rectifier 87, *88*
  voltage-gated 87–88
potassium (K$^+$) leak current 187, 189, **191**
PPLANE 20
progesterone 286, *287*, 293–294
  bolus challenge in GnRH pulse regime *301*, 302
  induced GnRH surge blockade 298–300
  luteal deficiency 298, *299*
  priming GnRH surge amplitude 297–298
prolactin (PRL) network *207*, 220–223
pro-opiomelanocortin gene 82
protein kinase A (PKA) 101, 102–103
pseudo-plateau bursting 80, 130–132
pulse-coupled network 244

random network 211–213
rapid equilibrium approximation 85–86, 87, 88, 89, 90
refractory period 175, *231*, 232
repetitive firing *43*
repolarization 4
repulsion, sign of *k* determining 70
resting potential 3, 93
reversal potentials 9, 12–13, *14*
Roper model, vasopressin neurons 186, 187
ryanodine receptor 135

saddle 53, *54*
  collision with stable node 61
  eigenvalues 72
saddle-node bifurcation (SN)
  Ca^{2+} oscillations 127, 128, 133

of equilibria 53
  homoclinic bifurcation 61
saddle-node bifurcation (SN) of limit cycles
    46–47, 62
  HPA axis dynamics *263*, 264
saddle node on an invariant circle (SNIC)
    bifurcation 49, 50–55
  homoclinic bifurcation 61–62
sarco-endoplasmic reticulum calcium ATPase
    (SERCA)
  Ca^{2+} balance equations 114–116
  Ca^{2+} oscillations 116, 120, 129–130, 134
  GnRH model 145, *150*, 157, *159*
scale-free networks *212*, 213
secretory vesicles *see* vesicles, neurosecretory
separatrix 45
SERCA *see* sarco-endoplasmic reticulum
    calcium ATPase
serotonin 100
sex determining region Y-box 2 (SRY2 or
    SOX2) cells 206
shape parameters 84
single-scale networks *212*, 213–214
singular points 73–74
SK channels 90, *91*
  GnRH model 145, 148, 149, 156
  pituitary endocrine cells 96
slow-fast systems 289, 293
small-world networks *212*, 213, 247
SNIC *see* saddle node on an invariant circle
SNIC parameter set **18**, 50–51, 70–71
sodium (Na^+) channels 3, 4
  endocrine pituitary cells 93, 94–95
  GnRH model 145, 152
  voltage-gated 83–84, *85*
somatostatin 83, 100
somatotropes 82–83, 93
  ion channels 84, 91, 95
  network organization 206, 209
  pseudo-plateau bursting 130–131, *132–133*
  regulation of bursting 100, 101, 102, 104
  spontaneous bursting 80, *81*, 95, 99
spike-ordering effect 179
spike-response model *see* integrate-and-fire
    model
spike train analysis 174–176, 178–180
spiking 143
  Ca^{2+} oscillations and 124–126
  endocrine pituitary cells 93–95, *96*
  GnRH model *see* gonadotropin-releasing
    hormone model
  high baseline 50, *59*, 61
  Morris–Lecar model 39–43, 46–47, 48–50,
    62
  oxytocin neurons *167*, 168, 227–228
  SNIC bifurcation 51, 53, 54–55
  time-scale separation 56, *57*
  vasopressin neurons *167*, 168
spirals
  eigenvalues 73–74
  stable and unstable 52, *54*

square-wave bursting *see* plateau bursting
squid giant axon 6
stability
  eigenvalues and 68–76
  equilibria 34–35, 41–42, 52–53
  limit cycles 42, 44–46, 47
stable node 52, 53, *54*
  collision with saddle 61
  eigenvalues *69*, 73
  strong set 75
steady-state calcium theorem 115–116
steroids, ovarian
  challenges in pulsatile regime 301–302
  control of GnRH secretion 286–287,
    289–293, 297–302
  during ovarian cycle *287*
stochastic resonance 169
strange attractor 66
stress response 252, 271–280
strong sets 75
subcritical Hopf bifurcation 47, 131
supercritical Hopf bifurcation 47, 48
suprachiasmatic nucleus (SCN) 252, 255
supraoptic nucleus 166, 167–168, 227, 228,
    229
synaptic inputs
  oxytocin neurons 232, 233, *242*
  vasopressin neurons 168–169, 171–172
synchronized bursting, oxytocin neurons
    239–240
systems modeling approach
  HPA axis 256–261
  milk-ejection reflex 248–249

tetrodotoxin (TTX) 83, 93, *144*, 145, 157
thapsigargin 114–115
three-dimensional systems *64*, 65–68
thyrotropin-releasing hormone
    (TRH) 83, 256
thyrotropes 83, 93, 103
time-scale separation 56–58
trajectories *25*, 29–30, 32
transgenic animals 143, 206, 214
transient receptor potential (TRP) channels 89
  canonical (TRPC) 93, 102
TREK-1 (TWIK-related) channels 93
tri-stability 58, *59*
T-type Ca^{2+} channels 85, 86–87, 98–99
two-photon imaging 215, 218

UCL2077 158
ultradian HPA axis oscillations 254–256,
    280–281
  experimental studies of model predictions
    267–271
  mechanism 261–266
  modeling 256–261
  role in stress responsiveness 271–280
unstable equilibria 34–35
unstable node 52, 73
urocortin 1–3 82

Van Goor GnRH model 146, 147, 149
vasopressin neurons 166–203
    asynchronous bistability 170–171
    Hodgkin–Huxley-type models 186
    initial modeling of bursting 171–179
    inputs 168–169, 171–172
    in vivo vs *in vitro* activity 168–169
    modeling secretion 195–202
    outputs 170
    spiking model of bursting 179–193, *194*
    spontaneous firing pattern 166, *167*, 168
vasopressin secretion 181, 183, 195–202
    HPA axis 253–254
    population modeling 200–202
    single-cell modeling 195, 196–198, *199, 200*

stress response 272
vesicles, neurosecretory
    ACTH 254
    oxytocin 227, *230*, 233, *235*
    vasopressin 195
V-nullcline 33–34, 36–37
voltage clamp 6, *7*, 13
voltage dependence
    kinetics of K-channel gating
        16–17
    steady-state conductance 13, *14*
voltage-gated ion channels 83–89
W-nullcline 34, 35–36

XPP (XPP-Aut) 1, 19–76